Falk Symposium 169
May 15 and 16, 2009, Kiev

Inflammation in the Intestinal Tract: Pathogenesis and Treatment

Editors
H.J. Buhr, Berlin
N.V. Kharchenko, Kiev
B. Siegmund, Berlin
M.P. Zacharash, Kiev
M. Zeitz, Berlin

50 figures and 38 tables, 2009

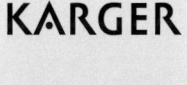

Basel · Freiburg · Paris · London · New York · Bangalore ·
Bangkok · Shanghai · Singapore · Tokyo · Sydney

Reprint of **Digestive Diseases** (ISSN 0257–2753)
Vol. 27, No. 4, 2009

Library of Congress Cataloging-in-Publication Data

Falk Symposium (169th : 2009 : Kiev, Ukraine)
 Inflammation in the intestinal tract : pathogenesis and treatment / Falk Symposium 169, May 15 and 16, 2009, Kiev ; editors, H.J. Buhr ... [et al.].
   p. ; cm.
 "Reprint of Digestive diseases (ISSN 0257-2753) vol. 27, no. 4, 2009"--T.p. verso.
 Includes bibliographical references and indexes.
 ISBN 978-3-8055-9348-9 (hard cover : alk. paper)
 1. Inflammatory bowel diseases--Pathogenesis--Congresses. 2. Inflammatory bowel diseases--Treatment--Congresses. I. Buhr, Heinz Johannes. II. Digestive diseases (Basel, Switzerland). III. Title.
  [DNLM: 1. Inflammatory Bowel Diseases--etiology--Congresses. 2. Inflammatory Bowel Diseases--therapy--Congresses. WI 420 F191ig 2009]
  RC862.I53F35 2009b
  616.3'44--dc22

                                                                          2009038889

S. Karger
Medical and Scientific Publishers
Basel • Freiburg • Paris • London •
New York • Bangalore • Bangkok •
Shanghai • Singapore • Tokyo • Sydney

Disclaimer
The statements, opinions and data contained in this publication are solely those of the individual authors and contributors and not of the publisher and the editor(s). The appearance of advertisements in the journal is not a warranty, endorsement, or approval of the products or services advertised or of their effectiveness, quality or safety. The publisher and the editor(s) disclaim responsibility for any injury to persons or property resulting from any ideas, methods, instructions or products referred to in the content or advertisements.

Drug Dosage
The authors and the publisher have exerted every effort to ensure that drug selection and dosage set forth in this text are in accord with current recommendations and practice at the time of publication. However, in view of ongoing research, changes in government regulations, and the constant flow of information relating to drug therapy and drug reactions, the reader is urged to check the package insert for each drug for any change in indications and dosage and for added warnings and precautions. This is particularly important when the recommended agent is a new and/or infrequently employed drug.

All rights reserved.
No part of this publication may be translated into other languages, reproduced or utilized in any form or by any means, electronic or mechanical, including photocopying, recording, microcopying, or by any information storage and retrieval system, without permission in writing from the publisher or, in the case of photocopying, direct payment of a specified fee to the Copyright Clearance Center (see 'General Information').

© Copyright 2009 by S. Karger AG,
P.O. Box, CH–4009 Basel (Switzerland)
Printed in Switzerland
on acid-free and non-aging paper (ISO 9706) by
Reinhardt Druck, Basel
ISBN 978–3–8055–9348–9

KARGER

Fax +41 61 306 12 34
E-Mail karger@karger.ch
www.karger.com

Contents

427 Preface
Zeitz, M. (Berlin)

Pathogenesis of IBD

428 The Genetic Basis of Inflammatory Bowel Disease
Cooney, R.; Jewell, D. (Oxford)

443 Mechanisms and Functional Implications of Intestinal Barrier Defects
Shen, L.; Su, L.; Turner, J.R. (Chicago, Ill.)

450 Therapeutic Options to Modulate Barrier Defects in Inflammatory Bowel Disease
Hering, N.A.; Schulzke, J.-D. (Berlin)

455 Inflammation in the Intestinal Tract: Pathogenesis and Treatment
Blumberg, R.S. (Boston, Mass.)

465 Targeted Therapies in Inflammatory Bowel Disease
Siegmund, B. (Berlin)

Diagnostic Approach in IBD

470 Mucosal Healing: Impact on the Natural Course or Therapeutic Strategies
Vatn, M.H. (Lørenskog/Oslo)

476 Diagnostic Approach to Small Bowel Involvement in Inflammatory Bowel Disease: View of the Endoscopist
Papadakis, K.A. (Heraklion)

482 Significance of Abdominal Ultrasound in Inflammatory Bowel Disease
Dietrich, C.F. (Bad Mergentheim)

Differential Diagnosis of Chronic Diarrhea

494 New Insights into Whipple's Disease – A Rare Intestinal Inflammatory Disorder
Marth, T. (Daun)

Clinical Manifestation of IBD

502 Joint Extraintestinal Manifestations in Ulcerative Colitis
Dorofeyev, A.E.; Vasilenko, I.V.; Rassokhina, O.A. (Donetsk)

511 Joint Involvement Associated with Inflammatory Bowel Disease
De Vos, M. (Ghent)

516 Can We Modulate the Clinical Course of Inflammatory Bowel Diseases by Our Current Treatment Strategies?
Cosnes, J. (Paris)

522 Primary Sclerosing Cholangitis: A Clinical Case
Gubergrits, N.B. (Donetsk)

526 Surveillance and Screening of Primary Sclerosing Cholangitis
El Fouly, A.E.; Dêchene, A.; Gerken, G. (Essen)

Treatment Algorithms in IBD (1)

536 Medical Management of Crohn's Disease: Treatment Algorithms 2009
Hanauer, S.B. (Chicago, Ill.)

542 Medical Management of Ulcerative Colitis
Rogler, G. (Zürich)

550 Diagnostic and Treatment Algorithms of Ulcerative Colitis in Ukraine
Skrypnyk, I.N. (Poltava)

555 Therapy- and Non-Therapy-Dependent Infectious Complications in Inflammatory Bowel Disease
Epple, H.-J. (Berlin)

Treatment Algorithms in IBD (2)

560 Laparoscopic Management of Inflammatory Bowel Disease
Rosenthal, R.J.; Bashankaev, B.; Wexner, S.D. (Weston, Fla.)

565 Treatment Algorithms in the Case of Perianal Complications of Crohn's Disease
Lozynskyy, Y.S. (Lviv)

Malignant Transformation in IBD: Prevention – Surveillance – Treatment

571 Malignant Transformation in Inflammatory Bowel Disease: Prevention, Surveillance and Treatment – New Techniques in Endoscopy
Bojarski, C. (Berlin)

576 Diagnostic Standards in the Pathology of Inflammatory Bowel Disease
Loddenkemper, C. (Berlin)

584 Malignant Transformation in Inflammatory Bowel Disease – Surveillance Guide
Stallmach, A.; Bielecki, C.; Schmidt, C. (Jena)

591 Falk Symposium Series

594 Author Index
595 Subject Index

Preface

Our knowledge of the etiology and pathogenesis of inflammatory diseases of the gastrointestinal tract has made major advances over the past several decades. The clinical phenotype of chronic inflammatory intestinal diseases is highly variable, the most common forms being ulcerative colitis and Crohn's disease. These diseases – inflammatory bowel diseases (IBDs) – represent a relevant group within medicine. Treatment is often demanding since young patients are often affected with severe clinical manifestations, and treatment modalities become more and more complex.

Advances in understanding IBDs have arisen from research involving experimental models of intestinal inflammation or the study of tissues and cells obtained from patients. Data from clinical studies of patients and their responses to various forms of treatment as well as from environmental and genetic studies of large patient cohorts likewise contributed to this knowledge. These advances have led to a deeper understanding of the genetic basis of the disease, the relationship of the disease to the intestinal microflora, and the role of epithelial cells and the mucosal immune system in disease pathogenesis. On this basis a general theory of disease causation is emerging, interpreting IBD as a multifactorial disturbance of mucosal homeostasis leading to hyperresponsiveness of both the innate and the adaptive elements of the mucosal immune system. In addition, on this basis more specific and effective therapy options have been developed.

In May 2009, the Falk Foundation provided the framework for an international Symposium entitled 'Inflammation in the Intestinal Tract: Pathogenesis and Treatment' that was dedicated to an in-depth review of current research and clinical management of inflammatory diseases of the intestinal tract. The organizers were gastroenterologists and surgeons from Germany and the Ukraine, and internationally well-known basic and clinical scientists were invited to contribute and present their latest results. The Falk Symposium 169 took place in the historic city of Kiev, Ukraine. The presented work addressed each of the major areas of current IBD research. The symposium covered all the significant advances in this field. This publication contains the papers submitted by the participating scientists and, as such, presents an excellent review of what is known about IBD and its clinical management.

Martin Zeitz, Berlin
for the organizers of the Falk Symposium 169

The Genetic Basis of Inflammatory Bowel Disease

Rachel Cooney   Derek Jewell

Nuffield Department of Medicine, Oxford University, Oxford, UK

Key Words

Linkage regions · Genome-wide association studies · NOD2 · Autophagy · IL-23R

Abstract

Twin studies and large-scale population studies have confirmed an increased sibling risk for both Crohn's disease (CD) and ulcerative colitis (UC). Unlike single gene disorders, CD and UC are thought to result from a complex interplay of multiple genes and environmental factors. The confirmation of *CARD15/NOD2* as a CD susceptibility gene in the late 1990s caused much excitement in the field of complex diseases in general and since then, the rapid rate of progress in molecular genetics, with the advent of large-scale affordable genotyping techniques, has resulted in large collaborations and the identification of over 30 inflammatory bowel disease (IBD)-associated genes. In particular, the importance of the innate immune system has been reaffirmed with the identification of *IRGM* and *ATG16L1* genes in the autophagy pathway as CD susceptibility genes. Disturbance in the adaptive immune system, in particular the IL-23/Th17 axis, has also shown to be of importance for IBD overall. In this era of genome-wide association studies it may be possible to, at last, identify the multiple genes involved in IBD and thus improve our understanding of the genotype-phenotype correlation and improve treatment.

Copyright © 2009 S. Karger AG, Basel

Introduction

The two main forms of inflammatory bowel disease (IBD) – Crohn's disease (CD) and ulcerative colitis (UC) – are thought to result from an aberrant intestinal immune response to bacterial microflora in a genetically susceptible individual [1]. It has long been appreciated that genetic factors play a role in IBD pathogenesis, however the identification of specific genes has been difficult due to complex disease genetics (the involvement of multiple genes and lack of mendelian pattern of inheritance) and the interplay of microbial and environmental factors. Recent development of large hypothesis-free, genome-wide association studies (GWAS) has confirmed previously recognised associations as well as revealing novel disease pathways. In this chapter the major findings of IBD genetic research will be discussed and arbitrarily divided into 'pre-GWAS' era and 'GWAS' era findings.

Pre-Genome-Wide Association Studies

Genetic Epidemiology
Burrill B. Crohn himself first observed familial clustering of disease in the early 1930s [2]. A classical mendelian inheritance attributable to a single gene locus is not exhibited but rather a more complex polygenic mode of inheritance [3]. Population studies have shown that 10–

29% of patients with IBD have a positive family history [4, 5]. The genetic basis for IBD is seen in the twin concordance rates; in CD the monozygotic concordance rate is up to 50% with a dizygotic rate of 10%, whereas in UC the monozygotic concordance rate is 18% and 4% for dizygotic twins [6]. Although the importance of genetic factors is confirmed in these twin studies, the disease concordance is significantly lower than 100%, highlighting a major role for environmental and developmental factors. Genetic factors not only influence disease onset but also disease phenotype and course. Monozygotic twins concordant for CD status when compared to non-identical twin CD patients have significantly greater similarity in CD age of onset, disease location, and disease behaviour at diagnosis and 10 years post-diagnosis [7]. Studies of first-degree relatives of patients with disease have shown that the λs (ratio of the risk of siblings to the reported population prevalence, used as a quantitative measure of familial clustering) of a patient with CD has been estimated at between 13 and 42 and in UC between 7 and 17 [8, 9]. Equivalent figures in type 1 diabetes, schizophrenia and cystic fibrosis are 15, 8.6 and 40, respectively.

There are also ethnic variations in disease prevalence. Studies have consistently shown an elevated prevalence of CD in Jewish populations, in particular the Ashkenazi people, and this is irrespective of geographical location [10, 11]. However, an increase risk of IBD seen in Asian migrants as compared to other UK residents, when the risk in non-immigrant Asians is low, highlights the interplay between genetic and environmental factors [12].

The risk of IBD is greater if more than one first-degree relative has the condition [13]. Of multiply affected families with IBD, 75% are concordant for disease type, with the 25% being 'mixed' (having 1 member with UC and 1 with CD) [9, 14, 15]. These data support the existence of some genetic variants that are specific for CD or UC and others that are common for both diseases, the phenotypic expression being influenced by environmental factors.

Genetic variants also impact on disease location, particularly in CD where the percentage of familial cases is lower in CD confined to the colon than in ileal disease [16]. Familial cases have an average age of onset about 5 years younger than sporadic cases (22–23 vs. 27–28 years), suggesting the presence of an 'early-onset gene' [10, 17, 18]. In series of familial CD, an earlier age of onset is consistently seen in affected children than affected parents [19]. Genetic anticipation is an alternative explanation, whereby a decrease in the age of onset and an increase in severity of disease are seen in subsequent generations as in the case with Huntington's disease. However, these findings are open to bias as an increased awareness of diagnosis may lead to diagnosis at an earlier age.

Genome-Wide Linkage Studies in Inflammatory Bowel Disease

Much effort has been made to determine the underlying susceptibility genes as this can assist our understanding of the underlying disease process, and thus aid our efforts to develop improved therapies. Two main types of genetic studies have been used in IBD research, namely genetic linkage and association studies, which includes candidate gene studies. In linkage studies a large cohort of affected relative pairs (e.g. affected sibling pairs) are typed for microsatellite markers spaced throughout the genome. Affected relative pairs indicate relatives that share a common disease trait. Microsatellite markers are highly informative tri- or tetranucleotide repeats and maps that cover 90% of the human genome became available in 1992 [20]. If one identifies a particular genetic marker in which more that 50% allelic sharing is observed within the affected relative pair, this would imply that a disease-associated gene resides in this general area. The extent by which allelic sharing between individuals is greater than would be expected by chance is expressed as a logarithm of the odds (LOD) score. Due to the problems of multiple testing, strict criteria have been developed to define a significant degree of linkage. Lander and Kruglyak [21] determined that a LOD score >3.6 was required for genome-wide significance of a marker, which equates to one false positive in every 20 genome-wide scans. A LOD score >2.2 is suggestive of linkage.

Once linkage is identified, the specific underlying gene can be identified through genetic association studies and fine mapping approaches. Potential candidate genes are identified and, in general, differences in allelic frequencies in cases compared to controls are sought. Family-based cohorts can also be used in a similar way comparing unaffected parents to affected siblings using transmission disequilibrium testing (TdT), the advantage being that a family association avoids many potentially confounding factors that can occur in case-control studies.

Since 1996, twelve genome-wide linkage studies on IBD from Europe and North America have been published. These resulted in the identification of a total of nine disease loci designated IBD1–9, and figure 1 highlights these regions. Five loci (IBD1, 2, 4–6) meet the stringent LOD >3.6 criteria, whereas IBD3 and IBD7 did not meet these criteria, although there is other supportive

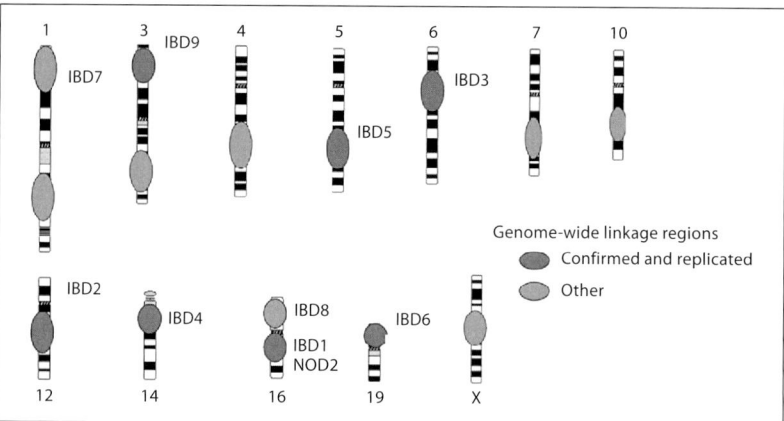

Fig. 1. IBD linkage regions. Chromosomal location of the IBD linkage loci 1–6. Some loci have either LOD scores >3.6 and/or have had their linkage replicated in two or more studies. Other loci with suggestive linkage have significance levels defined as per Lander and Kruglyak [21]. Adapted from Ahmad et al. [26], with permission.

evidence for them to be designated IBD loci [22–24]. A meta-analysis of 10 genome-wide linkage studies showed evidence of linkage to chromosome (Chr) 2q, 3q, 5q, 7q and 16 for IBD overall; Chr 2q, 3q, 6p, 16, 17q and 19p for CD, and 2q for UC [25].

The NIDDK/IBD genetics consortium gathered phenotypic data from four previous genome-wide linkage scans to assess phenotypic associations with the major IBD susceptibility loci. The cohort consisted of 904 affected individuals thereby having adequate power for meaningful subset analyses. They found the following: IBD1 (CARD15) increases the risk of small intestine CD; IBD2 increases risk of colonic CD; IBD2 has a strong link to extensive UC, which is a novel finding, and IBD3 and Chr 3q linkage regions contribute to both small intestinal and colonic CD [27].

CARD15/NOD2

The identification of *CARD15* (also known as *NOD2*) in the IBD1 locus on Chr 16 as a CD susceptibility gene was a major breakthrough for IBD research specifically and polygenic diseases in general. Hugot et al. [28] fine mapped the IBD1 linkage locus and identified *CARD15* as the underlying gene in 2001. At the same time, two separate investigators using a candidate gene approach also identified *CARD15* [29, 30]. 30 non-conservative polymorphisms have been identified within this gene, but three single nucleotide polymorphisms (SNPs) (G908R, 1007fsCins, R702W) account for approximately 82% of the mutated alleles [31]. Replication studies have confirmed that these three SNPs are independently associated with disease [32–34]. A gene dosing effect is seen in most studies with carriage of one copy of the risk allele increasing the risk of developing CD 2- to 4-fold and carriage of two copies of risk alleles increases the risk of disease 20- to 40-fold in adults. Studies from France, Germany, the UK and USA have shown that up to 40% of patients with CD (vs. 14% of controls) will have one or more of these mutations [31, 32]. However, allelic frequency is much lower in other countries, e.g. Ireland, Scotland, Scandinavia and Iceland (8–15%), and *NOD2* mutations are not found in patients with CD in Japan, Korea or China [35–37]. A population-attributable risk for CD of 26% in non-Jewish Caucasians has been calculated from meta-analysis of the three *CARD15* mutations in 29 studies [38]. Jewish patients, who tend to have the highest frequency of mutations, have an even greater population-attributable risk [39]. The prevalence of the different types of *NOD2* mutation also varies; the most prevalent *NOD2* mutation in non-Jewish Caucasian CD patients is the R702 mutation, whereas the G908R mutation is the most prevalent in the Ashkenazi Jewish CD patients (18% in children and 11% in adults) [40].

CARD15 mutations are particularly associated with ileal CD rather than colonic disease [31–33, 41]. The majority of studies have shown no association with UC [30]. Ileal involvement is associated with an earlier presentation of CD and two of these studies also found an association between mutation of both *CARD15* alleles and earlier age onset of adult CD (16.9–23 vs. 19.8–29 years, respectively) [31, 41]. Many but not all studies show an association with stricturing disease, which may be explained by the tendency for ileal disease to stricture [31, 42, 43]. Analysis of disease behaviour is complicated by changes in disease behaviour with time and inconsistencies in classification schemes between groups [44].

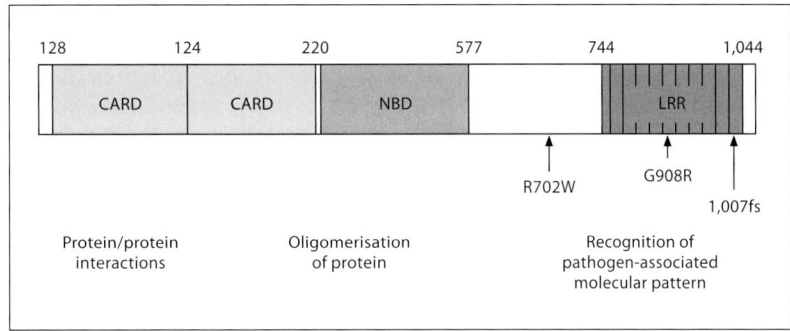

Fig. 2. Functional domains of NOD2/CARD15 protein.

CARD15/NOD2 gene encodes for a protein expressed constitutively in Paneth cells, a subset of epithelial cells at the base of intestinal crypts predominantly in the terminal ileum [45–49]. It is also expressed in the cytoplasm of monocytes and tissue macrophages, and expression can be induced on intestinal epithelial cells [50]. Figure 2 demonstrates the structural domains of CARD15, highlighting the function of each domain. CARD15 is a member of the caterpillar group of proteins, implicated in pathogen recognition in both plants and animals. A rare monogenic dominant disorder called BLAU syndrome (characterised by uveitis, arthritis with granuloma formation and rashes) is caused by mutations in the nucleotide-binding region (NBD) of CARD15. However, in CD the majority of mutations occur in the leucine-rich repeat domain (LRR). The LRR is of particular importance as it serves as a receptor for muramyl dipeptide (MDP), a small molecule derived from the cell wall peptidoglycan of Gram-positive and Gram-negative bacteria [51]. When MDP binds to the LRR, a conformational change occurs in the molecule resulting in downstream activation of NF-κB via RICK/RIP2 and of caspase 3 via the CARD domains.

Our knowledge of the function of NOD2/CARD15 is rapidly expanding and it has become apparent that experimental results are dependent on the model used. Epithelial cell lines transfected with the mutated NOD2/CARD15 fail to upregulate NF-κB, and hence gene transcription, in response to MDP compared with cells transfected with the wild-type NOD2/CARD15. Furthermore, intracellular killing of *Salmonella* is impaired in cell lines expressing the mutated gene [47]. This decrease in NF-κB activity is contrary to the inflammatory profile observed clinically.

Genetically engineered mice deficient in the *NOD2/CARD15* gene are healthy and have no intestinal inflammation. However, compared with mice expressing wild-type NOD2/CARD15, the deficient mice are more susceptible to infection with *Listeria monocytogenes* when administered intragastrically (but not intravenously or via the peritoneum). In those mice infected in this manner, more organisms were present in the liver and the spleen than in the wild-type mice, but no intestinal inflammation was observed. Interestingly, the expression of certain cryptidins was low in the mice containing the mutated gene and was even lower following infection [52]. Cryptidins (equivalent to human defensins) are antimicrobial peptides, secreted upon recognition of MDP, to protect the host from invasion.

Maeda et al. [53] created a 'knock-in' mouse model whereby the wild-type NOD2 was replaced with a homologue of the most common NOD2 mutation *(3020insC)*. These mutant mice exhibited elevated NF-κB activation in response to MDP and increased secretion of the proinflammatory cytokine interleukin (IL)-1β. They then induced colitis using dextran sodium sulphate and found that the mutant mice had more severe colitis, increased macrophage apoptosis and levels of IL-1β.

In humans, peripheral blood mononuclear cells produce several cytokines (TNF, IL-1β) in response to activating toll-like receptors with their appropriate ligands. This response is augmented in the presence of MDP in individuals with wild-type *NOD2/CARD15* genotype, but not in individuals who possess one or more mutations. It has been shown that Paneth cells fail to secrete much α-defensin 5 and 6 in biopsy specimens from patients with NOD mutations – a finding analogous to NOD-deficient mice [54].

In summary, the identification of *NOD2/CARD15* mutations in many patients with ileal CD and the association with a deficient antimicrobial defence has provided insight into the complex balance between tolerance to food antigens and commensal bacteria and the rigorous immune response to foreign pathogens occurring at the luminal wall, so much that CD has been described as the archetypal inflammatory barrier disease [55].

Chromosome 5q/IBD5 Cytokine Cluster
Multiple linkage studies show evidence for the IBD5 locus on Chr 5q31 [56, 57], and there are now ten GWAS confirming this association [58]. A Canadian group used linkage disequilibrium (LD) mapping to define a 250-kb haplotype spanning the Chr 5 cytokine cluster. This 250-kb interval is defined by 11 SNPs that are in almost complete LD with each other. Heterozygous carriage of the risk alleles increases the risk of CD 2-fold compared to a 6-fold increase with homozygous carriage [59, 60]. The Chr 5q31 region contains a cluster of cytokine genes involved in immune response but, due to the tight LD in this region, it has been difficult to dissect out a disease-causing gene from the many potential candidate genes. The organic cation transporter gene cluster (OCTN) genes are attractive candidate genes in this region that has been associated with other chronic inflammatory disorders [61]. *Solute carrier family 22 member 4 (SLC22A4)* and *SLC22A5* encode OCTN1 and 2 respectively, which play an important role in the energy supply to epithelial cells. They are known to mediate the transport of carnitine and many other organic cations and have recently been identified as the ergothioneine transporter [62, 63].

In 2004, Peltekova et al. [64], after resequencing five genes in the IBD5 interval, reported association between CD and polymorphisms in the *SLC22A4* and *SLC22A5* genes as well as a two-locus haplotype (*SLC22A4* 1672T/*SLC22A5*–207C), the two allele (TC) risk haplotype. They performed functional studies suggesting that the 1672C→T missense substitution in *SLC22A4* and the –207G→C transversion in the *SLC22A5* promoter resulted in impaired transporter or transcription function of the OCTNs, respectively. Based on their functional work and their observation that the OCTN variants were significantly associated with CD even in the absence of IBD5 risk haplotypes, Peltokova et al. suggested that *SLC22A5* 1672T and –207C variants per se were causative for CD. Despite initial studies confirming these findings [65, 66], controversy continued as other well-designed relatively large studies were unable to establish an effect for OCTN1/2 independent from the IBD5 risk haplotype, and therefore the role for other candidate genes within this extended haplotype could not be excluded [66–75]. Findings from GWAS suggest that *SLC22A4* is the susceptibility gene at this locus [76–78].

Studies on a Japanese population failed to show any association, however, again highlighting the population-specific variations in genetic susceptibility to IBD [71, 79, 80]. No evidence has been found for an association between IBD5 haplotype and CD in the high-risk Jewish population [65, 71].

IBD5 haplotype epistasis has been shown with *CARD15* in CD [64, 65, 70, 73]. Mirza et al. [70] found that, when they stratified the CD offspring in their large TdT sample (511 affected offspring) and a case-control group (n = 943), the association with 5q31 risk haplotype was present only in cases with at least one of the known *CARD15* disease susceptibility alleles. They determined that the combined population-attributable risk for the *CARD15* and IBD5 haplotype alleles was 33%. Other studies have found that *CARD15* and IBD5 haplotype act independently of each other but perhaps they were underpowered to detect a relationship [34, 59, 69, 71, 72, 81]. In a genome-wide scan, Van Heel et al. [82] found evidence for epistasis between Chr 19 (IBD6) and CD pairs possessing one or two copies of the IBD5 risk haplotype (p = 0.0005).

IBD5 haplotype is associated with perianal CD and in some studies, an earlier age of disease onset [83, 84].

IBD2/Chromosome 12
Evidence for linkage on this region to IBD was first shown in a UK genome-wide linkage scan (LOD score of 5.4) and has been replicated in various populations [85–89]. This region shows strongest linkage with UC with weaker linkage with CD and IBD in general. Like other susceptibility loci, there is variation across populations with no association found in the Flemish population and significant variation across African-American and Jewish-Caucasian populations [90, 91]. Data from 904 phenotyped cases showed that the IBD2 locus is associated with extensive UC and because of this suggested that this form of UC should be considered a pathophysiologic subset of disease [27]. STAT6, a key transcription factor involved in IL-4- and IL-13-mediated Th2 responses [92], is an attractive candidate gene in this region, but positive association has not been confirmed [87, 93]. To date, GWAS have not identified specific disease-causing mutations in this region.

IBD3/Chromosome 6
The major histocompatibility complex (MHC) region on Chr 6p21.1–23 is one of the most extensively studied regions in IBD. Linkage studies have clearly established that this region contributes to IBD pathogenesis (both CD and UC). Linkage has been consistently replicated

across different populations, which may suggest that there are several susceptibility factors in the extended MHC [24, 25, 94]. Calculations derived from studies of HLA allele sharing within families suggest that this region contributes between 10 and 33% of the total genetic risk of CD and 65 and 100% of the total genetic risk of UC [95, 96]. Association studies into candidate genes have not been so successful due to the strong LD, high gene density and extensive polymorphism in this region. HLA proteins present peptides to T-cell receptors. Class I proteins are present on all cell types and consist of a single heavy chain encoded by three polymorphic genes (HLA-A, -B, -C). In contrast, class II molecules are normally only expressed on specialised immune cells and are composed of α and β chains encoded by three genes (HLA-DP, -DQ, -DR). The most consistently replicated association with UC is with the rare allele HLA-DRB1*0103. This rare variant is present in 0.2–3.2% of the population, 6–10% of all UC cases and 15.8% of extensive UC cases and 14.1–25% of severe UC requiring colectomy [96–98]. HLA-DRB1*0103 is also associated with isolated colonic CD [99]. The odds ratios for isolated colonic disease range from 5.1 to 18.5 in non-Jewish Caucasians [41, 100]. Despite the strength of this association, Ahmad et al. [101] noted that this allele was present in no more than 32% of patients with isolated colonic CD, indicating that whilst the marker has a high positive likelihood ratio, the negative likelihood ratio limits its clinical application.

The most consistent association of CD is with the common HLA allele, HLA-DRB1*0701. Three studies from the UK (n = 244), Spain (n = 210), Canada (n = 432) showed that this association was specifically for subjects with ileal involvement [41, 100, 102], and in the UK and Canadian study the association was only found in patients who did not possess any of the three common CARD15 mutations. The classic autoimmune haplotype A1-B8-DR3 is associated with colonic disease, although large replication studies are needed to look at the LD with other disease-associated alleles [41].

The Oxford group have looked extensively at genotypes associated with extraintestinal manifestations of disease. Type 1 peripheral arthropathy, which affects fewer than five joints, with one large joint usually involved and is associated with disease activity, is associated with HLA-B27, HLA-B35 and HLA-DRB1*0103. Type 2 is characterised by non-destructive inflammation of the small joints, is not associated with disease activity and has been found to be associated with HLA-B44 [103].

TNF is an important candidate gene located within the IBD3 linkage region. No association has been found with SNPs within the coding region of the gene. However, SNP –857C in the promoter region has been reported to be associated equally with UC and CD in both family-based and case-control studies, with conflicting data on CARD15 epistasis [104, 105]. Orchard et al. [106] have found a strong association between another polymorphism in the promoter region of the TNF-α gene (–1031C) and the risk of developing erythema nodosum.

Genome-Wide Association Studies

The combination of progress in high throughput genotyping technology and growing knowledge about the human genome through the International HapMap Project and the Human Genome Project has enabled the development of GWA studies for several complex diseases. The first GWAS in CD was published in 2005 and since then a further nine IBD studies have been published [76–78, 107–113]. In contrast to candidate gene association studies, GWA scans are 'hypothesis-free', simply seeking statistical evidence for association between variants distributed across the genome and disease susceptibility. Although there is growing focus on the application of GWA methodologies to population-based cohorts, most published GWA studies until now have featured case-control designs [114], and to date there have been approximately 205 published GWA studies which have more than 100,000 SNP assays [115]. In GWA studies, large panels of well-defined cases and controls are required to provide adequate power, necessitating large multicentre collaborations. Other requirements for GWA studies include: the genotyping of several hundreds of thousands of markers in order to capture a majority of the common genomic variations; stringent quality control criteria for the processing of genotype and phenotype data, and replication in independent datasets on a different genotyping platform to confirm robust, true signals [114, 116, 117].

In CD, the number of risk loci has risen to 32 in this new GWA era [118] (table 1). The finding of multiple genes with high population frequencies being associated with disease supports the 'frequent disease, frequent variant' hypothesis proposed by Pritchard and Cox [119] in 2002. Another novel finding from GWA scans is that several loci predispose to more than one autoimmune disease as highlighted in table 1 [118].

Autophagy and Crohn's Disease
The hypothesis-free approach of genetic GWAS has brought the association between autophagy and CD to

Table 1. GWAS studies

Reference	Initial GWAS sample size, cases/controls	Replication sample size, cases/controls; trios	Chromosomal region	Relevant gene	Autoimmune disease associated with gene
Duerr et al. [109]	547/548	401/433; 883	1p31	IL-23R	UC, psoriasis, AS
Raelson et al. [78]	382 trios	750/828; 828		IL-23R haplotype	
Hampe et al. [76]	735/368	498/1,032; 380	2q37	ATG16L1	
Libioulle et al. [111]	547/928	1,266/559; 428	5p13.1	PTGER4	UC
Rioux et al. [110]	946/977	353/207; 530	10q21 4 22 16q24	Intergenic/ZNF365 Phox2B NCF4 FAM92B	GD, T1D
WTCCC [77, 112]	1,748/2,938	1,182/2,024	3p21 5q33 10q24 18p11	MST1 IRGM NKX2-3 PTPN2	UC, GD, RA, SLE, T1D psoriasis UC
Barrett et al. [107]	3,230/4,829	2,325/1,809; 1,339	1p13 1q23 1q24 5q33.3 6p22 6q21 6q27 7p12 8q24 9p24 10p11 11q13 12q12 13q13 17q21.2 21q21 21q22	PTPN22 ITNLN1 IL-12B CDKAL1 unknown CCR6 JAK2 C11orf30 LRRK2, Muc19 ORMDL3, STAT3 ICOSLG	 UC UC

SLE = Systemic lupus erythematosus; T1D = type 1 diabetes; GD = Grave's disease; RA = rheumatoid arthritis; AS = ankylosing spondylitis.

light [116]. In the genome-wide association scans (GWAS) on CD cohorts published since 2007, two of the strongest associations were with ATG16L1 and IRGM, genes critical to the autophagy process. In a British study [77] of 3,000 controls and 2,000 cases, the ATG16L1 association had an impressive p value of 6.5×10^{-13}. A German study [76] had a smaller cohort (735 CD patients and 368 controls) and a p value of 4×10^{-8}, whereas in an American study using an ileal CD cohort and two independent replication cohorts [110], there was a similar p value of $<10^{-10}$. Independent replication studies in German, Italian, British, Scottish and Dutch cohorts have confirmed the association between CD and ATG16L1 polymorphisms [112, 120–124]. This polymorphism results in a change from A to G allele, with GG being the disease-associated genotype. Interestingly, GG allele occurs in 51.3% of controls versus 58.1% of CD patients [123]. The high incidence of GG in the control population is a factor that must be taken into consideration when investigating the function of the altered protein.

As regards association with IRGM, the original WTCCC study was the first to report an association with a SNP upstream of this gene. Parkes et al. [112] then went on to sequence the gene and confirm association in

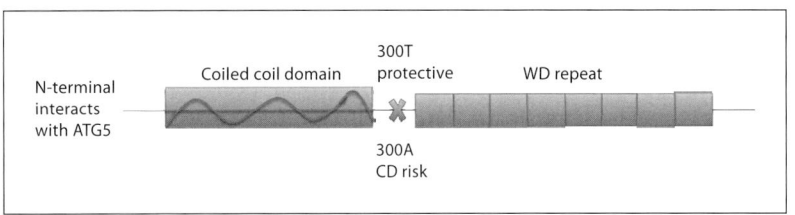

Fig. 3. Schematic of ATG16L1 structure. The WD repeat domain and the site of the disease-associated polymorphism (indicated with an 'x') are not present in yeast. The CCD is conserved and mediates self-multimerisation [145]. Amino acid alteration at position 300 does not affect dimerisation or ATG5 interaction [146].

an independent CD cohort (combined p value = 2.1 × 10^{-10}), which has since been replicated [125].

GWAS published on cohorts of UC patients have not shown any association with autophagy genes [113, 126].

The *ATG16L1* gene is located on Chr 2q37.1 and IRGM on 5q33.1. The genetic signal from *ATG16L1* appears to come entirely from a non-synonymous SNP, rs2241880, which results in a change from a polar threonine to non-polar alanine (T300A). Atg16L1 is a 400-kDa protein (607 amino acids) and the human form contains an N-terminal domain coiled-coiled domain that interacts with Atg5 and eight C-terminal WD repeats [76, 127] (fig. 3). The T300A variation is in the evolutionarily conserved N-terminus of the WD repeat domain. WD domains are structural motifs found in all eukaryotic cells, which have no intrinsic catalytic activity but are thought to act as a stable surface for protein/protein interactions [128, 129]. Hampe et al. [76], using various protein structure software tools, predict that the WD repeat domains form an eight-bladed β-propeller-like structure and, by comparing to similar structures, speculated that the WD domain of Atg16L1 is involved in actin regulation. Atg16L1 is expressed in a wide range of cells including intestinal epithelial cells, CD4+, CD8+ and CD19+ T cells and antigen presenting cells [76, 110]. ATG16L1 is homologous with the yeast autophagy gene ATG16 and has been definitively shown to be an autophagy gene in mouse cell lines. Atg16 binds to the Atg5/12 complex. Atg5 is first conjugated to Atg12 and then Atg16L binds to this complex via its N-terminal domain forming an 800-kDa protein complex [130]. Arg35 and Phe46 of Atg16 are crucial for this interaction and the entire multimeric complex has recently been crystallised [127, 131]. In yeast and mammalian cells, this complex is essential for autophagosome formation, and it is proposed that Atg16/Atg5/Atg12 complex functions as a scaffold for recruiting the LC3-Atg3 during the elongation of the isolation membrane [127, 130, 132–134]. Localisation of Atg12/5/16L complex is symmetric, with most of the molecules being associated with the outer side of the isolation membrane. The mechanism by which Atg16L recognises the isolation membrane is unknown. Rab33 is a Golgi-resident membrane trafficking protein and has been recently found to interact with the coiled-coil domain of Atg16L and may act to tether the complex to the isolation membrane [135, 136]. There has been little work published on the function of the disease-associated Atg16L1 gene product. However, two excellent studies have recently been published in *Nature* [137, 138].

Saitoh et al. [137] generated a mouse with ATG16L1 coiled coil domain (CCD)-deleted, *ΔCCD* mice. These mice died within 1 day of birth. Subsequently they tested various specific cell types and found that fetal liver-derived macrophages produced elevated IL-1β in response to LPS and *ΔCCD* macrophages exposed to commensal bacteria such as *Escherichia coli* elicited abnormally high IL-1β processing. Finally, lethally irradiated mouse chimeras reconstituted with *ΔCCD* embryonic liver cells were given dextran sulphate to induce colitis. The *ATG16L1 ΔCCD* chimeras all died by day 10, showing distal colitis and elevated IL-1β and IL-18. The importance of these cytokines was demonstrated by reversal of pathology with IL-1β and IL-18 reversing antibodies [137, 139].

Cadwell et al. [138] generated mice hypomorphic for Atg16L1 protein expression by gene-trap vector technology. This vector disrupts the *ATG16L1* gene by insertions into intronic regions. They found decreased autophagy in the ileum of these mice, and although the overall morphology of the ileum and colon was normal, there were obvious abnormalities in Paneth cells, with disorganised granules, decreased granule numbers, and frequent absence of apical microvilli. The granules were found intact in the lumen, but there was decreased lysosyme in the mucus layer suggesting a defect in the Paneth cell granule exocytosis pathway. Interestingly, these abnormalities were all found in *ATG5 flox/flox villin-cre* mice that do not express *ATG5* in their intestinal mucosa, suggesting that Paneth cells are uniquely sensitive to autophagy gene disruption. Transcriptional change as detected by microarray analysis of Atg16L1-deficient Paneth cells showed increased expression of genes involved in PPAR (peroxisome proliferator-activated receptor) pathways and additionally adipocytokines for example leptin and adiponectin. Analysis of deficient T cells confirmed the specificity of these findings to Paneth cells. The findings of this study are supported by previous work that described increased leptin and adiponectin in CD patients [140]. They also found increased cytoplasmic vesicles in Paneth cells of Atg16L1 hypomorphic cells on electron microscopy, a finding that has been previously reported in CD patients [141]. The findings of this study were validated by retrospective analysis of uninflamed resection margins of patients with the homozygous for the *ATG16L1* mutation but wild-type *NOD2* and *IL-23R*. They found abnormal Paneth cells with disordered granules and diffuse lysosyme cytoplasmic staining and increased staining for leptin protein when compared to control.

This study indicates that deficiency in Atg16L1 may result in very specific effects on a single cell lineage in CD, and although response to *L. monocytogenes* was unchanged in this study, alteration in Paneth cell function due to *ATG16L1* polymorphisms may effect the microbiome in other, as yet to be investigated ways.

Even less is known about the possible functional significance of *IRGM* gene polymorphisms and CD. The SNPs associated with CD are upstream of *IRGM* and are not coding-sequence variants. McCarroll et al. [142] found a 20-kb deletion polymorphism immediately upstream of *IRGM* that is in perfect LD with the most strongly CD-associated SNPs and altered IRGM expression levels. *IRGM* encodes a protein belonging to the p47 immunity-related guanosine triphosphatase family. Its murine analogue LRG-47 is an interferon-γ-inducible gene that stimulates autophagy. Mice deficient in LRG-47 have an impaired capacity to eliminate intracellular pathogens such as *L. monocytogenes* and *Toxoplasma gondii* [143]. Although the human IRGM lacks the interferon-γ response element, gene knockdown experiments have demonstrated the importance of *IRGM* in autophagy and the clearance of *M. tuberculosis* from human macrophages [144]. It has been proposed that a primary defect in the intracellular processing of bacteria in CD could result in the compensatory increase in the activity of Th1 cells observed in the lamina propria of CD patients but not those with UC [1].

IL-23R and IBD

The first GWAS in CD with broad genome-wide coverage identified an association with a SNP on Chr 1p in the *IL-23R* gene [109]. Subsequent GWAS and replication studies have confirmed this association [77, 78].

IL-23R is also a heterodimer, which consists of an IL-12Rb1 subunit that is shared with the IL-12 receptor, and a novel IL-23R subunit. Activated T cells and myeloid cells express IL-23R. IL-23 has the ability to promote Th17 cells, a subset of CD4+ T cells that produce IL-17 [147, 148]. IL-6 and TGF-β drive the differentiation of Th17 cells from naive T cells and induce their expression of IL-23R [148, 149]. IL-17 can activate stromal, endothelial and epithelial cells to produce cytokines and chemokines, leading to increased neutrophil recruitment into tissues, and also induces inflammatory cytokine production by macrophages [150]. Levels of IL-17 are increased in the intestine and serum of patients with active UC and CD, being undetectable in individuals with infectious colitis and controls [151]. However, neutralization of IL-17 is not sufficient to inhibit colitis in IL-10-deficient mice, and this suggests that in the intestine IL-23 may drive IL-17-independent inflammatory pathways [152, 153]. In contrast, two trials in patients with active CD, using an IL-12 p40 monoclonal antibody that neutralises IL-12 and IL-23, have shown efficacy [154, 155]. IL-23 is required for murine experimental colitis and promotes activation of T cells and perpetuation of organ-specific responses [152, 156].

GWAS of UC Patients

With regard UC, two large GWAS have been published in addition to a study which examined 53 significant SNPS from a CD GWAS in a large UC cohort [126, 157, 158]. The first published examined 10,886 non-synonymous SNPs, whereas the second examined used a 500K chip [126, 157]. There is reassuring concordance between these studies, with *IL-23R*, *NKX2-3*, 3p21 and *IL-12B* regions identified as contributing to both UC and CD [126, 158, 159]. In addition, Fisher et al. [126] report a novel association with the *ECM1* (extracellular matrix 1) locus that appears to be unique to UC [160]. *ECM1* is of particular interest as a candidate gene in that it is intestinally express and involved in the activation of NF-κB signalling as well as having a potential role in epithelial function. In Franke et al.'s [158] 500K genome-wide study, three independent UC cohorts were used to replicate the top 20 markers which resulted in 4 significant markers, the most significant of which flanks the IL-10 gene on Chr 1q32.1.

It is interesting to note that some of the most important CD susceptibility genes are not associated with UC, i.e. *NOD2*, *ATG16L1* and *IRGM*, which may suggest that an abnormal intracellular handling of microbial antigens is specifically involved in CD, but not UC pathogenesis [161].

Conclusions

Since the first genome-wide study in 1996, considerable advances in our understanding of the genetics of IBD have occurred. However, we are still far from understanding the complex interaction between multiple susceptibility and disease-modifying genes and environmental factors occurring within the gut mucosa. In recent years, new genes involving both the innate and the adaptive immune system have been identified renewing enthusiasm in this field. Advances in technology such as gene chips allowing thousands of SNPs to be tested on large cohorts as well as new computational and statistical techniques to analyse the results greatly increases the potential for future discoveries. Such advances may allow a molecular classification of IBD and even individualise patient treatment accordingly.

Disclosure Statement

The authors declare that no financial or other conflict of interest exists in relation to the content of the article.

References

1 Cho JH: The genetics and immunopathogenesis of inflammatory bowel disease. Nat Rev Immunol 2008;8:458–466.
2 Crohn G: Regional ileitis: a pathologic and clinical entity. JAMA 1932;99:1323–1329.
3 Forabosco P, Collins A, Latiano A, Annese V, Clementi M, Andriulli A, Fortina P, Devoto M, Morton NE: Combined segregation and linkage analysis of inflammatory bowel disease in the IBD1 region using severity to characterise Crohn's disease and ulcerative colitis. On behalf of the GISC. Eur J Hum Genet 2000;8:846–852.
4 Farmer RG, Michener WM, Mortimer EA: Studies of family history among patients with inflammatory bowel disease. Clin Gastroenterol 1980;9:271–277.
5 Monsen U, Brostrom O, Nordenvall B, Sorstad J, Hellers G: Prevalence of inflammatory bowel disease among relatives of patients with ulcerative colitis. Scand J Gastroenterol 1987;22:214–218.
6 Halme L, Paavola-Sakki P, Turunen U, Lappalainen M, Farkkila M, Kontula K: Family and twin studies in inflammatory bowel disease. World J Gastroenterol 2006;12:3668–3672.
7 Halfvarson J, Jess T, Bodin L, Jarnerot G, Munkholm P, Binder V, Tysk C: Longitudinal concordance for clinical characteristics in a Swedish-Danish twin population with inflammatory bowel disease. Inflamm Bowel Dis 2007;13:1536–1544.
8 Ahmad T, Satsangi J, McGovern D, Bunce M, Jewell DP: The genetics of inflammatory bowel disease. Aliment Pharmacol Ther 2001;15:731–748.
9 Orholm M, Munkholm P, Langholz E, Nielsen OH, Sorensen TI, Binder V: Familial occurrence of inflammatory bowel disease. N Engl J Med 1991;324:84–88.
10 Yang H, McElree C, Roth MP, Shanahan F, Targan SR, Rotter JI: Familial empirical risks for inflammatory bowel disease: differences between Jews and non-Jews. Gut 1993;34:517–524.
11 Roth MP, Petersen GM, McElree C, Feldman E, Rotter JI: Geographic origins of Jewish patients with inflammatory bowel disease. Gastroenterology 1989;97:900–904.
12 Montgomery SM, Morris DL, Pounder RE, Wakefield AJ: Asian ethnic origin and the risk of inflammatory bowel disease. Eur J Gastroenterol Hepatol 1999;11:543–546.
13 Russell RK, Satsangi J: IBD: a family affair. Best Pract Res Clin Gastroenterol 2004;18:525–539.
14 Meucci G, Vecchi M, Torgano G, Arrigoni M, Prada A, Rocca F, Curzio M, Pera A, de Franchis R: Familial aggregation of inflammatory bowel disease in northern Italy: a multicenter study. The Gruppo di Studio per le Malattie Infiammatorie Intestinali (IBD Study Group). Gastroenterology 1992;103:514–519.
15 Binder V: Genetic epidemiology of inflammatory bowel disease. Dig Dis 1998;16:351–355.
16 Cottone M, Brignola C, Rosselli M, Oliva L, Belloli C, Cipolla C, Orlando A, De Simone G, Aiala MR, Di Mitri R, Gatto G, Buccellato A: Relationship between site of disease and familial occurrence in Crohn's disease. Dig Dis Sci 1997;42:129–132.
17 Colombel JF, Grandbastien B, Gower-Rousseau C, Plegat S, Evrard JP, Dupas JL, Gendre JP, Modigliani R, Belaiche J, Hostein J, Hugot JP, van Kruiningen H, Cortot A: Clinical characteristics of Crohn's disease in 72 families. Gastroenterology 1996;111:604–607.
18 Polito JM 2nd, Childs B, Mellits ED, Tokayer AZ, Harris ML, Bayless TM: Crohn's disease: influence of age at diagnosis on site and clinical type of disease. Gastroenterology 1996;111:580–586.
19 Polito JM 2nd, Rees RC, Childs B, Mendeloff AI, Harris ML, Bayless TM: Preliminary evidence for genetic anticipation in Crohn's disease. Lancet 1996;347:798–800.
20 Weissenbach J, Gyapay G, Dib C, Vignal A, Morissette J, Millasseau P, Vaysseix G, Lathrop M: A second-generation linkage map of the human genome. Nature 1992;359:794–801.
21 Lander E, Kruglyak L: Genetic dissection of complex traits: guidelines for interpreting and reporting linkage results. Nat Genet 1995;11:241–247.
22 Cho JH, Nicolae DL, Ramos R, Fields CT, Rabenau K, Corradino S, Brant SR, Espinosa R, LeBeau M, Hanauer SB, Bodzin J, Bonen DK: Linkage and linkage disequilibrium in chromosome band 1p36 in American Chaldeans with inflammatory bowel disease. Hum Mol Genet 2000;9:1425–1432.
23 Cho J: Linkage of inflammatory bowel disease to human chromosome 6p. Inflamm Bowel Dis 2000;6:259–261.
24 Hampe J, Shaw SH, Saiz R, Leysens N, Lantermann A, Mascheretti S, Lynch NJ, MacPherson AJ, Bridger S, van Deventer S, Stokkers P, Morin P, Mirza MM, Forbes A, Lennard-Jones JE, Mathew CG, Curran ME, Schreiber S: Linkage of inflammatory bowel disease to human chromosome 6p. Am J Hum Genet 1999;65:1647–1655.
25 Van Heel DA, Fisher SA, Kirby A, Daly MJ, Rioux JD, Lewis CM: Inflammatory bowel disease susceptibility loci defined by genome scan meta-analysis of 1,952 affected relative pairs. Hum Mol Genet 2004;13:763–770.
26 Ahmad T, Tamboli CP, Jewell D, Colombel JF: Clinical relevance of advances in genetics and pharmacogenetics of IBD. Gastroenterology 2004;126:1533–1549.
27 Achkar JP, Dassopoulos T, Silverberg MS, Tuvlin JA, Duerr RH, Brant SR, Siminovitch K, Reddy D, Datta LW, Bayless TM, Zhang L, Barmada MM, Rioux JD, Steinhart AH, McLeod RS, Griffiths AM, Cohen Z, Yang H, Bromfield GP, Schumm P, Hanauer SB, Cho JH, Nicolae DL: Phenotype-stratified genetic linkage study demonstrates that IBD2 is an extensive ulcerative colitis locus. Am J Gastroenterol 2006;101:572–580.

28 Hugot JP, Chamaillard M, Zouali H, Lesage S, Cezard JP, Belaiche J, Almer S, Tysk C, O'Morain CA, Gassull M, Binder V, Finkel Y, Cortot A, Modigliani R, Laurent-Puig P, Gower-Rousseau C, Macry J, Colombel JF, Sahbatou M, Thomas G: Association of NOD2 leucine-rich repeat variants with susceptibility to Crohn's disease. Nature 2001; 411:599–603.

29 Ogura Y, Bonen DK, Inohara N, Nicolae DL, Chen FF, Ramos R, Britton H, Moran T, Karaliuskas R, Duerr RH, Achkar JP, Brant SR, Bayless TM, Kirschner BS, Hanauer SB, Nunez G, Cho JH: A frameshift mutation in NOD2 associated with susceptibility to Crohn's disease. Nature 2001;411:603–606.

30 Hampe J, Cuthbert A, Croucher PJ, Mirza MM, Mascheretti S, Fisher S, Frenzel H, King K, Hasselmeyer A, MacPherson AJ, Bridger S, van Deventer S, Forbes A, Nikolaus S, Lennard-Jones JE, Foelsch UR, Krawczak M, Lewis C, Schreiber S, Mathew CG: Association between insertion mutation in NOD2 gene and Crohn's disease in German and British populations. Lancet 2001;357: 1925–1928.

31 Lesage S, Zouali H, Cezard JP, Colombel JF, Belaiche J, Almer S, Tysk C, O'Morain C, Gassull M, Binder V, Finkel Y, Modigliani R, Gower-Rousseau C, Macry J, Merlin F, Chamaillard M, Jannot AS, Thomas G, Hugot JP: CARD15/NOD2 mutational analysis and genotype-phenotype correlation in 612 patients with inflammatory bowel disease. Am J Hum Genet 2002;70:845–857.

32 Cuthbert AP, Fisher SA, Mirza MM, King K, Hampe J, Croucher PJ, Mascheretti S, Sanderson J, Forbes A, Mansfield J, Schreiber S, Lewis CM, Mathew CG: The contribution of NOD2 gene mutations to the risk and site of disease in inflammatory bowel disease. Gastroenterology 2002;122:867–874.

33 Hampe J, Grebe J, Nikolaus S, Solberg C, Croucher PJ, Mascheretti S, Jahnsen J, Moum B, Klump B, Krawczak M, Mirza MM, Foelsch UR, Vatn M, Schreiber S: Association of NOD2 (CARD15) genotype with clinical course of Crohn's disease: a cohort study. Lancet 2002;359:1661–1665.

34 Vermeire S, Wild G, Kocher K, Cousineau J, Dufresne L, Bitton A, Langelier D, Pare P, Lapointe G, Cohen A, Daly MJ, Rioux JD: CARD15 genetic variation in a Quebec population: prevalence, genotype-phenotype relationship, and haplotype structure. Am J Hum Genet 2002;71:74–83.

35 Arnott ID, Nimmo ER, Drummond HE, Fennell J, Smith BR, MacKinlay E, Morecroft J, Anderson N, Kelleher D, O'Sullivan M, McManus R, Satsangi J: NOD2/CARD15, TLR4 and CD14 mutations in Scottish and Irish Crohn's disease patients: evidence for genetic heterogeneity within Europe? Genes Immun 2004;5:417–425.

36 Croucher PJ, Mascheretti S, Hampe J, Huse K, Frenzel H, Stoll M, Lu T, Nikolaus S, Yang SK, Krawczak M, Kim WH, Schreiber S: Haplotype structure and association to Crohn's disease of CARD15 mutations in two ethnically divergent populations. Eur J Hum Genet 2003;11:6–16.

37 Guo QS, Xia B, Jiang Y, Qu Y, Li J: NOD2 3020insC frameshift mutation is not associated with inflammatory bowel disease in Chinese patients of Han nationality. World J Gastroenterol 2004;10:1069–1071.

38 Mathew CG, Lewis CM: Genetics of inflammatory bowel disease: progress and prospects. Hum Mol Genet 2004;13(Spec No 1): R161–R168.

39 Bonen DK, Ogura Y, Nicolae DL, Inohara N, Saab L, Tanabe T, Chen FF, Foster SJ, Duerr RH, Brant SR, Cho JH, Nunez G: Crohn's disease-associated NOD2 variants share a signaling defect in response to lipopolysaccharide and peptidoglycan. Gastroenterology 2003;124:140–146.

40 Weiss B, Shamir R, Bujanover Y, Waterman M, Hartman C, Fradkin A, Berkowitz D, Weintraub I, Eliakim R, Karban A: NOD2/CARD15 mutation analysis and genotype-phenotype correlation in Jewish pediatric patients compared with adults with Crohn's disease. J Pediatr 2004;145:208–212.

41 Ahmad T, Armuzzi A, Bunce M, Mulcahy-Hawes K, Marshall SE, Orchard TR, Crawshaw J, Large O, de Silva A, Cook JT, Barnardo M, Cullen P, Welsh KI, Jewell DP: The molecular classification of the clinical manifestations of Crohn's disease. Gastroenterology 2002;122:854–866.

42 Langmead L, Rampton DS: Plain abdominal radiographic features are not reliable markers of disease extent in active ulcerative colitis. Am J Gastroenterol 2002;97:354–359.

43 Bjarnason I, Helgason KO, Geirsson AJ, Sigthorsson G, Reynisdottir I, Gudbjartsson D, Einarsdottir AS, Sherwood R, Kristjansson K, Kjartansson O, Thjodleifsson B: Subclinical intestinal inflammation and sacroiliac changes in relatives of patients with ankylosing spondylitis. Gastroenterology 2003;125: 1598–1605.

44 Louis E, Michel V, Hugot JP, Reenaers C, Fontaine F, Delforge M, El Yafi F, Colombel JF, Belaiche J: Early development of stricturing or penetrating pattern in Crohn's disease is influenced by disease location, number of flares, and smoking but not by NOD2/CARD15 genotype. Gut 2003;52:552–557.

45 Ogura Y, Inohara N, Benito A, Chen FF, Yamaoka S, Nunez G: NOD2, a NOD1/APAF-1 family member that is restricted to monocytes and activates NF-κB. J Biol Chem 2001;276:4812–4818.

46 Lala S, Ogura Y, Osborne C, Hor SY, Bromfield A, Davies S, Ogunbiyi O, Nunez G, Keshav S: Crohn's disease and the NOD2 gene: a role for Paneth cells. Gastroenterology 2003;125:47–57.

47 Hisamatsu T, Suzuki M, Reinecker HC, Nadeau WJ, McCormick BA, Podolsky DK: CARD15/NOD2 functions as an antibacterial factor in human intestinal epithelial cells. Gastroenterology 2003;124:993–1000.

48 Ogura Y, Lala S, Xin W, Smith E, Dowds TA, Chen FF, Zimmermann E, Tretiakova M, Cho JH, Hart J, Greenson JK, Keshav S, Nunez G: Expression of NOD2 in Paneth cells: a possible link to Crohn's ileitis. Gut 2003;52:1591–1597.

49 Tanabe T, Chamaillard M, Ogura Y, Zhu L, Qiu S, Masumoto J, Ghosh P, Moran A, Predergast MM, Tromp G, Williams CJ, Inohara N, Nunez G: Regulatory regions and critical residues of NOD2 involved in muramyl dipeptide recognition. EMBO J 2004;23:1587–1597.

50 Begue B, Dumant C, Bambou JC, Beaulieu JF, Chamaillard M, Hugot JP, Goulet O, Schmitz J, Philpott DJ, Cerf-Bensussan N, Ruemmele FM: Microbial induction of CARD15 expression in intestinal epithelial cells via toll-like receptor 5 triggers an antibacterial response loop. J Cell Physiol 2006; 209:241–252.

51 Inohara N, Ogura Y, Fontalba A, Gutierrez O, Pons F, Crespo J, Fukase K, Inamura S, Kusumoto S, Hashimoto M, Foster SJ, Moran AP, Fernandez-Luna JL, Nunez G: Host recognition of bacterial muramyl dipeptide mediated through NOD2. Implications for Crohn's disease. J Biol Chem 2003;278:5509–5512.

52 Kobayashi KS, Chamaillard M, Ogura Y, Henegariu O, Inohara N, Nunez G, Flavell RA: NOD2-dependent regulation of innate and adaptive immunity in the intestinal tract. Science 2005;307:731–734.

53 Maeda S, Hsu LC, Liu H, Bankston LA, Iimura M, Kagnoff MF, Eckmann L, Karin M: NOD2 mutation in Crohn's disease potentiates NF-κB activity and IL-1β processing. Science 2005;307:734–738.

54 Wehkamp J, Harder J, Weichenthal M, Schwab M, Schaffeler E, Schlee M, Herrlinger KR, Stallmach A, Noack F, Fritz P, Schroder JM, Bevins CL, Fellermann K, Stange EF: NOD2 (CARD15) mutations in Crohn's disease are associated with diminished mucosal α-defensin expression. Gut 2004;53:1658–1664.

55 Schreiber S, Rosenstiel P, Albrecht M, Hampe J, Krawczak M: Genetics of Crohn's disease, an archetypal inflammatory barrier disease. Nat Rev Genet 2005;6:376–388.

56 Rioux JD, Silverberg MS, Daly MJ, Steinhart AH, McLeod RS, Griffiths AM, Green T, Brettin TS, Stone V, Bull SB, Bitton A, Williams CN, Greenberg GR, Cohen Z, Lander ES, Hudson TJ, Siminovitch KA: Genome-wide search in Canadian families with inflammatory bowel disease reveals two novel susceptibility loci. Am J Hum Genet 2000; 66:1863–1870.

57 Ma Y, Ohmen JD, Li Z, Bentley LG, McElree C, Pressman S, Targan SR, Fischel-Ghodsian N, Rotter JI, Yang H: A genome-wide search identifies potential new susceptibility loci for Crohn's disease. Inflamm Bowel Dis 1999;5:271–278.

58 Achkar JP, Duerr R: The expanding universe of inflammatory bowel disease genetics. Curr Opin Gastroenterol 2008;24:429–434.

59 Rioux JD, Daly MJ, Silverberg MS, Lindblad K, Steinhart H, Cohen Z, Delmonte T, Kocher K, Miller K, Guschwan S, Kulbokas EJ, O'Leary S, Winchester E, Dewar K, Green T, Stone V, Chow C, Cohen A, Langelier D, Lapointe G, Gaudet D, Faith J, Branco N, Bull SB, McLeod RS, Griffiths AM, Bitton A, Greenberg GR, Lander ES, Siminovitch KA, Hudson TJ: Genetic variation in the 5q31 cytokine gene cluster confers susceptibility to Crohn disease. Nat Genet 2001;29:223–228.

60 Daly MJ, Rioux JD, Schaffner SF, Hudson TJ, Lander ES: High-resolution haplotype structure in the human genome. Nat Genet 2001; 29:229–232.

61 Tokuhiro S, Yamada R, Chang X, Suzuki A, Kochi Y, Sawada T, Suzuki M, Nagasaki M, Ohtsuki M, Ono M, Furukawa H, Nagashima M, Yoshino S, Mabuchi A, Sekine A, Saito S, Takahashi A, Tsunoda T, Nakamura Y, Yamamoto K: An intronic SNP in a RUNX1 binding site of SLC22A4, encoding an organic cation transporter, is associated with rheumatoid arthritis. Nat Genet 2003; 35:341–348.

62 Burckhardt G, Wolff NA: Structure of renal organic anion and cation transporters. Am J Physiol Renal Physiol 2000;278:F853–F866.

63 Grundemann D, Harlfinger S, Golz S, Geerts A, Lazar A, Berkels R, Jung N, Rubbert A, Schomig E: Discovery of the ergothioneine transporter. Proc Natl Acad Sci USA 2005; 102:5256–5261.

64 Peltekova VD, Wintle RF, Rubin LA, Amos CI, Huang Q, Gu X, Newman B, Van Oene M, Cescon D, Greenberg G, Griffiths AM, St George-Hyslop PH, Siminovitch KA: Functional variants of OCTN cation transporter genes are associated with Crohn's disease. Nat Genet 2004;36:471–475.

65 Newman B, Gu X, Wintle R, Cescon D, Yazdanpanah M, Liu X, Peltekova V, Van Oene M, Amos CI, Siminovitch KA: A risk haplotype in the solute carrier family 22A4/ 22A5 gene cluster influences phenotypic expression of Crohn's disease. Gastroenterology 2005;128:260–269.

66 Torok HP, Glas J, Tonenchi L, Lohse P, Muller-Myhsok B, Limbersky O, Neugebauer C, Schnitzler F, Seiderer J, Tillack C, Brand S, Brunnler G, Jagiello P, Epplen JT, Griga T, Klein W, Schiemann U, Folwaczny M, Ochsenkuhn T, Folwaczny C: Polymorphisms in the DLG5 and OCTN cation transporter genes in Crohn's disease. Gut 2005;54:1421–1427.

67 Fisher SA, Hampe J, Onnie CM, Daly MJ, Curley C, Purcell S, Sanderson J, Mansfield J, Annese V, Forbes A, Lewis CM, Schreiber S, Rioux JD, Mathew CG: Direct or indirect association in a complex disease: The role of SLC22A4 and SLC22A5 functional variants in Crohn disease. Hum Mutat 2006;27:778–785.

68 Noble CL, Nimmo ER, Drummond H, Ho GT, Tenesa A, Smith L, Anderson N, Arnott ID, Satsangi J: The contribution of OCTN1/2 variants within the IBD5 locus to disease susceptibility and severity in Crohn's disease. Gastroenterology 2005;129:1854–1864.

69 Waller S, Tremelling M, Bredin F, Godfrey L, Howson J, Parkes M: Evidence for association of OCTN genes and IBD5 with ulcerative colitis. Gut 2006;55:809–814.

70 Mirza MM, Fisher SA, King K, Cuthbert AP, Hampe J, Sanderson J, Mansfield J, Donaldson P, Macpherson AJ, Forbes A, Schreiber S, Lewis CM, Mathew CG: Genetic evidence for interaction of the 5q31 cytokine locus and the CARD15 gene in Crohn disease. Am J Hum Genet 2003;72:1018–1022.

71 Negoro K, McGovern DP, Kinouchi Y, Takahashi S, Lench NJ, Shimosegawa T, Carey A, Cardon LR, Jewell DP, van Heel DA: Analysis of the IBD5 locus and potential gene-gene interactions in Crohn's disease. Gut 2003;52: 541–546.

72 Giallourakis C, Stoll M, Miller K, Hampe J, Lander ES, Daly MJ, Schreiber S, Rioux JD: IBD5 is a general risk factor for inflammatory bowel disease: replication of association with Crohn's disease and identification of a novel association with ulcerative colitis. Am J Hum Genet 2003;73:205–211.

73 Latiano A, Palmieri O, Valvano RM, D'Inca R, Vecchi M, Ferraris A, Sturniolo GC, Spina L, Lombardi G, Dallapiccola B, Andriulli A, Devoto M, Annese V: Contribution of IBD5 locus to clinical features of IBD patients. Am J Gastroenterol 2006;101:318–325.

74 Gazouli M, Mantzaris G, Archimandritis AJ, Nasioulas G, Anagnou NP: Single nucleotide polymorphisms of OCTN1, OCTN2, and DLG5 genes in Greek patients with Crohn's disease. World J Gastroenterol 2005;11: 7525–7530.

75 Silverberg MS, Duerr RH, Brant SR, Bromfield G, Datta LW, Jani N, Kane SV, Rotter JI, Philip Schumm L, Hillary Steinhart A, Taylor KD, Yang H, Cho JH, Rioux JD, Daly MJ: Refined genomic localization and ethnic differences observed for the IBD5 association with Crohn's disease. Eur J Hum Genet 2007; 15:328–335.

76 Hampe J, Franke A, Rosenstiel P, Till A, Teuber M, Huse K, Albrecht M, Mayr G, De La Vega FM, Briggs J, Gunther S, Prescott NJ, Onnie CM, Hasler R, Sipos B, Folsch UR, Lengauer T, Platzer M, Mathew CG, Krawczak M, Schreiber S: A genome-wide association scan of nonsynonymous SNPS identifies a susceptibility variant for Crohn disease in Atg16L1. Nat Genet 2007;39:207–211.

77 Genome-wide association study of 14,000 cases of seven common diseases and 3,000 shared controls. Nature 2007;447:661–678.

78 Raelson JV, Little RD, Ruether A, Fournier H, Paquin B, Van Eerdewegh P, Bradley WE, Croteau P, Nguyen-Huu Q, Segal J, Debrus S, Allard R, Rosenstiel P, Franke A, Jacobs G, Nikolaus S, Vidal JM, Szego P, Laplante N, Clark HF, Paulussen RJ, Hooper JW, Keith TP, Belouchi A, Schreiber S: Genome-wide association study for Crohn's disease in the Quebec founder population identifies multiple validated disease loci. Proc Natl Acad Sci USA 2007;104:14747–14752.

79 Tosa M, Negoro K, Kinouchi Y, Abe H, Nomura E, Takagi S, Aihara H, Oomori S, Sugimura M, Takahashi K, Hiwatashi N, Takahashi S, Shimosegawa T: Lack of association between IBD5 and Crohn's disease in Japanese patients demonstrates population-specific differences in inflammatory bowel disease. Scand J Gastroenterol 2006;41:48–53.

80 Yamazaki K, Takazoe M, Tanaka T, Ichimori T, Saito S, Iida A, Onouchi Y, Hata A, Nakamura Y: Association analysis of SLC22A4, SLC22A5 and DLG5 in Japanese patients with Crohn disease. J Hum Genet 2004;49: 664–668.

81 Palmieri O, Latiano A, Valvano R, D'Inca R, Vecchi M, Sturniolo GC, Saibeni S, Peyvandi F, Bossa F, Zagaria C, Andriulli A, Devoto M, Annese V: Variants of OCTN1-2 cation transporter genes are associated with both Crohn's disease and ulcerative colitis. Aliment Pharmacol Ther 2006;23:497–506.

82 Van Heel DA, Dechairo BM, Dawson G, McGovern DP, Negoro K, Carey AH, Cardon LR, Mackay I, Jewell DP, Lench NJ: The IBD6 Crohn's disease locus demonstrates complex interactions with CARD15 and IBD5 disease-associated variants. Hum Mol Genet 2003;12:2569–2575.

83 Armuzzi A, Ahmad T, Ling KL, de Silva A, Cullen S, van Heel D, Orchard TR, Welsh KI, Marshall SE, Jewell DP: Genotype-phenotype analysis of the Crohn's disease susceptibility haplotype on chromosome 5q31. Gut 2003;52:1133–1139.

84 Onnie CM, Fisher SA, Prescott NJ, Mirza MM, Green P, Sanderson J, Forbes A, Lewis CM, Mathew CG: Diverse effects of the CARD15 and IBD5 loci on clinical phenotype in 630 patients with Crohn's disease. Eur J Gastroenterol Hepatol 2008;20:37–45.

85 Satsangi J, Parkes M, Jewell DP, Bell JI: Genetics of inflammatory bowel disease. Clin Sci (Lond) 1998;94:473–478.

86 Satsangi J, Parkes M, Louis E, Hashimoto L, Kato N, Welsh K, Terwilliger JD, Lathrop GM, Bell JI, Jewell DP: Two stage genome-wide search in inflammatory bowel disease provides evidence for susceptibility loci on chromosomes 3, 7 and 12. Nat Genet 1996; 14:199–202.

87 Klein W, Tromm A, Folwaczny C, Hagedorn M, Duerig N, Epplen J, Schmiegel W, Griga T: The G2964A polymorphism of the STAT6 gene in inflammatory bowel disease. Dig Liver Dis 2005;37:159–161.

88 Duerr RH, Barmada MM, Zhang L, Davis S, Preston RA, Chensny LJ, Brown JL, Ehrlich GD, Weeks DE, Aston CE: Linkage and association between inflammatory bowel disease and a locus on chromosome 12. Am J Hum Genet 1998;63:95–100.

89 Curran ME, Lau KF, Hampe J, Schreiber S, Bridger S, Macpherson AJ, Cardon LR, Sakul H, Harris TJ, Stokkers P, Van Deventer SJ, Mirza M, Raedler A, Kruis W, Meckler U, Theuer D, Herrmann T, Gionchetti P, Lee J, Mathew C, Lennard-Jones J: Genetic analysis of inflammatory bowel disease in a large European cohort supports linkage to chromosomes 12 and 16. Gastroenterology 1998; 115:1066–1071.

90 Uthoff SM, Crawford NP, Eichenberger MR, Hamilton CJ, Petras RE, Martin ER, Galandiuk S: Association of ulcerative colitis with the inflammatory bowel disease susceptibility locus IBD2 in non-Jewish Caucasians and evidence of genetic heterogeneity among racial and ethnic populations with Crohn disease. Am J Med Genet 2002;113:242–249.

91 Vermeire S, Rutgeerts P, Van Steen K, Joossens S, Claessens G, Pierik M, Peeters M, Vlietinck R: Genome-wide association scan in a Flemish inflammatory bowel disease population: support for the IBD4 locus, population heterogeneity, and epistasis. Gut 2004;53:980–986.

92 Schreiber S, Rosenstiel P, Hampe J, Nikolaus S, Groessner B, Schottelius A, Kuhbacher T, Hamling J, Folsch UR, Seegert D: Activation of signal transducer and activator of transcription (STAT) 1 in human chronic inflammatory bowel disease. Gut 2002;51:379–385.

93 De Jong DJ, Franke B, Naber AH, Willemen JJ, Heister AJ, Brunner HG, de Kovel CG, Hol FA: No evidence for involvement of IL-4r and CD11b from the IBD1 region and STAT6 in the IBD2 region in Crohn's disease. Eur J Hum Genet 2003;11:884–887.

94 Nomura E, Kinouchi Y, Negoro K, Kojima Y, Oomori S, Sugimura M, Hiroki M, Takagi S, Aihara H, Takahashi S, Hiwatashi N, Shimosegawa T: Mapping of a disease susceptibility locus in chromosome 6p in Japanese patients with ulcerative colitis. Genes Immun 2004;5:477–483.

95 Yang H, Plevy SE, Taylor K, Tyan D, Fischel-Ghodsian N, McElree C, Targan SR, Rotter JI: Linkage of Crohn's disease to the major histocompatibility complex region is detected by multiple non-parametric analyses. Gut 1999;44:519–526.

96 Satsangi J, Welsh KI, Bunce M, Julier C, Farrant JM, Bell JI, Jewell DP: Contribution of genes of the major histocompatibility complex to susceptibility and disease phenotype in inflammatory bowel disease. Lancet 1996; 347:1212–1217.

97 De la Concha EG, Fernandez-Arquero M, Martinez A, Vigil P, Vidal F, Lopez-Nava G, Diaz-Rubio M, Garcia-Paredes J: Amino acid polymorphism at residue 71 in HLA-DRβ chain plays a critical role in susceptibility to ulcerative colitis. Dig Dis Sci 1999; 44:2324–2329.

98 Roussomoustakaki M, Satsangi J, Welsh K, Louis E, Fanning G, Targan S, Landers C, Jewell DP: Genetic markers may predict disease behavior in patients with ulcerative colitis. Gastroenterology 1997;112:1845–1853.

99 Hancock L, Beckly J, Geremia A, Cooney R, Cummings F, Pathan S, Guo C, Warren BF, Mortensen N, Ahmad T, Jewell D: Clinical and molecular characteristics of isolated colonic Crohn's disease. Inflamm Bowel Dis 2008;14:1667–1677.

100 Fernandez L, Mendoza JL, Martinez A, Urcelay E, Fernandez-Arquero M, Garcia-Paredes J, Pena AS, Diaz-Rubio M, de la Concha EG: IBD1 and IBD3 determine location of Crohn's disease in the Spanish population. Inflamm Bowel Dis 2004;10: 715–722.

101 Ahmad T, Marshall SE, Jewell D: Genetics of inflammatory bowel disease: the role of the HLA complex. World J Gastroenterol 2006;12:3628–3635.

102 Newman B, Silverberg MS, Gu X, Zhang Q, Lazaro A, Steinhart AH, Greenberg GR, Griffiths AM, McLeod RS, Cohen Z, Fernandez-Vina M, Amos CI, Siminovitch K: CARD15 and HLA-DRB1 alleles influence susceptibility and disease localization in Crohn's disease. Am J Gastroenterol 2004; 99:306–315.

103 Orchard TR, Thiyagaraja S, Welsh KI, Wordsworth BP, Hill Gaston JS, Jewell DP: Clinical phenotype is related to HLA genotype in the peripheral arthropathies of inflammatory bowel disease. Gastroenterology 2000;118:274–278.

104 Van Heel DA, Udalova IA, De Silva AP, McGovern DP, Kinouchi Y, Hull J, Lench NJ, Cardon LR, Carey AH, Jewell DP, Kwiatkowski D: Inflammatory bowel disease is associated with a TNF polymorphism that affects an interaction between the OCT1 and NF-κB transcription factors. Hum Mol Genet 2002;11:1281–1289.

105 Tremelling M, Waller S, Bredin F, Greenfield S, Parkes M: Genetic variants in TNF-α but not DLG5 are associated with inflammatory bowel disease in a large United Kingdom cohort. Inflamm Bowel Dis 2006; 12:178–184.

106 Orchard TR, Chua CN, Ahmad T, Cheng H, Welsh KI, Jewell DP: Uveitis and erythema nodosum in inflammatory bowel disease: clinical features and the role of HLA genes. Gastroenterology 2002;123:714–718.

107 Barrett JC, Hansoul S, Nicolae DL, Cho JH, Duerr RH, Rioux JD, Brant SR, Silverberg MS, Taylor KD, Barmada MM, Bitton A, Dassopoulos T, Datta LW, Green T, Griffiths AM, Kistner EO, Murtha MT, Regueiro MD, Rotter JI, Schumm LP, Steinhart AH, Targan SR, Xavier RJ, Libioulle C, Sandor C, Lathrop M, Belaiche J, Dewit O, Gut I, Heath S, Laukens D, Mni M, Rutgeerts P, Van Gossum A, Zelenika D, Franchimont D, Hugot JP, de Vos M, Vermeire S, Louis E, Cardon LR, Anderson CA, Drummond H, Nimmo E, Ahmad T, Prescott NJ, Onnie CM, Fisher SA, Marchini J, Ghori J, Bumpstead S, Gwilliam R, Tremelling M, Deloukas P, Mansfield J, Jewell D, Satsangi J, Mathew CG, Parkes M, Georges M, Daly MJ: Genome-wide association defines more than 30 distinct susceptibility loci for Crohn's disease. Nat Genet 2008;40:955–962.

108 Yamazaki K, McGovern D, Ragoussis J, Paolucci M, Butler H, Jewell D, Cardon L, Takazoe M, Tanaka T, Ichimori T, Saito S, Sekine A, Iida A, Takahashi A, Tsunoda T, Lathrop M, Nakamura Y: Single nucleotide polymorphisms in TNFSF15 confer susceptibility to Crohn's disease. Hum Mol Genet 2005;14:3499–3506.

109 Duerr RH, Taylor KD, Brant SR, Rioux JD, Silverberg MS, Daly MJ, Steinhart AH, Abraham C, Regueiro M, Griffiths A, Dassopoulos T, Bitton A, Yang H, Targan S, Datta LW, Kistner EO, Schumm LP, Lee AT, Gregersen PK, Barmada MM, Rotter JI, Nicolae DL, Cho JH: A genome-wide association study identifies IL-23R as an inflammatory bowel disease gene. Science 2006;314:1461–1463.

110 Rioux JD, Xavier RJ, Taylor KD, Silverberg MS, Goyette P, Huett A, Green T, Kuballa P, Barmada MM, Datta LW, Shugart YY, Griffiths AM, Targan SR, Ippoliti AF, Bernard EJ, Mei L, Nicolae DL, Regueiro M, Schumm LP, Steinhart AH, Rotter JI, Duerr RH, Cho JH, Daly MJ, Brant SR: Genome-wide association study identifies new susceptibility loci for Crohn disease and implicates autophagy in disease pathogenesis. Nat Genet 2007;39:596–604.

111 Libioulle C, Louis E, Hansoul S, Sandor C, Farnir F, Franchimont D, Vermeire S, Dewit O, de Vos M, Dixon A, Demarche B, Gut I, Heath S, Foglio M, Liang L, Laukens D, Mni M, Zelenika D, Van Gossum A, Rutgeerts P, Belaiche J, Lathrop M, Georges M: Novel Crohn's disease locus identified by genome-wide association maps to a gene desert on 5p13.1 and modulates expression of PTGER4. PLoS Genet 2007;3:e58.

112 Parkes M, Barrett JC, Prescott NJ, Tremelling M, Anderson CA, Fisher SA, Roberts RG, Nimmo ER, Cummings FR, Soars D, Drummond H, Lees CW, Khawaja SA, Bagnall R, Burke DA, Todhunter CE, Ahmad T, Onnie CM, McArdle W, Strachan D, Bethel G, Bryan C, Lewis CM, Deloukas P, Forbes A, Sanderson J, Jewell DP, Satsangi J, Mansfield JC, Cardon L, Mathew CG: Sequence variants in the autophagy gene IRGM and multiple other replicating loci contribute to Crohn's disease susceptibility. Nat Genet 2007;39:830–832.

113 Franke A, Balschun T, Karlsen TH, Sventoraityte J, Nikolaus S, Mayr G, Domingues FS, Albrecht M, Nothnagel M, Ellinghaus D, Sina C, Onnie CM, Weersma RK, Stokkers PC, Wijmenga C, Gazouli M, Strachan D, McArdle WL, Vermeire S, Rutgeerts P, Rosenstiel P, Krawczak M, Vatn MH, Mathew CG, Schreiber S: Sequence variants in IL-10, ARPC2 and multiple other loci contribute to ulcerative colitis susceptibility. Nat Genet 2008;40:1319–1323.

114 McCarthy MI, Abecasis GR, Cardon LR, Goldstein DB, Little J, Ioannidis JP, Hirschhorn JN: Genome-wide association studies for complex traits: consensus, uncertainty and challenges. Nat Rev Genet 2008;9:356–369.

115 Hindorff LA, Sethupathy P, Junkins HA, Ramos EM, Mehta JP, Collins FS, Manolio TA: Potential etiologic and functional implications of genome-wide association loci for human diseases and traits. Proc Natl Acad Sci USA 2009;106:9362–9367.

116 Massey DC, Parkes M: Genome-wide association scanning highlights two autophagy genes, Atg16L1 and IRGM, as being significantly associated with Crohn's disease. Autophagy 2007;3:649–651.

117 Chanock SJ, Manolio T, Boehnke M, Boerwinkle E, Hunter DJ, Thomas G, Hirschhorn JN, Abecasis G, Altshuler D, Bailey-Wilson JE, Brooks LD, Cardon LR, Daly M, Donnelly P, Fraumeni JF Jr, Freimer NB, Gerhard DS, Gunter C, Guttmacher AE, Guyer MS, Harris EL, Hoh J, Hoover R, Kong CA, Merikangas KR, Morton CC, Palmer LJ, Phimister EG, Rice JP, Roberts J, Rotimi C, Tucker MA, Vogan KJ, Wacholder S, Wijsman EM, Winn DM, Collins FS: Replicating genotype-phenotype associations. Nature 2007;447:655–660.

118 Lettre G, Rioux JD: Autoimmune diseases: Insights from genome-wide association studies. Hum Mol Genet 2008;17:R116–R121.

119 Pritchard JK, Cox NJ: The allelic architecture of human disease genes: common disease-common variant ... or not? Hum Mol Genet 2002;11:2417–2423.

120 Glas J, Konrad S, Schmechel S, Dambacher J, Seiderer J, Schroff F, Wetzke M, Roeske D, Torok HP, Tonenchi L, Pfennig S, Haller D, Griga T, Klein W, Epplen JT, Folwaczny C, Lohse P, Goke B, Ochsenkuhn T, Mussack T, Folwaczny M, Muller-Myhsok B, Brand S: The Atg16L1 gene variants rs2241879 and rs2241880 (T300A) are strongly associated with susceptibility to Crohn's disease in the German population. Am J Gastroenterol 2008;103:682–691.

121 Latiano A, Palmieri O, Valvano MR, D'Inca R, Cucchiara S, Riegler G, Staiano AM, Ardizzone S, Accomando S, de Angelis GL, Corritore G, Bossa F, Annese V: Replication of interleukin-23 receptor and autophagy-related 16-like 1 association in adult- and pediatric-onset inflammatory bowel disease in Italy. World J Gastroenterol 2008; 14:4643–4651.

122 Van Limbergen J, Russell RK, Nimmo ER, Drummond HE, Smith L, Anderson NH, Davies G, Gillett PM, McGrogan P, Weaver LT, Bisset WM, Mahdi G, Arnott ID, Wilson DC, Satsangi J: Autophagy gene Atg16L1 influences susceptibility and disease location but not childhood-onset in Crohn's disease in Northern Europe. Inflamm Bowel Dis 2008;14:338–346.

123 Prescott NJ, Fisher SA, Franke A, Hampe J, Onnie CM, Soars D, Bagnall R, Mirza MM, Sanderson J, Forbes A, Mansfield JC, Lewis CM, Schreiber S, Mathew CG: A nonsynonymous SNP in ATG16I1 predisposes to ileal Crohn's disease and is independent of CARD15 and IBD5. Gastroenterology 2007; 132:1665–1671.

124 Weersma RK, Zhernakova A, Nolte IM, Lefebvre C, Rioux JD, Mulder F, van Dullemen HM, Kleibeuker JH, Wijmenga C, Dijkstra G: Atg16L1 and IL-23R are associated with inflammatory bowel diseases but not with celiac disease in the Netherlands. Am J Gastroenterol 2008;103:621–627.

125 Roberts RL, Hollis-Moffatt JE, Gearry RB, Kennedy MA, Barclay ML, Merriman TR: Confirmation of association of IRGM and NCF4 with ileal Crohn's disease in a population-based cohort. Genes Immun 2008;9: 561–565.

126 Fisher SA, Tremelling M, Anderson CA, Gwilliam R, Bumpstead S, Prescott NJ, Nimmo ER, Massey D, Berzuini C, Johnson C, Barrett JC, Cummings FR, Drummond H, Lees CW, Onnie CM, Hanson CE, Blaszczyk K, Inouye M, Ewels P, Ravindrarajah R, Keniry A, Hunt S, Carter M, Watkins N, Ouwehand W, Lewis CM, Cardon L, Lobo A, Forbes A, Sanderson J, Jewell DP, Mansfield JC, Deloukas P, Mathew CG, Parkes M, Satsangi J: Genetic determinants of ulcerative colitis include the ECM1 locus and five loci implicated in Crohn's disease. Nat Genet 2008;40:710–712.

127 Matsushita M, Suzuki NN, Obara K, Fujioka Y, Ohsumi Y, Inagaki F: Structure of Atg5.Atg16, a complex essential for autophagy. J Biol Chem 2007;282:6763–6772.

128 Lambright DG, Sondek J, Bohm A, Skiba NP, Hamm HE, Sigler PB: The 2.0 Å crystal structure of a heterotrimeric g protein. Nature 1996;379:311–319.

129 Smith TF, Gaitatzes C, Saxena K, Neer EJ: The WD repeat: a common architecture for diverse functions. Trends Biochem Sci 1999;24:181–185.

130 Kuma A, Mizushima N, Ishihara N, Ohsumi Y: Formation of the approximately 350-kDa Apg12-Apg5.Apg16 multimeric complex, mediated by Apg16 oligomerization, is essential for autophagy in yeast. J Biol Chem 2002;277:18619–18625.

131 Noda NN, Fujioka Y, Ohsumi Y, Inagaki F: Crystallization of the Atg12-Atg5 conjugate bound to Atg16 by the free-interface diffusion method. J Synchrotron Radiat 2008;15:266–268.

132 Matsushita M, Suzuki NN, Fujioka Y, Ohsumi Y, Inagaki F: Expression, purification and crystallization of the Atg5-Atg16 complex essential for autophagy. Acta Crystallograph Sect F Struct Biol Cryst Commun 2006;62:1021–1023.

133 Hanada T, Ohsumi Y: Structure-function relationship of ATG12, a ubiquitin-like modifier essential for autophagy. Autophagy 2005;1:110–118.

134 Fujita N, Itoh T, Omori H, Fukuda M, Noda T, Yoshimori T: The Atg16L complex specifies the site of LC3 lipidation for membrane biogenesis in autophagy. Mol Biol Cell 2008;19:2092–2100.

135 Fukuda M, Itoh T: Direct link between ATG protein and small GTPase Rab: Atg16L functions as a potential Rab33 effector in mammals. Autophagy 2008;4:824–826.

136 Itoh T, Fujita N, Kanno E, Yamamoto A, Yoshimori T, Fukuda M: Golgi-resident small GTPase Rab33B interacts with Atg16L and modulates autophagosome formation. Mol Biol Cell 2008;19:2916–2925.

137 Saitoh T, Fujita N, Jang MH, Uematsu S, Yang BG, Satoh T, Omori H, Noda T, Yamamoto N, Komatsu M, Tanaka K, Kawai T, Tsujimura T, Takeuchi O, Yoshimori T, Akira S: Loss of the autophagy protein Atg16L1 enhances endotoxin-induced IL-1β production. Nature 2008;456:264–268.

138 Cadwell K, Liu JY, Brown SL, Miyoshi H, Loh J, Lennerz JK, Kishi C, Kc W, Carrero JA, Hunt S, Stone CD, Brunt EM, Xavier RJ, Sleckman BP, Li E, Mizushima N, Stappenbeck TS, Virgin HW 4th: A key role for autophagy and the autophagy gene Atg16L1 in mouse and human intestinal Paneth cells. Nature 2008;456:259–263.

139 Deretic V, Master S, Singh S: Autophagy gives a nod and a wink to the inflammasome and Paneth cells in Crohn's disease. Dev Cell 2008;15:641–642.

140 Yamamoto K, Kiyohara T, Murayama Y, Kihara S, Okamoto Y, Funahashi T, Ito T, Nezu R, Tsutsui S, Miyagawa JI, Tamura S, Matsuzawa Y, Shimomura I, Shinomura Y: Production of adiponectin, an anti-inflammatory protein, in mesenteric adipose tissue in Crohn's disease. Gut 2005;54:789–796.

141 Dvorak AM, Dickersin GR: Crohn's disease: transmission electron microscopic studies. I. Barrier function. Possible changes related to alterations of cell coat, mucous coat, epithelial cells, and Paneth cells. Hum Pathol 1980;11:561–571.

142 McCarroll SA, Huett A, Kuballa P, Chilewski SD, Landry A, Goyette P, Zody MC, Hall JL, Brant SR, Cho JH, Duerr RH, Silverberg MS, Taylor KD, Rioux JD, Altshuler D, Daly MJ, Xavier RJ: Deletion polymorphism upstream of IRGM associated with altered IRGM expression and Crohn's disease. Nat Genet 2008;40:1107–1112.

143 Collazo CM, Yap GS, Sempowski GD, Lusby KC, Tessarollo L, Woude GF, Sher A, Taylor GA: Inactivation of LRG-47 and IRG-47 reveals a family of interferon-γ-inducible genes with essential, pathogen-specific roles in resistance to infection. J Exp Med 2001;194:181–188.

144 Singh SB, Davis AS, Taylor GA, Deretic V: Human IRGM induces autophagy to eliminate intracellular mycobacteria. Science 2006;313:1438–1441.

145 Mizushima N, Kuma A, Kobayashi Y, Yamamoto A, Matsubae M, Takao T, Natsume T, Ohsumi Y, Yoshimori T: Mouse APG16L, a novel WD-repeat protein, targets to the autophagic isolation membrane with the Apg12-Apg5 conjugate. J Cell Sci 2003;116:1679–1688.

146 Kuballa P, Huett A, Rioux JD, Daly MJ, Xavier RJ: Impaired autophagy of an intracellular pathogen induced by a Crohn's disease associated Atg16L1 variant. PLoS One 2008;3:e3391.

147 Aggarwal S, Ghilardi N, Xie MH, de Sauvage FJ, Gurney AL: Interleukin-23 promotes a distinct CD4 T-cell activation state characterized by the production of interleukin-17. J Biol Chem 2003;278:1910–1914.

148 Harrington LE, Hatton RD, Mangan PR, Turner H, Murphy TL, Murphy KM, Weaver CT: Interleukin-17-producing CD4+ effector T cells develop via a lineage distinct from the T-helper type 1 and 2 lineages. Nat Immunol 2005;6:1123–1132.

149 Veldhoen M, Hocking RJ, Atkins CJ, Locksley RM, Stockinger B: TGF-β in the context of an inflammatory cytokine milieu supports de novo differentiation of IL-17-producing T cells. Immunity 2006;24:179–189.

150 Kolls JK, Linden A: Interleukin-17 family members and inflammation. Immunity 2004;21:467–476.

151 Fujino S, Andoh A, Bamba S, Ogawa A, Hata K, Araki Y, Bamba T, Fujiyama Y: Increased expression of interleukin-17 in inflammatory bowel disease. Gut 2003;52:65–70.

152 Yen D, Cheung J, Scheerens H, Poulet F, McClanahan T, McKenzie B, Kleinschek MA, Owyang A, Mattson J, Blumenschein W, Murphy E, Sathe M, Cua DJ, Kastelein RA, Rennick D: IL-23 is essential for T cell-mediated colitis and promotes inflammation via IL-17 and IL-6. J Clin Invest 2006;116:1310–1316.

153 McGovern D, Powrie F: The IL-23 axis plays a key role in the pathogenesis of IBD. Gut 2007;56:1333–1336.

154 Mannon PJ, Fuss IJ, Mayer L, Elson CO, Sandborn WJ, Present D, Dolin B, Goodman N, Groden C, Hornung RL, Quezado M, Yang Z, Neurath MF, Salfeld J, Veldman GM, Schwertschlag U, Strober W: Anti-interleukin-12 antibody for active Crohn's disease. N Engl J Med 2004;351:2069–2079.

155 Sandborn WJ, Feagan BG, Fedorak RN, Scherl E, Fleisher MR, Katz S, Johanns J, Blank M, Rutgeerts P: A randomized trial of ustekinumab, a human interleukin-12/23 monoclonal antibody, in patients with moderate-to-severe Crohn's disease. Gastroenterology 2008;135:1130–1141.

156 Wiekowski MT, Leach MW, Evans EW, Sullivan L, Chen SC, Vassileva G, Bazan JF, Gorman DM, Kastelein RA, Narula S, Lira SA: Ubiquitous transgenic expression of the IL-23 subunit p19 induces multiorgan inflammation, runting, infertility, and premature death. J Immunol 2001;166:7563–7570.

157 Franke A, Balschun T, Karlsen TH, Sventoraityte J, Nikolaus S, Mayr G, Domingues FS, Albrecht M, Nothnagel M, Ellinghaus D, Sina C, Onnie CM, Weersma RK, Stokkers PC, Wijmenga C, Gazouli M, Strachan D, McArdle WL, Vermeire S, Rutgeerts P, Rosenstiel P, Krawczak M, Vatn MH, Mathew CG, Schreiber S: Sequence variants in IL-10, ARPC2 and multiple other loci contribute to ulcerative colitis susceptibility. Nat Genet 2008;40:1319–1323.

158 Franke A, Balschun T, Karlsen TH, Hedderich J, May S, Lu T, Schuldt D, Nikolaus S, Rosenstiel P, Krawczak M, Schreiber S: Replication of signals from recent studies of Crohn's disease identifies previously unknown disease loci for ulcerative colitis. Nat Genet 2008;40:713–715.

159 Dubois PC, van Heel DA: New susceptibility genes for ulcerative colitis. Nat Genet 2008;40:686–688.

160 Anderson CA, Massey DC, Barrett JC, Prescott NJ, Tremelling M, Fisher SA, Gwilliam R, Jacob J, Nimmo ER, Drummond H, Lees CW, Onnie CM, Hanson C, Blaszczyk K, Ravindrarajah R, Hunt S, Varma D, Hammond N, Lewis G, Attlesey H, Watkins N, Ouwehand W, Strachan D, McArdle W, Lewis CM, Lobo A, Sanderson J, Jewell DP, Deloukas P, Mansfield JC, Mathew CG, Satsangi J, Parkes M: Investigation of Crohn's disease risk loci in ulcerative colitis further defines their molecular relationship. Gastroenterology 2009;136:523–529.

161 Sans M, Castells A: Ulcerative colitis and Crohn's disease genetics: more similar than we thought? Gastroenterology 2008;135:1796–1798.

Mechanisms and Functional Implications of Intestinal Barrier Defects

Le Shen   Liping Su   Jerrold R. Turner

Department of Pathology, The University of Chicago, Chicago, Ill., USA

Key Words

Tight junction · Crohn's disease · Inflammatory bowel disease · Occludin · Myosin light chain kinase · Claudin

Abstract

Intestinal epithelial barrier defects, or increased paracellular permeability, were first reported in patients with Crohn's disease (CD) over 25 years ago. Although increased permeability may herald relapse to active disease, suggesting that impaired barrier function may contribute to progression, limited understanding of the mechanisms that create barrier defects in CD has made it impossible to determine whether increased permeability is a cause or effect of disease. It is now clear that inflammatory cytokines trigger intestinal barrier defects acutely, by cytoskeletal contraction, or chronically, via modulation of tight junction protein expression. Both mechanisms cause barrier dysfunction, but their effects on paracellular size and charge selectivity differ. The clinical ramifications of this distinction are not yet clear. Recent data using in vivo models demonstrate that cytoskeletally mediated barrier dysfunction is sufficient to activate innate and adaptive components of mucosal immunity. Consistent with the presence of increased permeability in some healthy first-degree relatives of CD patients, these barrier defects are insufficient to cause disease in the absence of other stimuli. However, cytoskeletally mediated barrier defects are sufficient to accelerate onset and increase severity of experimental inflammatory bowel disease. Thus, inflammatory cytokines can cause barrier defects and, conversely, barrier defects can activate the mucosal immune system. This raises the possibility that restoration of barrier function may be therapeutic in CD. Consistent with this hypothesis, emerging data indicate that inhibition of cytoskeletally mediated barrier dysfunction may be able to prevent disease progression. Barrier restoration may, therefore, represent a non-immunosuppressive approach to achieving or maintaining disease remission.

Copyright © 2009 S. Karger AG, Basel

The intestinal mucosa is charged with the complex tasks of absorbing nutrients and secreting waste products [1]. The successful completion of these tasks requires a semi-permeable barrier that limits back-diffusion of actively absorbed or secreted materials into the lumen or lamina propria, respectively. The barrier also supports paracellular transport, a passive process driven by concentration gradients, while preventing luminal microbes and their products from contaminating the internal milieu. Regulation and dysregulation of the barrier and the impact of these events on health and disease are the focus of this review.

The Intestinal Mucosal Barrier

The barrier is composed of cellular as well as extracellular components. The latter include the presence of an aqueous unstirred layer of as much as 800 μm in thickness and a layer of mucins that form a viscous hydrated gel. These extracellular barriers limit exposure of the monolayer of intestinal epithelial cells to sheer forces and other physical trauma from particles within the lumen and may also limit direct contact of the epithelium with microorganisms.

The cellular components of the intestinal barrier consist of the complete array of epithelial cell types present within the intestine. These cells are polarized with a luminal, or apical, surface membrane composition that is distinct from the basolateral membranes. For example, the nutrient transporters found on the apical membrane, many of which use cotransport of Na^+ ions to provide the energy and directionality of transport, are typically absent on basolateral membrane. In contrast, the Na^+,K^+-ATPase, which establishes the Na^+ electrochemical gradient, is present on basolateral, but not apical membranes. In addition, the lipid composition of the membrane domains differs; the apical membrane is enriched in sphingolipids and cholesterol relative to the basolateral membrane. One result of this polarization of proteins and lipids is that the apical membranes of intestinal epithelial cells are generally impermeable to hydrophilic solutes in the absence of specific transporters. Thus, the mere presence of epithelial cells, particularly the apical membranes, contributes significantly to the mucosal barrier. Their absence, as occurs in mucosal erosions, leads to marked barrier defects whose magnitude correlates directly with the surface area involved.

While the intestinal epithelial cell membranes are essential to mucosal barrier function, the paracellular space between adjacent cells must also be sealed. This function is served by the apical junctional complex that is composed of tight junctions, adherens junctions, and desmosomes. The tight junctions, which form the paracellular barrier, are located most apically, and define the boundary between apical and basolateral plasma membrane domains [2]. The subjacent adherens junctions and desmosomes serve important structural and signaling roles, but are not thought to contribute directly to paracellular barrier function.

Tight Junction Barrier Properties

Tight junctions have been categorized as 'leaky' and 'tight' [3]. Tight junctions within urinary bladder epithelium are 'tight', meaning that they are highly impermeant to even small solutes, such as ions as well as macromolecules. In contrast, tight junctions established by intestinal epithelia are leaky and allow some amount of paracellular flux. In either case, the tight junctions are the rate-limiting determinants of paracellular transport. In addition, because of the marked difference in permeabilities of the apical plasma membrane and tight junction in leaky epithelia, the tight junction is the primary determinant of mucosal permeability in the presence of an intact epithelium.

Gastrointestinal tight junctions demonstrate both ion and size selectivity. For example, intestinal epithelial tight junctions are typically more permeable to Na^+ than to Cl^-. However, this ion selectivity can be modified by altering tight junction protein expression patterns [4, 5]. Size selectivity of the tight junction barrier also varies along the villus-crypt axis. Studies of jejunal tight junction structure and paracellular flux suggest that pores within crypt tight junctions are permeable to molecules with radii as large as 50 Å, while pores within villus tight junctions allow only molecules with radii of <6 Å [6, 7]. In addition, the number of these pores is subject to acute regulation, with Na^+ nutrient cotransport triggering an increase in the number of small, but not large, pores [6, 8, 9]. While the functional significance of this regulation has been a topic of controversy [10–12], available data suggest that increased tight junction permeability allows for paracellular amplification of water and nutrient absorption when the transcellular pathway is saturated [13–16].

Barrier Defects in Crohn's Disease

Increased paracellular permeability was reported in patients with Crohn's disease (CD) over 25 years ago [17, 18]. Although such barrier loss may be caused by erosions that occur in active disease, some approaches used to measure permeability partially excluded this possibility by normalizing absorption of the inert sugar lactulose to that of the smaller, and more easily absorbed, inert sugar mannitol [17, 18]. The implication that increased permeability in CD reflects abnormal tight junction permeability was supported by transmission and scanning electron microscopy studies showing a reduction in the number of tight junction contacts as well as disruption of the normal anastomosing strand pattern seen by freeze fracture electron microscopy [19, 20]. Subsequent work showed that, in addition to being present in CD patients, increased paracellular permeability was also present in a subset of their healthy first-degree relatives [21, 22]. This suggested that barrier defects could be a cause of CD [23, 24], and more recent work has linked barrier defects in healthy relatives to specific mutations in *NOD2/CARD15* [25]. Unfortunately, the contribution of barrier defects to risk of developing disease in healthy relatives of CD patients has not been assessed. One case report has described a subject who had increased intestinal permeability at age 13, but no evidence of CD, and went on to develop disease 8 years later [26]. However, this patient had 2 first-degree relatives with CD and, therefore, was at increased risk of developing disease regardless of intestinal permeability. Nonetheless, this case does demonstrate a barrier defect prior to onset of CD and, therefore, supports the hypothesis that increased permeability may be an early step in the pathogenesis of this disorder.

Additional circumstantial evidence supporting a role for barrier defects in CD pathogenesis comes from a series of studies examining patients during remission. These analyses showed that patients with increased intestinal permeability were at greater risk of relapse over the subsequent year [27–29]. It should, however, be noted that one more recent study failed to reproduce these data [30]. In that study, reduced psychosocial stress correlated with decreased rates of relapse. The implications of this observation are of interest in terms of treatment and pathogenesis and may relate to barrier function, as stress can induce increases in small intestinal permeability [31]. Notably, the more recent work also identified the presence of colonic disease as an independent predictor of disease relapse [30]. This is particularly significant, since the probes used to assess permeability in that study, lactulose and mannitol, are degraded by colonic bacteria. Thus, an alternative explanation for the absence of a correlation between disease relapse and permeability in that study is that subclinical disease was present in the colon. The fact that lactulose and mannitol, as well as other commonly used paracellular probes, are degraded by colonic bacteria is the principle reason why the data above apply primarily to CD. However, it should be noted that some of the observations described above, included abnormal tight junction ultrastructure [32], have been demonstrated in ulcerative colitis. Further analysis of these issues in ulcerative colitis patients may now be possible, as newer probes able to assess colonic paracellular permeability have become available [33].

Tight Junction Alterations in Inflammatory Bowel Disease

As mentioned above, tight junction structure and function are abnormal in CD and ulcerative colitis. Recent advances in our understanding of tight junction proteins components have made it possible to directly assess these events in human specimens. Remarkably, both epithelial cells from CD and ulcerative colitis patients demonstrate increased expression of claudin-2 [34, 35]. Claudin-2 expression in cell culture models increases Na^+ conductance across the tight junction and also increases the number of small tight junction pores [4, 5, 36]. However, this may not be sufficient to explain the increased permeability to lactulose seen in CD patients. One potential explanation for observed increases in permeability of lactulose and other large molecules may be the removal of claudin-5, claudin-8, and occludin from the tight junction as well as degradation of these proteins in CD patients [37]. However, it may also be that acute cytokine-dependent tight junction regulation plays a critical role. For example, the tumor necrosis factor (TNF)-neutralizing antibody infliximab, which is remarkably effective in CD and some ulcerative colitis patients [38–40], also restores the intestinal barrier in CD patients [41]. While these effects may be secondary effects of reduced inflammatory activity after infliximab treatment, a direct role of tumor necrosis in regulating barrier function must be considered.

Tumor Necrosis Factor-Dependent Tight Junction Regulation

TNF causes barrier loss in cultured intestinal epithelial monolayers [42, 43]. Given the ability of infliximab to restore barrier function in human patients, the means by which TNF causes increased paracellular permeability is of considerable interest. A major advance in understanding this process came from the observation that myosin light chain kinase inhibition was able to acutely restore barrier function in TNF-treated intestinal epithelial monolayers [44]. In addition to providing insight into TNF-dependent tight junction regulation, this result suggests that the underlying mechanism may overlap with those responsible for physiological barrier regulation by Na^+-nutrient cotransport, which also requires myosin light chain kinase activity [9]. Further studies showed that acute TNF treatment resulted in increased myosin light chain kinase expression [43, 45], as a result of transcriptional activation [46], in vitro and in vivo. Consistent with a role in barrier loss in human disease, further study revealed increases in myosin light chain kinase expression and activity in intestinal epithelia from ulcerative colitis and CD patients [47]. Thus, it was hypothesized that TNF-dependent myosin light chain kinase activation might be a critical mechanism of barrier dysfunction in inflammatory bowel disease.

Myosin Light Chain Kinase Activity Is Required for TNF-Induced Acute Diarrhea

An in vivo model was required to better define the role of TNF in barrier loss and diarrheal disease. This model was established by treating mice with either an anti-CD3 monoclonal antibody, to activate T cells, or by injecting purified recombinant TNF [48–50]. These treatments cause an acute, self-limited diarrhea that can be prevented by infliximab [48, 49]. Moreover, treatment of human subjects with anti-CD3 monoclonal antibody induces an acute, self-limited diarrhea that, like inflammatory bowel disease, can be treated with corticosteroids [51–53]. Thus, while the mouse model does not cause chronic disease, it has pathophysiological relevance to human inflammatory bowel disease.

T-cell activation induced increases in jejunal paracellular permeability within hours [49]. This was accompanied by jejunal epithelial myosin II regulatory light chain phosphorylation, consistent with myosin light chain kinase activation [49]. Moreover, myosin II regulatory light chain phosphorylation waxed and waned in parallel with the development and resolution of diarrhea and both phosphorylation and increased paracellular permeability were prevented by infliximab [49]. This suggested that TNF-dependent myosin light chain kinase activation might be required for in vivo barrier loss and diarrhea. To test this hypothesis, the response of mice lacking the long myosin light chain kinase [54], the only form expressed in intestinal epithelia [55], to T-cell activation was assessed. Mucosal cytokine production induced by T cell activation was similar in wild-type and long myosin light chain kinase knockout mice. However, intestinal epithelial myosin II regulatory light chain phosphorylation did not increase, there was no increase in paracellular permeability, and diarrhea was prevented [49]. In addition, the most prominent morphological correlate of tight junction dysregulation, endocytosis of the tight junction protein occludin, did not occur in long myosin light chain kinase knockout mice. Similarly, treatment of mice with a specific peptide inhibitor of myosin light chain kinase prevented myosin II regulatory light chain phosphorylation, occludin endocytosis, barrier loss, and diarrhea. Thus, the TNF-dependent diarrhea that occurs after T-cell activation requires long myosin light chain kinase-mediated myosin II regulatory light chain phosphorylation [56].

Constitutive Myosin Light Chain Kinase Activation Accelerates Onset and Increases Severity of Experimental Inflammatory Bowel Disease

The data presented thus far demonstrate that (1) myosin light chain kinase activation is necessary for acute TNF-induced barrier loss and diarrhea, (2) myosin light chain kinase expression and activity are increased in inflammatory bowel disease patients, (3) barrier loss is present in some first-degree relatives of CD patients, and (4) barrier loss precedes and may be a marker of impending disease reactivation. In addition, in vitro work has shown that expression of a constitutively active truncated myosin light chain kinase in cultured intestinal epithelial monolayers is sufficient to increase tight junction permeability [57]. Thus, to test the hypothesis that increases in tight junction permeability, similar to those detected in CD patients and a subset of their relatives, a transgenic mouse expressing the constitutively active truncated myosin light chain kinase within the intestinal epithelium was developed [58]. As expected, this mouse displayed increased myosin II regulatory light chain phosphorylation within intestinal epithelia and increased paracellular permeability within the small intestine and colon [58]. However, the mice developed, gained weight, and reproduced normally under standard specific pathogen-free housing. While some might consider this to indicate that the model was poorly executed, the absence of spontaneous disease in these mice actually recapitulates human data. Healthy first-degree relatives of CD patients with increased permeability are notable because they are healthy; with no evidence of disease. Many of these relatives will never develop disease. Thus, the transgenic mice expressing constitutively active myosin light chain kinase represent a unique opportunity to probe the mechanisms that maintain mucosal homeostasis despite the presence of barrier defects and to ask if such defects predispose an individual to inflammatory bowel disease.

Detailed analysis of the constitutively active myosin light chain kinase transgenic mice showed that TNF, interferon-γ, and interleukin-10 expression were increased within the colonic mucosa [58]. Interestingly, these increases were not present prior to weaning, raising the possibility that the rapid changes in luminal microbiota composition that accompany weaning may contribute to the observed mucosal immune activation. The transgenic mice also demonstrated a marked increase in the number of lamina propria T cells and a repositioning of CD11c+ dendritic cells to a subepithelial location. It will be a great interest in the future to determine what immune mechanisms prevent disease in these mice.

To determine if increased intestinal paracellular permeability could contribute to disease progression, the transgenic mice were studied using the CD4+CD45Rb^{hi} adoptive transfer model of colitis, which shares many biochemical, immune, and morphological characteristics of human inflammatory bowel disease [59–62]. When constitutively active myosin light chain kinase transgenic mice were challenged with CD4+CD45Rb^{hi} T cells, they developed colitis more rapidly than their non-transgenic littermates. Weight loss occurred earlier, mucosal cytokine expression was higher, and histologic damage more advanced in the transgenic mice. As disease progressed, weight loss in transgenic mice and non-transgenic littermates became similar, but mucosal cytokine expression remained higher and histologic damage more severe in the transgenic mice. In addition, survival of transgenic mice was reduced relative to non-transgenic littermates. Thus, pathophysiologically relevant regulation of intestinal epithelial tight junctions induces mucosal immune activation and, while insufficient to cause disease, can contribute to development and progression of colitis.

Conclusion

The tight junction is a critical determinant of mucosal barrier function. In the absence of mucin deficiency or gross epithelial damage, the tight junction is the primary determinant of paracellular permeability. Increases in intestinal permeability are present in healthy individuals and have been reported at increased frequency in first-degree relatives of CD patients. A role of barrier loss in CD pathogenesis is further suggested by the observation that increased intestinal permeability correlates with increased risk of relapse from remission. Finally, studies using pre-clinical animal models have demonstrated that TNF induces cytoskeletally mediated tight junction dysregulation. Conversely, cytoskeletally mediated tight junction dysregulation is able to increase mucosal TNF production, suggesting the presence of a cycle linking immune activation and epithelial barrier dysfunction. These data suggest that restoration of the intestinal epithelial barrier is an appropriate therapeutic target that may be an effective, non-immunosuppressive means of achieving or maintaining disease remission.

Acknowledgements

Supported by the NIH (grants R01DK61931, R01DK68271, and P01DK67887) and a Research Fellowship Award from the Crohn's and Colitis Foundation of America sponsored by Laura McAteer Hoffman (to L. Shen).

Disclosure Statement

The authors declare that no financial or other conflict of interest exists in relation to the content of this article.

References

1 Turner JR, Madara JL: Epithelia: biological principles of organization; in Yamada T, Alpers DH, Kalloo AN, Kaplowitz N, Owyang C, Powell DW (eds): Textbook of Gastroenterology, ed 5. New York, Blackwell Publishing, 2009, pp 169–186.
2 Machen TE, Erlij D, Wooding FB: Permeable junctional complexes. The movement of lanthanum across rabbit gallbladder and intestine. J Cell Biol 1972;54:302–312.
3 Claude P, Goodenough DA: Fracture faces of zonulae occludentes from 'tight' and 'leaky' epithelia. J Cell Biol 1973;58:390–400.
4 Furuse M, Furuse K, Sasaki H, Tsukita S: Conversion of zonulae occludentes from tight to leaky strand type by introducing claudin-2 into Madin-Darby canine kidney I cells. J Cell Biol 2001;153:263–272.
5 Amasheh S, Meiri N, Gitter AH, Schoneberg T, Mankertz J, Schulzke JD, et al: Claudin-2 expression induces cation-selective channels in tight junctions of epithelial cells. J Cell Sci 2002;115:4969–4976.
6 Fihn BM, Sjoqvist A, Jodal M: Permeability of the rat small intestinal epithelium along the villus-crypt axis: effects of glucose transport. Gastroenterology 2000;119:1029–1036.
7 Marcial MA, Carlson SL, Madara JL: Partitioning of paracellular conductance along the ileal crypt-villus axis: a hypothesis based on structural analysis with detailed consideration of tight junction structure-function relationships. J Membr Biol 1984; 80:59–70.

8 Madara JL, Pappenheimer JR: Structural basis for physiological regulation of paracellular pathways in intestinal epithelia. J Membr Biol 1987;100:149–164.
9 Turner JR, Rill BK, Carlson SL, Carnes D, Kerner R, Mrsny RJ, et al: Physiological regulation of epithelial tight junctions is associated with myosin light-chain phosphorylation. Am J Physiol 1997;273:C1378–C1385.
10 Fine KD, Santa Ana CA, Porter JL, Fordtran JS: Effect of D-glucose on intestinal permeability and its passive absorption in human small intestine in vivo. Gastroenterology 1993;105:1117–1125.
11 Madara JL: Sodium-glucose cotransport and epithelial permeability. Gastroenterology 1994;107:319–320.
12 Turner JR, Madara JL: Physiological regulation of intestinal epithelial tight junctions as a consequence of Na^+-coupled nutrient transport. Gastroenterology 1995;109:1391–1396.
13 Sadowski DC, Meddings JB: Luminal nutrients alter tight-junction permeability in the rat jejunum: an in vivo perfusion model. Can J Physiol Pharmacol 1993;71:835–839.
14 Turner JR, Cohen DE, Mrsny RJ, Madara JL: Noninvasive in vivo analysis of human small intestinal paracellular absorption: regulation by Na^+-glucose cotransport. Dig Dis Sci 2000;45:2122–2126.
15 Pappenheimer JR: Paracellular intestinal absorption of glucose, creatinine, and mannitol in normal animals: relation to body size. Am J Physiol 1990;259:G290–G299.
16 Pappenheimer JR: Physiological regulation of transepithelial impedance in the intestinal mucosa of rats and hamsters. J Membr Biol 1987;100:137–148.
17 Pearson AD, Eastham EJ, Laker MF, Craft AW, Nelson R: Intestinal permeability in children with Crohn's disease and coeliac disease. Br Med J (Clin Res Ed) 1982;285:20–21.
18 Ukabam SO, Clamp JR, Cooper BT: Abnormal small intestinal permeability to sugars in patients with Crohn's disease of the terminal ileum and colon. Digestion 1983;27:70–74.
19 Marin ML, Greenstein AJ, Geller SA, Gordon RE, Aufses AH Jr: A freeze fracture study of Crohn's disease of the terminal ileum: changes in epithelial tight junction organization. Am J Gastroenterol 1983;78:537–547.
20 Marin ML, Geller SA, Greenstein AJ, Marin RH, Gordon RE, Aufses AH Jr: Ultrastructural pathology of Crohn's disease: correlated transmission electron microscopy, scanning electron microscopy, and freeze fracture studies. Am J Gastroenterol 1983;78:355–364.

21 Hollander D, Vadheim CM, Brettholz E, Petersen GM, Delahunty T, Rotter JI: Increased intestinal permeability in patients with Crohn's disease and their relatives. A possible etiologic factor. Ann Intern Med 1986;105:883–885.
22 Katz KD, Hollander D, Vadheim CM, McElree C, Delahunty T, Dadufalza VD, et al: Intestinal permeability in patients with Crohn's disease and their healthy relatives. Gastroenterol 1989;97:927–931.
23 Hollander D: Is Crohn's a tight junction disease? Gut 1989;21:315–319.
24 Hollander D: Permeability in Crohn's disease: altered barrier functions in healthy relatives? Gastroenterology 1993;104:1848–1851.
25 Buhner S, Buning C, Genschel J, Kling K, Herrmann D, Dignass A, et al: Genetic basis for increased intestinal permeability in families with Crohn's disease: role of CARD15 3020insC mutation? Gut 2006;55:342–347.
26 Irvine EJ, Marshall JK: Increased intestinal permeability precedes the onset of Crohn's disease in a subject with familial risk. Gastroenterology 2000;119:1740–1744.
27 Wyatt J, Vogelsang H, Hubl W, Waldhoer T, Lochs H: Intestinal permeability and the prediction of relapse in Crohn's disease. Lancet 1993;341:1437–1439.
28 D'Inca R, Di Leo V, Corrao G, Martines D, D'Odorico A, Mestriner C, et al: Intestinal permeability test as a predictor of clinical course in Crohn's disease. Am J Gastroenterol 1999;94:2956–2960.
29 Arnott ID, Kingstone K, Ghosh S: Abnormal intestinal permeability predicts relapse in inactive Crohn's disease. Scand J Gastroenterol 2000;35:1163–1169.
30 Bitton A, Dobkin P, Edwardes MD, Sewitch M, Meddings J, Rawal S, et al: Predicting relapse in Crohn's disease: a biopsychosocial model. Gut 2008;57:1386–1392.
31 Meddings JB, Swain MG: Environmental stress-induced gastrointestinal permeability is mediated by endogenous glucocorticoids in the rat. Gastroenterology 2000;119:1019–1028.
32 Schmitz H, Barmeyer C, Fromm M, Runkel N, Foss HD, Bentzel CJ, et al: Altered tight junction structure contributes to the impaired epithelial barrier function in ulcerative colitis. Gastroenterology 1999;116:301–309.
33 Meddings JB, Gibbons I: Discrimination of site-specific alterations in gastrointestinal permeability in the rat. Gastroenterology 1998;114:83–92.
34 Heller F, Florian P, Bojarski C, Richter J, Christ M, Hillenbrand B, et al: Interleukin-13 is the key effector Th2 cytokine in ulcerative colitis that affects epithelial tight junctions, apoptosis, and cell restitution. Gastroenterology 2005;129:550–564.

35 Prasad S, Mingrino R, Kaukinen K, Hayes KL, Powell RM, MacDonald TT, et al: Inflammatory processes have differential effects on claudins 2, 3 and 4 in colonic epithelial cells. Lab Invest 2005;85:1139–1162.
36 Van Itallie CM, Holmes J, Bridges A, Gookin JL, Coccaro MR, Proctor W, et al: The density of small tight junction pores varies among cell types and is increased by expression of claudin-2. J Cell Sci 2008;121:298–305.
37 Zeissig S, Burgel N, Gunzel D, Richter J, Mankertz J, Wahnschaffe U, et al: Changes in expression and distribution of claudin 2, 5 and 8 lead to discontinuous tight junctions and barrier dysfunction in active Crohn's disease. Gut 2007;56:61–72.
38 Baert FJ, D'Haens GR, Peeters M, Hiele MI, Schaible TF, Shealy D, et al: Tumor necrosis factor-α antibody (infliximab) therapy profoundly down-regulates the inflammation in Crohn's ileocolitis. Gastroenterology 1999;116:22–28.
39 D'Haens G, Van Deventer S, Van Hogezand R, Chalmers D, Kothe C, Baert F, et al: Endoscopic and histological healing with infliximab anti-tumor necrosis factor antibodies in Crohn's disease: a European multicenter trial. Gastroenterology 1999;116:1029–1034.
40 Rutgeerts P, Sandborn WJ, Feagan BG, Reinisch W, Olson A, Johanns J, et al: Infliximab for induction and maintenance therapy for ulcerative colitis. N Engl J Med 2005;353:2462–2476.
41 Suenaert P, Bulteel V, Lemmens L, Noman M, Geypens B, Van Assche G, et al: Anti-tumor necrosis factor treatment restores the gut barrier in Crohn's disease. Am J Gastroenterol 2002;97:2000–2004.
42 Taylor CT, Dzus AL, Colgan SP: Autocrine regulation of epithelial permeability by hypoxia: role for polarized release of tumor necrosis factor-α. Gastroenterology 1998;114:657–668.
43 Wang F, Graham WV, Wang Y, Witkowski ED, Schwarz BT, Turner JR: Interferon-γ and tumor necrosis factor-α synergize to induce intestinal epithelial barrier dysfunction by up-regulating myosin light chain kinase expression. Am J Pathol 2005;166:409–419.
44 Zolotarevsky Y, Hecht G, Koutsouris A, Gonzalez DE, Quan C, Tom J, et al: A membrane-permeant peptide that inhibits MLC kinase restores barrier function in in vitro models of intestinal disease. Gastroenterology 2002;123:163–172.
45 Ma TY, Boivin MA, Ye D, Pedram A, Said HM: Mechanism of TNF-α modulation of Caco-2 intestinal epithelial tight junction barrier: role of myosin light-chain kinase protein expression. Am J Physiol 2005;288:G422–G430.

46 Graham WV, Wang F, Clayburgh DR, Cheng JX, Yoon B, Wang Y, et al: Tumor necrosis factor-induced long myosin light chain kinase transcription is regulated by differentiation-dependent signaling events. Characterization of the human long myosin light chain kinase promoter. J Biol Chem 2006; 281:26205–26215.

47 Blair SA, Kane SV, Clayburgh DR, Turner JR: Epithelial myosin light chain kinase expression and activity are upregulated in inflammatory bowel disease. Lab Invest 2006;86: 191–201.

48 Musch MW, Clarke LL, Mamah D, Gawenis LR, Zhang Z, Ellsworth W, et al: T-cell activation causes diarrhea by increasing intestinal permeability and inhibiting epithelial Na^+,K^+-ATPase. J Clin Invest 2002;110: 1739–1747.

49 Clayburgh DR, Barrett TA, Tang Y, Meddings JB, Van Eldik LJ, Watterson DM, et al: Epithelial myosin light chain kinase-dependent barrier dysfunction mediates T-cell activation-induced diarrhea in vivo. J Clin Invest 2005;115:2702–2715.

50 Clayburgh DR, Musch MW, Leitges M, Fu YX, Turner JR: Coordinated epithelial NHE3 inhibition and barrier dysfunction are required for TNF-mediated diarrhea in vivo. J Clin Invest 2006;116:2682–2694.

51 Ferran C, Dy M, Merite S, Sheehan K, Schreiber R, Leboulenger F, et al: Reduction of morbidity and cytokine release in anti-CD3 MoAb-treated mice by corticosteroids. Transplantation 1990;50:642–648.

52 Ferran C, Sheehan K, Dy M, Schreiber R, Merite S, Landais P, et al: Cytokine-related syndrome following injection of anti-CD3 monoclonal antibody: further evidence for transient in vivo T cell activation. Eur J Immunol 1990;20:509–515.

53 Abramowicz D, Crusiaux A, Goldman M: Anaphylactic shock after retreatment with OKT3 monoclonal antibody. N Engl J Med 1992;327:736.

54 Stull JT: Myosin minireview series. J Biol Chem 1996;271:15849.

55 Kamm KE, Stull JT: Dedicated myosin light chain kinases with diverse cellular functions. J Biol Chem 2001;276:4527–4530.

56 Turner JR: Molecular basis of epithelial barrier regulation: from basic mechanisms to clinical application. Am J Pathol 2006;169: 1901–1909.

57 Shen L, Black ED, Witkowski ED, Lencer WI, Guerriero V, Schneeberger EE, et al: Myosin light chain phosphorylation regulates barrier function by remodeling tight junction structure. J Cell Sci 2006;119:2095–2106.

58 Su L, Shen L, Clayburgh DR, Nalle SC, Sullivan EA, Meddings JB, et al: Targeted epithelial tight junction dysfunction causes immune activation and contributes to development of experimental colitis. Gastroenterology 2009;136:551–563.

59 Ostanin DV, Bao J, Koboziev I, Gray L, Robinson-Jackson SA, Kosloski-Davidson M, et al: T-cell transfer model of chronic colitis: concepts, considerations, and tricks of the trade. Am J Physiol 2009;296:G135–G146.

60 Te Velde AA, de Kort F, Sterrenburg E, Pronk I, ten Kate FJ, Hommes DW, et al: Comparative analysis of colonic gene expression of three experimental colitis models mimicking inflammatory bowel disease. Inflamm Bowel Dis 2007;13:325–330.

61 Powrie F, Correa-Oliveira R, Mauze S, Coffman RL: Regulatory interactions between $CD45RB^{high}$ and $CD45RB^{low}$ CD4+ T cells are important for the balance between protective and pathogenic cell-mediated immunity. J Exp Med 1994;179:589–600.

62 Powrie F, Leach MW, Mauze S, Caddle LB, Coffman RL: Phenotypically distinct subsets of CD4+ T cells induce or protect from chronic intestinal inflammation in C. B-17 scid mice. Int Immunol 1993;5:1461–1471.

Therapeutic Options to Modulate Barrier Defects in Inflammatory Bowel Disease

Nina A. Hering   Jörg-Dieter Schulzke

Department of General Medicine, Charité Center 10, Campus Benjamin Franklin, Berlin, Germany

Key Words

Apoptosis · Barrier function · Crohn's disease · Flavonoids · Glutamine · Inflammatory bowel disease · Probiotics · Tight junction · Ulcerative colitis · Zinc

Abstract

In inflammatory bowel disease (IBD), epithelial barrier function is impaired contributing to diarrhea by a leak flux mechanism and perpetuating inflammation by an increased luminal antigen uptake. This barrier of the intestinal epithelium is composed of the apical enterocyte membrane and the epithelial tight junction (TJ) and can be affected by TJ alterations, induction of epithelial apoptoses and appearance of gross lesions like erosions or ulcers as well as by accelerated transcytotic antigen uptake. TJ strands are reduced in Crohn's disease (CD) and strand breaks appear. Several of the 24 claudins are concerned in CD as e.g. claudin-2, -5 and -8. The epithelial apoptotic rate has also been shown to be elevated causing focal lesions. As far as regulation is concerned, Th1 cytokines like TNF-α and interferon-γ are important for CD, while Th2 responses are dominated by interleukin (IL)-13 and TNF-α in ulcerative colitis (UC). IL-13 does stimulate epithelial apoptosis as well as upregulates claudin-2 in UC. Together with an IL-13-dependent restitution arrest, this may explain why ulcer lesions are seen already early in UC but only in advanced stages of CD. Luminal antigen uptake occurs via TJ discontinuities, epithelial gross lesions and endocytotically. Therapeutically, anti-inflammatory remedies as e.g. TNF-α antibodies are most effective in improving active IBD and in parallel repairing barrier function. Again, this is assumed to be due to reduced cytokine release in active IBD, as a result of immune cell apoptosis. However, other agents can also directly affect barrier function. Glutamine is discussed as a candidate for barrier therapy but has never been shown to have a direct barrier influence in CD, although it is an important metabolic fuel for enterocytes and has been shown to preserve barrier functions in laboratory models. Also, probiotics and TGF-β and have beneficial effects in models, but no data exist on barrier repair in IBD. In contrast, zinc has been shown to improve barrier function in CD, although the inherent mechanisms are unknown. Finally, food components can strengthen the epithelial barrier as for example the flavonoid quercetin which has been shown to upregulate claudin-4 within the epithelial TJ.

Copyright © 2009 S. Karger AG, Basel

Introduction

Intestinal inflammation is accompanied by altered epithelial barrier function in small and large intestine. This has two main consequences. First, ions and water can passively diffuse from the circulation to the intestinal lumen and cause *leak flux diarrhea*. The second consequence regards antigens and macromolecules, which under normal conditions cross the epithelial barrier only in very limited amounts. However, if the barrier function is

Table 1. Barrier function, TJs and apoptosis in CD

	Epithelial resistance	TJ strand count	Strand discontinuities	Apoptotic rate
Control	$39 \pm 4\ \Omega \cdot cm^2$ (10)	7.2 ± 0.2 (6)	0.2 ± 0.1 (6)	$1.0 \pm 0.1\%$ (10)
CD	$23 \pm 3\ \Omega \cdot cm^2$ (10)**	4.7 ± 0.2 (6)***	2.9 ± 0.6 (6)***	$2.8 \pm 0.3\%$ (8)***

In sigmoid colon of controls and patients with CD, epithelial resistance was measured by impedance spectroscopy. Epithelial TJs were characterized by measuring the number of horizontally oriented strands in the main compact meshwork of the TJ (strand count) and the frequency of strand discontinuities (per μm strand length) by freeze fracture electron microscopy. Finally, apoptotic rate was determined within the epithelium using TUNEL staining. All values are means ± SEM, number of patients is given in parentheses.
** $p < 0.01$ vs. control; *** $p < 0.001$ vs. control.

disturbed, uptake of antigens is increased and aggravates or even initiates chronic intestinal inflammation. Besides tight junction (TJ) changes, also other structural alterations in the epithelium as epithelial cell apoptosis, induction of erosions or ulcer lesions and transcytosis can play a role. In some regions along the gastrointestinal tract M-cells, the follicle-associated epithelium above Peyer's patches and transepithelial extrusions of antigen-presenting cells can contribute to the passage of antigens through the epithelial barrier. Thus, the present work gives an overview over changes of these barrier properties in inflammatory bowel disease (IBD) and the actual therapeutic options which can target epithelial dysfunction.

Epithelial Barrier Function in Inflammatory Bowel Disease

The autoimmune disease Crohn's disease (CD) goes along with segmental inflammation of the small and/or large intestinal mucosa which finally leads to diarrhea. The inherent mechanisms comprise reduced absorption and a defect in epithelial barrier function. Therefore, epithelial barrier function as well as TJ structure and epithelial apoptosis were studied in forceps biopsies obtained during endoscopy from the inflamed sigmoid colon of CD patients. Biopsy sites were chosen with mild to moderate disease activity which endoscopically appeared with hyperemia, edema and granularity and a histological score indicating an intact epithelium without erosions or ulcer-type lesions. Impedance spectroscopy was used to determine the epithelial resistance. The discrimination between epithelial and subepithelial resistance contributions is crucial, since both can change in the opposite direction. Epithelial resistance decreased by 41% which in conventional Ussing experiments would have been masked by the increase of subepithelial resistance due to inflammatory cell infiltration and submucosal edema. Thus, the inflamed colonic mucosa in CD is characterized by a significant disturbance of barrier function.

A possible structural correlate would be altered TJ structure within the epithelium. Here, large differences in resistance have been found to be associated with only small differences in the number of horizontally oriented TJ strands following a logarithmic correlation [1]. This held true also for CD, where the pronounced decrease in epithelial resistance was paralleled by a rather small reduction in epithelial cell TJ strands (table 1). Perhaps even more important, TJ strand discontinuities were more frequent in CD than in controls (table 1). Strand discontinuities are important for enabling macromolecules including food antigens to pass the epithelial barrier. To get insight into the molecular structure of the changes in TJ strands in CD, we have analyzed TJ proteins by Western blotting and densitometry in plasma membrane fractions prepared from endoscopic biopsies of the distal large intestine. It turned out that occludin, claudin-5 and claudin-8 were downregulated in CD, while claudin-1 and -4 were almost unchanged. In addition, claudin-2 which represents a pore-forming TJ protein was increased in CD. Finally, claudin-5 and -8 were distributed off the TJ in confocal laser scanning microscopy (data not shown).

In addition to changes in epithelial TJs, there was evidence for upregulation of epithelial apoptosis in CD (table 1). However, epithelial lesions like erosions were not observed (data not shown) which is in sharp contrast to our previous investigation in ulcerative colitis [2] and may explain why the extent of barrier disturbance is more pronounced in ulcerative colitis than in CD.

There is now increasing evidence that antigens or even bacteria can be taken up to a significant amount through the transcellular route by endocytosis and subsequent transcytotic extrusion over the basolateral enterocyte membrane. This mechanism is intensified in CD as indicated by electron microscope studies using ovalbumin and horseradish peroxidase [3, 4]. The mechanisms which regulate this transport during inflammation, however, are still unknown. The relative contribution of these different barrier defects to the overall barrier impairment in CD, however, may also vary and may as well depend on the severity of the inflammation and needs further experimental exploration in the future.

Effect of Therapeutic Agents on Intestinal Barrier Function

Our gain of information on intestinal barrier function at cellular and molecular level has raised the expectation that repair of barrier function becomes possible in IBD as the result of therapeutic intervention. This is indeed the case with anti-inflammatory therapy strategies which can heal the inflamed mucosa. That anti-inflammatory therapy can improve epithelial barrier function is in principle true for every therapeutic agent of this group of therapeutics, and it can be assumed that there is a direct correlation of barrier improvement with the anti-inflammatory efficacy. Data to support this have usually been obtained using in vivo permeability tests with drinking solutions containing various permeability markers including lactulose/rhamnose ratio, PEG400 or ^{51}Cr-EDTA. This is indicated by a correlation of CD activity and intestinal permeability [5, 6]. On the other hand, this is supported by data from patients with active CD either before and after steroid therapy or before and after application of elemental diets [7, 8]. Along this line of evidence, there is now also direct evidence for anti-TNF-α antibodies to improve epithelial barrier function in CD [9]. While TJ structure was not affected, apoptotic rate almost completely recovered towards normal in most of the patients 2 weeks after a single infusion of Remicade® (infliximab). As a result of this change in apoptotic rate, epithelial resistance as measured by impedance spectroscopy was also improved in endoscopic biopsies from these CD patients.

On the other hand, several distinct agents have been proposed to improve barrier function (table 2). Any piece of evidence for their efficacy in IBD, however, is usually

Table 2. Barrier-affecting agents in IBD

Agent	Barrier effect in models	Effect on IBD	Barrier effect in IBD	Ref.
L-Glutamine	+	–	–	10–13
Probiotics	+	+	–	14–16
TGF-β	+	–	–	17–19
Zinc	–	–	+	20
Quercetin	+	–	–	21

either lacking or was only arrived at inflammatory models either in cell cultures or animal models. This latter group of agents is summarized in table 2 and comprises L-glutamine, probiotics, TGF-β, zinc and food components like the flavonoid quercetin.

L-Glutamine has been shown to have direct short-term effects on intestinal barrier properties, namely to reduce bacterial translocation in animal and cell culture models including mice after a skin burn injury [10] and in rats on total parenteral nutrition [11]. However, no effect could be identified in CD patients with total parenteral nutrition when supplemented with glutamine [12] or when giving L-glutamine orally to CD patients in a long-term intervention study [13]. A possible explanation for this discrepancy could be that L-glutamine acts as an important source of energy for the enterocytes and that there is in contrast to the other experimental conditions no metabolic fuel deficiency in IBD. However, it could also be that the effect is not that pronounced and may be undetectable in a small group of IBD patients in an intervention design.

Another therapeutic approach in IBD which has been hypothesized to affect epithelial barrier function is probiotics. This assumption is mainly based on experimental studies performed in animal or cell line models. For example, *Saccharomyces boulardii* improved epithelial barrier function and diminished the translocation of enteropathogenic *Escherichia coli* in infected T84 cell monolayers [14], the probiotic compound VSL#3 attenuated *Salmonella* invasion in T84 cells [15] and *Lactobacillus acidophilus* reduced the aspirin-induced barrier disturbance in HT-29/B6 cells [16]. Although this seems to support the hypothesis of a barrier-preserving effect, direct experimental evidence for a short-term influence on the disturbed intestinal barrier function in IBD and putative inherent mechanisms has not been presented yet. However, since the probiotic *E. coli* Nissle 1917 has been shown to be as effective as mesalazine in keeping ulcerative colitis patients in remission and since VSL#3 normalized epithelial barrier function of the inflamed intestine in interleukin-10-deficient mouse model, it seems reasonable to conclude that an anti-inflammatory effect of (some) probiotics is very likely. Since this does subsequently also improve barrier properties, it will be very difficult to detect distinct direct barrier effects of probiotics as part of their therapeutic efficacy. Nevertheless, probiotics are today a prominent candidate within the remedies directed against intestinal barrier disturbances in IBD.

Another potential target therapeutics for barrier disturbances is the growth factor TGF-β. It has been demonstrated to stabilize epithelial barrier function in T84 cells after exposure to interferon-γ [17], to increase restitution velocity in injured T84 monolayers [18] and to improve epithelial barrier function in T84 infected with *E. coli* O157:H7 [19]. Thus, the common barrier-affecting mechanism of TGF-β is the increase in epithelial restitution velocity which is an important component of barrier function in the intestine against the appearance of apoptotic leaks and erosions. However, a final piece of evidence for a barrier effect in IBD tissue as part of a general therapeutic effect is still lacking. Again, this may also be difficult to work out in small and usually heterogeneous group of IBD patients. Thus, a certain potential for a barrier influence in IBD remains.

A further therapeutic option is zinc. In a direct intervention protocol, a beneficial effect of oral zinc supplementation has indeed been reported using lactulose-mannitol-permeability-ratio measurements in the urine after oral ingestion of the test sugars in 12 CD patients under 110 mg zinc three times daily [20]. As the only limitation of this finding, this effect of zinc could also be due to the recovery of a preexisting zinc deficiency in these CD patients and may be absent in other CD patients with a normal nutrition status. This could also explain that no direct barrier-affecting mechanisms of zinc have been reported. Thus, it is too early to draw a final conclusion on the role of zinc in IBD barrier repair.

As a final candidate within this paper, the flavonoid quercetin will be discussed. Quercetin is a secondary food component which is found in vegetables as apple and onion. It is absorbed from the lumen and has a direct barrier effect on Caco-2 cells which is due to a transcriptional upregulation of the TJ protein claudin-4 (promoter activity and mRNA level increased), as a consequence of which more barrier-forming claudin-4 is inserted into TJ strands as indicated by confocal laser scanning microscopy [21]. While this is strong laboratory data in support of a barrier-preserving function of flavonoids, direct evidence for a beneficial role in IBD is still lacking.

Taken together, a lot of barrier-affecting agents exist which could in a multimodal concept help to preserve barrier properties in IBD. More important, however, seems to be at present an effective anti-inflammatory strategy in IBD as e.g. anti-TNF-α antibodies which include in addition to many other targets within the inflamed intestinal wall also pronounced barrier effects in the epithelium.

Disclosure Statement

The authors declare that no financial or other conflict of interest exists in relation to the content of this article.

References

1 Claude P: Morphological factors influencing transepithelial permeability: a model for the resistance of the zonula occludens. J Membr Biol 1978;39:219–232.
2 Gitter AH, Wullstein F, Fromm M, Schulzke JD: Epithelial barrier defects in ulcerative colitis: characterization and quantification by electrophysiological imaging. Gastroenterology 2001;121:1320–1328.
3 Schurmann G, Bruwer M, Klotz A, Schmid KW, Senninger N, Zimmer KP: Transepithelial transport processes at the intestinal mucosa in inflammatory bowel disease. Int J Colorectal Dis 1999;14:41–46.
4 Soderholm JD, Streutker C, Yang PC, Paterson C, Singh PK, McKay DM, Sherman PM, Croitoru K, Perdue MH: Increased epithelial uptake of protein antigens in the ileum of Crohn's disease mediated by tumour necrosis factor-α. Gut 2004;53:1817–1824.
5 Andre F, Andre C, Emery Y, Forichon J, Descos L, Minaire Y: Assessment of the lactulose-mannitol test in Crohn's disease. Gut 1988;29:511–515.
6 Adenis A, Colombel JF, Lecouffe P, Wallaert B, Hecquet B, Marchandise X, Cortot A: Increased pulmonary and intestinal permeability in Crohn's disease. Gut 1992;33:678–682.
7 Sanderson IR, Boulton P, Menzies I, Walker-Smith JA: Improvement of abnormal lactulose/rhamnose permeability in active Crohn's disease of the small bowel by an elemental diet. Gut 1987;28:1073–1076.
8 Zoli G, Care M, Parazza M, Spano C, Biagi PL, Bernardi M, Gasbarrini G: A randomized controlled study comparing elemental diet and steroid treatment in Crohn's disease. Aliment Pharmacol Ther 1997;11:735–740.

9 Zeissig S, Bojarski C, Buergel N, Mankertz J, Zeitz M, Fromm M, Schulzke JD: Downregulation of epithelial apoptosis and barrier repair in active Crohn's disease by tumour necrosis factor-α antibody treatment. Gut 2004;53:1295–1302.
10 Gennari R, Alexander JW: Arginine, glutamine, and dehydroepiandrosterone reverse the immunosuppressive effect of prednisone during gut-derived sepsis. Crit Care Med 1997;25:1207–1214.
11 Li J, Langkamp-Henken B, Suzuki K, Stahlgren LH: Glutamine prevents parenteral nutrition-induced increases in intestinal permeability. JPEN J Parenter Enteral Nutr 1994;18:303–307.
12 Akobeng AK, Miller V, Stanton J, Elbadri AM, Thomas AG: Double-blind randomized controlled trial of glutamine-enriched polymeric diet in the treatment of active Crohn's disease. J Pediatr Gastroenterol Nutr 2000; 30:78–84.
13 Den Hond E, Hiele M, Peeters M, Ghoos Y, Rutgeerts P: Effect of long-term oral glutamine supplements on small intestinal permeability in patients with Crohn's disease. JPEN J Parenter Enteral Nutr 1999;23:7–11.
14 Czerucka D, Dahan S, Mograbi B, Rossi B, Rampal P: Saccharomyces boulardii preserves the barrier function and modulates the signal transduction pathway induced in enteropathogenic *Escherichia coli*-infected T84 cells. Infect Immun 2000;68:5998–6004.
15 Madsen K, Cornish A, Soper P, McKaigney C, Jijon H, Yachimec C, Doyle J, Jewell L, De Simone C: Probiotic bacteria enhance murine and human intestinal epithelial barrier function. Gastroenterology 2001;121:580–591.
16 Montalto M, Maggiano N, Ricci R, Curigliano V, Santoro L, Di Nicuolo F, Vecchio FM, Gasbarrini A, Gasbarrini G: *Lactobacillus acidophilus* protects tight junctions from aspirin damage in HT-29 cells. Digestion 2004; 69:225–228.
17 Planchon SM, Martins CA, Guerrant RL, Roche JK: Regulation of intestinal epithelial barrier function by TGF-$β_1$. Evidence for its role in abrogating the effect of a T-cell cytokine. J Immunol 1994;153:5730–5739.
18 McKaig BC, Makh SS, Hawkey CJ, Podolsky DK, Mahida YR: Normal human colonic subepithelial myofibroblasts enhance epithelial migration (restitution) via TGF-$β_3$. Am J Physiol 1999;276:G1087–G1093.
19 Howe KL, Reardon C, Wang A, Nazli A, McKay DM: Transforming growth factor-β regulation of epithelial tight junction proteins enhances barrier function and blocks enterohemorrhagic *Escherichia coli* O157: H7-induced increased permeability. Am J Pathol 2005;167:1587–1597.
20 Sturniolo GC, Di Leo V, Ferronato A, D'Odorico A, D'Inca R: Zinc supplementation tightens 'leaky gut' in Crohn's disease. Inflamm Bowel Dis 2001;7:94–98.
21 Amasheh M, Schlichter S, Amasheh S, Mankertz J, Zeitz M, Fromm M, Schulzke JD: Quercetin enhances epithelial barrier function and increases claudin-4 expression in Caco-2 cells. J Nutr 2008;138:1067–1073.

Inflammation in the Intestinal Tract: Pathogenesis and Treatment

Richard S. Blumberg

Gastroenterology Division, Brigham and Women's Hospital, Harvard Medical School, Boston, Mass., USA

Key Words

Inflammatory bowel disease · Innate immunity · Adaptive immunity · Inflammation · Intestines

Abstract

Over the past decade a major hypothesis has emerged for the etiopathogenesis of inflammatory bowel disease (IBD). This hypothesis proposes that IBD represents a dysregulated mucosal immune response to antigens derived from the commensal microbiota in a genetically susceptible host that initially derives from innate immune abnormalities leading to an excessive proinflammatory cytokine derived from CD4+ T cells (T-helper 1, T-helper 2, and T-helper 17 cytokines) over and above the response that is normally associated with tolerance and immunoregulation derived from T-regulatory cells. Given that the genetic predisposition has increasingly been recognized to affect the regulation of innate and adaptive immunity, intestinal epithelial cell physiologic barrier function and the potential inappropriate access of antigens to the mucosal immune system through this dysfunctional barrier function, a key point in understanding IBD pathophysiology is to understand the immunoregulatory pathways associated with the intestinal immune system as they apply to IBD. Therefore, immunogenetic pathways associated with innate and adaptive immunity, the cytokines secreted by innate and adaptive immune cells, the epithelial factors and leukocyte factors that are associated with inflammation and structures on the endothelium that regulate the recruitment of leukocytes define potential pathways that may be amenable to therapeutic manipulation in IBD.

Copyright © 2009 S. Karger AG, Basel

Introduction

Recent studies on the immunologic, microbiologic and genetic basis of both forms of inflammatory bowel disease (IBD), Crohn's disease (CD) and ulcerative colitis (UC) have provided an important blueprint for understanding the pathogenesis of these disorders and directing the development of new types of therapies. In this model (fig. 1), which is now well supported by a large body of evidence, IBD represents the dysregulated mucosal immune response to the normal commensal microbial antigens in a genetically susceptible host. It is clear that the genetic basis for this disease is centered on genetic factors that regulate the components of the innate and adaptive immune responses as well as the regulation of intestinal epithelial cell barrier function and interestingly the composition of the normal commensal microbiota itself within the intestines. This state of genetic susceptibility for the development of IBD is further modified by a variety of environmental factors which together affect the probability that either form

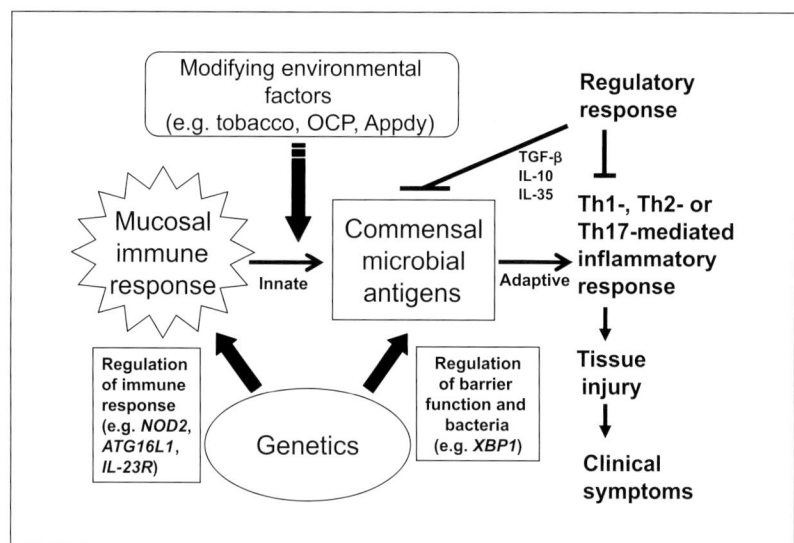

Fig. 1. Model for pathogenesis of IBD (see text for details).

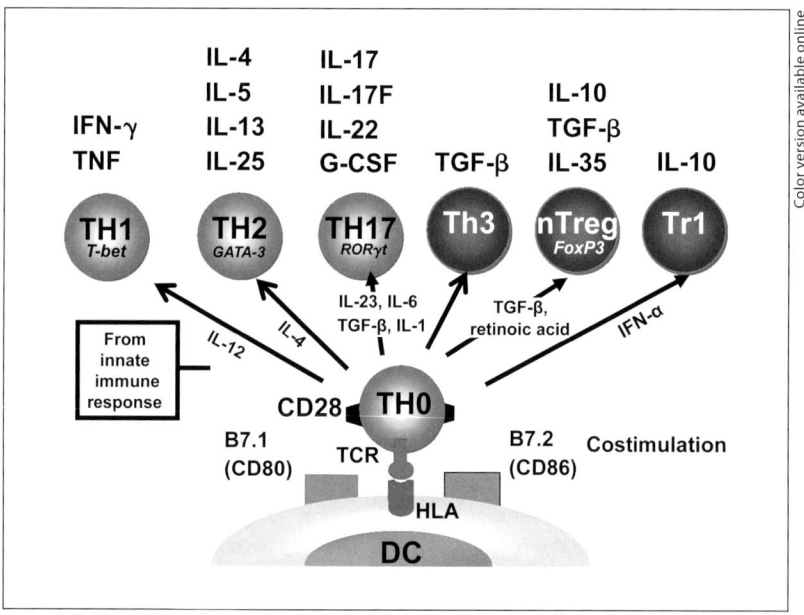

Fig. 2. Generation of T-helper cell subtypes based upon cytokine secretion. An APC such as a dendritic cell (DC) provides factors derived from the innate immune response to naive T cells (TH0) together with antigenic peptides in the context of MHC class II molecules to the TCR which is associated with the CD3 protein complex as well as secondary so-called co-stimulatory signals (e.g. B7-1 and B7-2 on the APC and CD28 on the T cells) that ultimately lead to polarized T-cell responses. These T-cell responses are regulated by transcription factors (e.g. T-bet in the case of TH1 cells) and either promote inflammation (TH1, TH2, TH17) or inhibit inflammation (Treg) making each of these cytokines or cell surface molecules a potential therapeutic target (see text for details).

of IBD will develop. The environmental factors that have been supported by epidemiologic studies to be important in modifying the risk for developing IBD include tobacco, appendectomy, antibiotics, oral contraceptive pills and likely non-steroidal anti-inflammatory agents. These environmental factors can be assumed to be important to the development of IBD through their ability to regulate the immune response of the host, the physiologic functions of the intestinal epithelial cell barrier and likely the composition and function of the commensal microbiota.

IBD is determined by the genetically defined, innate immune responsiveness of intestinal tissues to components of the commensal microbiota. Once initiated, the disease distills into a final common pathway that is characterized by an exaggerated adaptive immune response as expressed by the properties of aggressive T cells and B cells through their production of IgG antibodies that drive a state of chronic inflammation. The T cells that cause the inflammation associated with IBD are T cells that have been polarized to secrete distinct patterns of cytokines under the influence from factors derived from innate immune cells (fig. 2). Such polarized T cells are highly differentiated cell types that are defined as either T-helper 1 (TH1), TH2 or TH17. TH1 cells primarily secrete cytokines such as interferon-γ and tumor necrosis factor (TNF). TH2 cells are primarily those T cells that secrete interleukin (IL)-4, IL-5 and IL-13, and TH17 cells are those that primarily secrete IL-6, IL-22, and IL-17. The polarization of T cells to these types of cytokine-secreting cells which are in general highly inflammatory are regulated by particular transcription factors that include T-bet in the case of TH1 cells, GATA-3 in the case of TH2 cells and ROR-γT in the case of TH17 cells. In the end, these inflammatory factors that derive from the initiating innate immune response and the consequential adaptive immune response result in tissue injury and the clinical symptoms that are characteristic of these disorders. It should be noted in concluding this introduction to these disorders that IBD is a highly regulated process which accounts for the relapsing and remitting nature of these disorders. Regulation in these disorders is provided primarily by unique subsets of lymphocytes that are so-called T-regulatory cells that secrete immunosuppressive cytokines such IL-10, IL-35 and tumor growth factor-β (TGF-β). A significant number of T-regulatory cells can be found in the inflamed intestine. Their ability to overcome the inflammatory response is hypothesized to be a major reason for remission and thus is a major goal of therapies which aim to enable the regulatory functions of these naturally immunosuppressive cells.

Innate versus Adaptive Immunity

The immune response can be defined into two basic components: innate and adaptive, respectively (fig. 3). Innate immunity represents a rapidly generated hard-wired process that enables particular types of cells within the immune system such as macrophages, dendritic cells and B cells to respond quickly to molecular patterns contained within particular types of bacterial antigens. The cells that are considered to be the major subtypes of cells that express these types of pattern recognition receptors (PRRs) are so-called antigen presenting cells (APC). Epi-

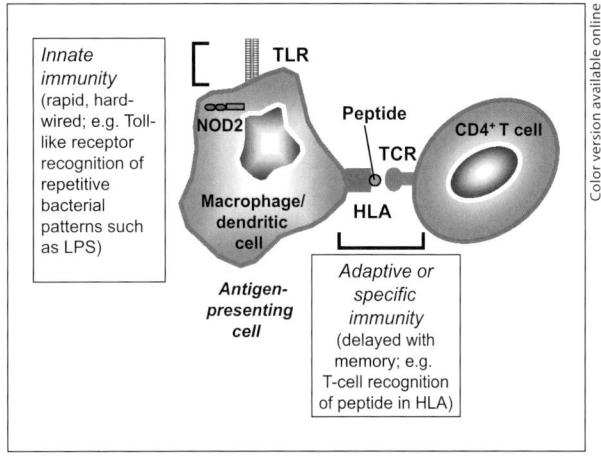

Fig. 3. Concept of innate and adaptive immune interactions between an APC and T cell (see text for details).

thelial cells of the intestine can also function as APC and express such PRRs. Another characteristic of an APC is, in addition to its expression of PRRs, its ability to internalize, process, and thus present antigens on the cell surface in the context of components of the major histocompatibility complex (MHC) encoded by genes on human chromosome 6. These MHC genes encode so-called human leukocyte antigens (HLA) that are either MHC class I (HLA-A, -B and -C) or MHC class II (HLA-DR, -DP and -DQ).

Examples of so-called PRRs are those receptors which can recognize and bind repetitive structural elements of bacteria, viruses and/or fungi. A classic example of this type of recognition is that associated with the lipopolysaccharide of Gram-negative bacteria which is bound by Toll-like receptor 4 (TLR-4). Another excellent example of pattern recognition is that associated with the so-called NOD like receptor (NLR) family such as NOD2 (or CARD15). NOD2 is an intracellular PRR that recognizes muramyl dipeptide derived from peptidoglycan contained within both Gram-positive and Gram-negative organisms. The interaction of an NLR or TLR by an APC occurs during the earliest phases of an immune response. The innate immune response to bacterial, viral or fungal antigens guides the subsequent responses of the T lymphocyte towards different types of differentiated fates that allow for a focused immune response appropriate to the antigenic encounter. Such a focusing of the T lymphocytes and especially particular CD4-positive lympho-

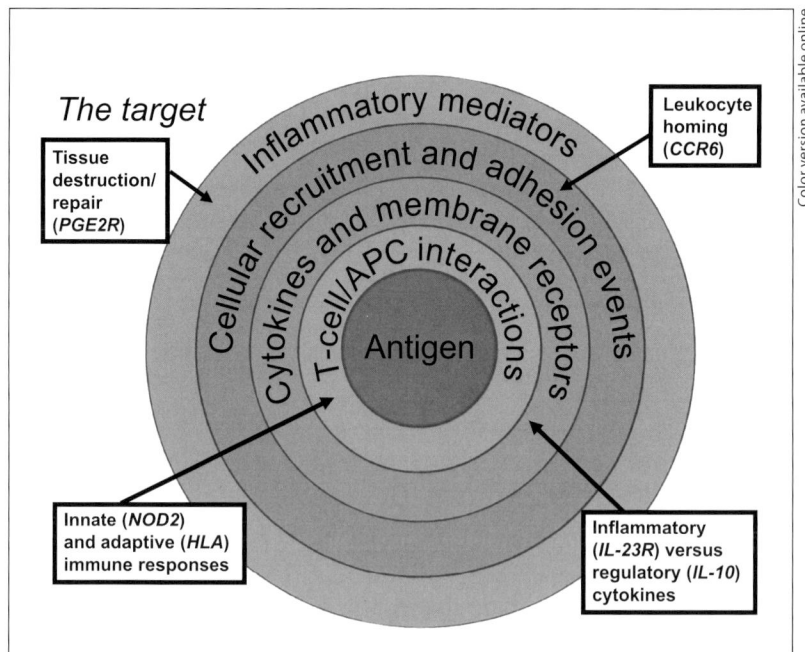

Fig. 4. Cascade of events associated with the development of an immune response. Each of these sequential steps is genetically regulated and subject to therapeutic manipulation. As such, the steps associated with inflammation represent a therapeutic target.

cytes or T-helper cells is associated with the so-called adaptive immune response that occurs over days to weeks and is thus delayed. Adaptive immunity is also characterized by memory for the antigen(s) that initiated the immune response. The major initial driving force for the development of an adaptive immune response is the presentation of a nominal (that is a small component antigen) antigen derived from a larger polypeptide or macromolecular structure via the HLA molecules to the T-cell receptor (TCR) that is expressed on the T-helper cell. T-cell recognition of these nominal peptides therefore in the context of HLA is the characteristic fingerprint of an initiating adaptive immune response (fig. 3). As a result of these processes, the adaptive T-cell response becomes focused into one of several different types of polarized classes of cytokine production as aforementioned: namely TH1, TH2 or TH17 or in the case of regulatory cells, T-reg.

In considering IBD, it is therefore important to understand the general development of immune response to an antigen (fig. 4). An immune response is initiated by the interactions between the innate immune system and an antigen. An inflammatory antigen characteristically has both innate and adaptive qualities. An excellent example of this is the flagellins of bacteria which are major antigenic drivers of CD. Flagellin has innate qualities through its repetitive structures that are able to bind TLR-5. Flagellin also is a polypeptide that upon internalization, processing and presentation by a professional APC such as a dendritic cell is able to generate nominal 14–22 amino acid peptides that are presented by MHC class II molecules (HLA-DR, -DP or -DQ) to CD4-positive T-helper cells. Thus the earliest phases of an immune response are dependent upon the recognition and interpretation of the antigenic composition of the milieu by a T cell and an APC as revealed by innate and adaptive immune responses. Subsequent to this interaction between the T cell, and APC in the context of an antigen, a series of events occur on both the T cell and APC that lead to the secretion of cytokines characteristic of each of these specific components as well as the upregulation of membrane receptors on the cell surface of the T cell and APC as a consequence of this activation. During this phase of an immune response the cytokines that are derived from these interactions can be either inflammatory (e.g. interferon-γ, IL-4, IL-13, TNF) or regulatory (IL-10, IL-35, TGF-β). These cytokines and membrane receptors also guide the responses of other cell types within the intestinal tissues or other tissues wherein an inflammatory response is initiated. This occurs through the effects of the cytokines and other soluble mediators on the endothelium that results in the activation of the endothelium and the recruitment of additional cells into the tissues through adhesion events between the circulating leukocytes within the peripheral blood and molecules on the cell surface of the endothelium. This process which is called *homing* is an important event in amplifying the immune response. As a consequence of inflammation of the endothelial lining, inflammatory mediators are produced that result in tissue destruction and consequently the inflammation that are associated with IBD. Each of these successive steps of the immune response is likely to be genetically regulated. Specifically, polymorphisms within genes associated with innate immunity *(NOD2)*, adaptive immunity *(HLA)*, inflammatory cytokine production and responses to inflammatory cytokines *(IL-23R)* production of regulatory cytokines *(IL-10)*, the homing of leukocytes through endothelium to the lamina propria *(CCR6)* and the development of tissue destruction secondary to responses to inflammatory mediators such as prostaglandins *(EP4R)* are all potentially genetically regulated pathways.

In summary therefore, IBD represents the interactions between genetic susceptibility and modifying environmental factors that culminate in mucosal immune dysregulation and consequently inflammation. At the foundation of this disease therefore is the genetic composition of the host and the susceptibility to IBD that is derived from this genetic composition. Thus, genes associated with innate immunity such as *NOD2* and *ATG16L1* that is specifically associated with autophagy, endoplasmic reticulum (ER) stress such as through polymorphisms in the gene that encodes the X-box binding protein 1 (XBP1) or responsiveness to inflammatory cytokines (e.g. *IL-23R*) regulate both the composition of the commensal microbiota as well as the immune response to the commensal microbiota.

Role of the Microbiota in IBD

The human gastrointestinal tract is the largest site of bacterial commensals in the human body. The concentrations of bacteria range from $<10^2$ colony-forming units per milliliter within the stomach to $>10^{12}$ colony-forming units of bacteria in the colon. In its totality, the numbers of bacteria in the human intestine achieve levels of 10^{13} to 10^{14} as compared to the number of cells within the human body which is only in the number of 10^{12} to 10^{13}. Thus there are more than ten times greater numbers of bacterial cells than human host cells in a normal individual. The normal microbiota achieve or comprise approximately 50% of fecal cellular material and are composed of more than 400 different species and a larger number of quasi species. Most of these bacteria are non-culturable. The normal bacteria are important for a wide variety of homeostatic processes. The normal bacteria provide approximately 40% of the normal energy metabolism associated with the host such that germ-free mice have less weight than normally colonized mice. The bacteria in the intestine fall largely within two major phyla namely Firmicutes that largely represent the Gram-positive bacteria and Bacteroidetes which mainly comprise the Gram-negative bacteria. In addition, the normal intestine contains many other life forms including viruses, protists, fungi, and archea as other life forms. Most of these are, as noted, contained within the normal colon. Consistent with this, IBD is mainly localized to the areas of the intestines in which most of the bacteria are congregated, namely, the distal small intestine or ileum, and the colon. This is consistent with the bacterial hypothesis that the commensal microbiota is the major environmental driver of IBD. In addition, recent genetic evidence that has revealed polymorphisms within genes associated with innate immune responses to bacteria such as *NOD2* in CD and autophagy-associated genes in CD (e.g. *ATG16L1* and *IRGM*) are also consistent with the bacterial hypothesis. Specifically, the bacterial hypothesis states that IBD represents the inappropriate response of the mucosal-associated immune system to the commensal microbiota in a genetically susceptible host such that removal of the commensal microbiota will prevent the development of IBD as supported by model systems for mice. Removal of the commensal bacteria from mouse models which are genetically susceptible for the development of intestinal inflammation that models IBD such as by establishing these mouse models under germ-free conditions or treatment of such mouse models with antibiotics will prevent the development of intestinal inflammation. Such animal models in which this has been achieved include mice which have genetic deletion of the *IL-2* gene which results in the loss of T-regulatory cells from the thymus or the *IL-10* gene or genes associated with other regulatory pathways. Similarly, treatment of humans, especially patients with CD, can result in diminution of intestinal inflammation in selected subjects. Thus in a genetically susceptible host the mucosal-associated immune system is responding to the commensal microbiota as if it were in fact a pathogen.

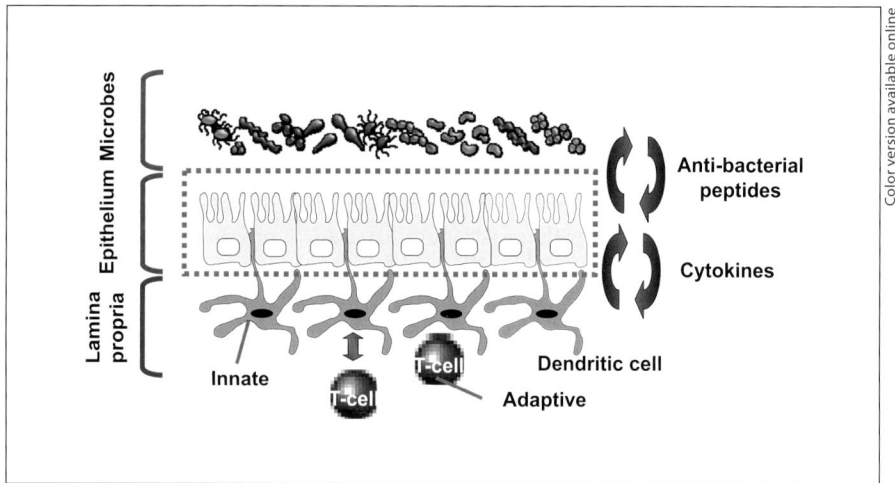

Fig. 5. Critical immunologic role of the IEC in IBD. There is a bidirectional cross-talk between the commensal microbiota and the IEC that regulates the function of the IEC and the composition of the commensal microbiota through the secretion of antimicrobial peptides. The IEC attracts innate and adaptive immune cells into the lamina propria and provides innate immune signals to dendritic cells that in turn regulate the activity of T cells which feeds back to the epithelium. ER stress within the epithelium can modify both of these important functions as described in the text. There is thus a tridirectional cross-talk between the microbes, intestinal epithelium and immune cells that are contained within the lamina propria.

The Intestinal Epithelial Cell in IBD

The fact that the commensal microbiota is a critical driver of the intestinal inflammation associated with IBD focuses attention on the special role of the intestinal epithelial cell in IBD. The intestinal epithelial cell (IEC) is uniquely located as a barrier between two totally distinct worlds (fig. 5). The IEC separates the outside world which contains the commensal microbiota from the inside world contained within the lamina propria that includes a complete set of immunologically responsive cells. The lamina propria in particular contains cells associated with innate immunity such as dendritic cells, macrophages and polymorphonuclear leukocytes as well as those that are associated with the adaptive immune system such as T lymphocytes, B lymphocytes and a unique set of lymphocytes that may be associated with UC; the so-called natural killer T cells (NKT cells). The epithelial cell is thus strategically located allowing for it to both regulate the composition of the commensal microbiota as well as respond to the commensal microbiota through the secretion of a variety of antibacterial peptides and other substances. In a similar manner, the IEC responds to bacterial factors such as through innate immune receptor signaling associated with PRRs resulting in the secretion of cytokines through the basal surface of the IEC that affects both the composition and the function of the subjacent immune cells. The epithelial cell for example in response to bacterial and other microbially associated sources leads to secretion of important regulatory molecules such as thymic stromal lymphopoietin that regulates the differentiation of T cells between TH1 and TH2 polarity by favoring the latter. The regulation of microbial composition and sensitivity to microbial products by the innate immune system of the intestines is therefore critical to the development of IBD in both forms of IBD.

IECs have therefore received a significant amount of attention in understanding IBD. IECs are derived from a common stem cell within the crypt that leads to the differentiation into four distinct lineages through the activity of specific transcription factors. These four lineages of cells include those which migrate to the apical cell surface of the villus tip (the mucus-secreting goblet cells, the hormone-secreting enteroendocrine cells and the cytokine-secreting absorptive epithelial cells) and a specialized lineage of cells that migrates deep into the crypt which is responsible for the secretion of antibacterial peptides (Paneth cell). The Paneth cell is a major site of production of antimicrobial peptides through secretion of molecules such as lysosyme and the α-defensins (so-called cryptdins). Paneth cells provide antibacterial protection and are primarily contained within the small intestine but not in the normal colon except during inflammation including the inflammation associated with bacterial infections and IBD. The Paneth cell has received a significant amount of attention because several different genetic risk factors have been observed to be associated with Paneth cell abnormalities in IBD – both CD and UC. Humans and mice with loss of either *NOD2* or *ATG16L1* function exhibit abnormalities in Paneth cell structure and function. These studies support the possibility that intracellular bacterial sensing through *NOD2* and the regulation of autophagy, an important housekeeping function of all cell types, is involved in the maintenance of Paneth cell function. Similarly, Paneth cells are significantly influenced by the functionality of genes associated with ER stress. ER stress is commonly observed in cells that are highly secretory such as Paneth cells. The ability of a highly secretory cell to manage ER stress through a pathway called the unfolded protein response (UPR) is of major importance to the development and function of such highly secretory cells. Deletion of at least one gene associated with the ER stress response, XBP1, has recently been linked to the functionality of Paneth cells as well as their presence in mouse models. Moreover, polymorphisms in XBP1 have been recently shown to be associated with genetic risk in humans with both CD and UC.

The UPR is a signaling pathway from the ER to the nucleus that protects cells from the stress caused by unfolded or misfolded proteins. As noted above, ER stress is quite common in highly secretory cells and may be particularly prominent in the intestine given that this is a highly stressful environment that has recently been appreciated to induce an UPR, especially in the small intestine as well as the colon. During an UPR in the context of cellular stress as would occur during the secretory requirements associated with inflammation, the cell activates a series of signaling pathways from the ER that regulate the transcription of factors that are able to compensate for the cellular stress within the ER. Studies in knockout mice have clearly shown that XBP1 is one such factor such that in the absence of XBP1 significant cellular stress to the epithelium is observed of such intensity that may lead in and of itself to primary intestinal inflammation [1].

Under normal homeostatic conditions, the IEC, given its important secretory function, maintains a UPR transcriptional program that provides for cellular vitality. In the context of hypomorphic XBP1 function as would occur in a genetically susceptible host, the IEC becomes highly subject to the stressful environment associated with the intestines. This stress in its worse case leads to the death of Paneth cells contained within the small intestine. It is possible that the Paneth cell metaplasia within the colon that characterizes IBD may also occur. As a result, there is decreased secretion of antimicrobial peptides into the lumen which may regulate the composition of the commensal microbiota. At the same time, IECs in the context of hypomorphic XBP1 function become exquisitely sensitive to PRR signaling such as that associated with TLRs leading to an exaggerated production of proinflammatory mediators such as chemokines that attract leukocytes into the gut as well as TNF. Thus, innate immune responses associated with abnormal ER stress within the epithelium as regulated by XBP1 can be an important means for the development of IBD. In fact, these recent studies suggest that intestinal inflammation associated with IBD may originate primarily from increased sensitivity of the intestinal epithelium to the environmental factors that are contained within the normal milieu per se as well as the milieu that is observed within the context of inflammation.

Taken together, a new model has emerged in which primary (genetic) and secondary (environmental factors) can drive ER stress in the intestinal epithelium and consequently either initiate and/or promote the development of inflammation. Primary genetic factors that appear to be important for the development of ER stress that may be linked to the development of intestinal inflammation include hypomorphic polymorphisms of the *XBP1* gene as well as genes such as *ATG16L1* and *IRGM* that are associated with autophagy. The reason for this is that ER stress is a major regulator of autophagy. Autophagy is a pathway of so-called 'self-eating' wherein degradative organelles contained within the cell ingest other organelles as a housekeeping function to maintain cell vitality. Autophagy is an important pathway in the maintenance of cell structure but is also important during conditions of starvation and the removal of ingested pathogens. It is therefore not surprising that hypomorphic autophagy function might be involved in the pathogenesis of IBD given the importance of microbial homeostasis in the underlying pathophysiology. It can be imagined therefore that that the concomitant inability of the host to both manage ER stress and autophagy could together serve as a particularly deleterious consequence for the host. In addition, it is also clear that a variety of secondary environmental factors can induce ER stress and theoretically promote intestinal inflammation. These secondary environmental factors include both those from bacteria which

Table 1. IBD – therapeutic implications

Target	Mechanism	Therapeutic
Antigen	Eliminate pathogenic bacterial strain	Antibiotic/probiotic (VSL #3®)
T-cell/APC interactions	Block innate immune signaling or manipulate co-stimulation	Anti-CD3 (Visilizumab®), CTLA4-Ig (Abatacept®), Azathioprine/6MP
Cytokines and membrane receptors	↓ Proinflammatory or ↑ anti-inflammatory cytokines	Anti-TNF (Remicaide®, Humira®, Certolizomab®), anti-IL-12p40, anti-TL1A, anti-IL-17, anti-IL-6R, anti-IL-13, IFN-β
Cellular recruitment	Block T-cell homing or endothelial cell addressins	Anti-α4β7 (Tysabri®, LDP-02®), anti-MadCAM1
Inflammatory mediators	Block inflammatory signaling	Protease inhibitors (TACEi), mesalamines
Barrier function and repair	↑ Epithelial barrier and restitution	Epidermal growth factor (?)

have been shown to inhibit XBP1 function for example such as factors from pathogenic bacteria, dietary factors such as high fat or glucose deprivation, inflammation and in particular hypoxia and cytokines such as TNF and potentially drugs or stress per se such as that due to neurogenic factors can all activate ER stress pathways. In a genetically susceptible host, such environmental factors may promote the development of intestinal inflammation and involve the IEC. Such models are currently under investigation and may be of particular relevance to IBD.

Innate and Adaptive Immune Interactions in the Development of IBD

These aforementioned comments lead to a pathophysiologic model in which a genetically susceptible host that is exposed to a particular set of environmental events that cause an alteration in the composition of microbial community associated with the intestines or the responsiveness or the level of responsiveness of the mucosal immune system can abnormally activate the innate and/or adaptive immune systems which will initiate intestinal inflammation. In this model, it can be imagined that an inability to appropriately manage ER stress or an inability to properly deal with intracellular bacterial challenges in the context of abnormal autophagy or PRR function may lead to an inappropriate innate immune response that would initiate the origins of IBD. In this model, pathogenic microorganisms may be particularly important because of their ability to cause dramatic alterations in the composition of the commensal microbiota as well as modify the immune response. Similarly, it can be imagined that antibiotics can in the genetically susceptible host create alterations to the microbiota that are also potentially deleterious. Another example is smoking which may be particularly deleterious in CD due to the ability for example of carbon monoxide to activate TH1 pathways as discussed further below. It can be further predicted that the genetically susceptible host will also have a genetically endowed abnormalities in the regulation of the adaptive immune system such that the adaptive immune system is overly responsive to factors derived from innate immune responses. An excellent example of this hypothesis is the description of polymorphisms in the IL-23 receptor that would predict the inappropriate responsiveness of T lymphocytes to IL-23 from innate cells such as dendritic cells. Thus it can be imagined that there is a pathogenic progression of IBD that begins with a series of environmental events in a genetically susceptible host that leads to an exaggerated innate immune response and/or overly reactive adaptive immune response that is unable to be downregulated.

Cytokines Associated with Adaptive Immunity

One of the greatest types of therapy that has been shown to be particularly important in the modern treatment of IBD is the use of biologic agents that target cytokines (table 1). It is therefore appropriate to conclude this discussion with consideration of the cytokines that are associated with transitioning from innate immunity to adaptive immunity. The exaggerated innate immune response that is believed to be associated with the development of IBD is characterized by the exaggerated secretion of cytokines derived from innate immune cells that are both proinflammatory and consequently important drivers of adaptive T-cell function. The former includes cytokines such as TNF and IL-6 both of which are important therapeutic targets in the treatment of IBD. Specifically antibodies directed at TNF or at the IL-6 receptor signaling pathways have revealed themselves to be important new approaches in the treatment of this disease [2–6]. Similarly, cytokines from innate immune cells such as IL-12 and IL-23 which are highly related to one another and which drive the development of inflammatory T cells and the inhibition of regulatory T cells have also been shown to be important therapeutic targets of CD. IL-12 and IL-23 are heterodimeric proteins. The IL-12p40 chain is shared in common between both the IL-12 and the IL-23 proteins and has shown itself to be an important potential new therapeutic target for these patients [7]. Finally, T cells under the influence of these factors from innate immune cells are forced to differentiate to either TH1 cells that secrete exaggerated amounts of interferon-γ or TH17 cells that secrete IL-17, especially in CD. Studies to evaluate the clinical responses of IBD patients to therapies that neutralize interferon-γ or IL-17 are underway and require additional evaluation [8]. In UC, there appears to be an inappropriate TH2-like cytokine response that may be associated with NKT cells and is characterized by excess IL-13 production through a less well characterized process, making IL-13 an interesting therapeutic target. Similarly, some subsets of dendritic cells and macrophages are able to induce T cells into a regulatory phenotype that inhibits inflammation through the secretion of TGF-β, IL-10 and IL-35. Thus it is the balance between regulatory T cells and proinflammatory T-helper cells that leads to the final determination of whether chronic inflammation or homeostasis will in fact occur.

Conclusion

From these comments, a common immunogenic pathway can be envisioned for the development of IBD. In this pathway, the genetically determined relationship between IECs and the commensal microbiota in the lumen and the immune cells within the lamina propria are a critical initial step in the pathogenesis of this disease. In this model, IECs are constantly secreting antimicrobial factors into the milieu of the lumen to regulate the composition of microbiota and are in turn continuously responding to components of the bacteria. In a genetically susceptible host such as one that possesses polymorphisms in the *XBP1* gene that regulates ER stress responses, the ability to manage the commensal microbiota and to respond appropriately to the intestinal microbiota is deranged. Similarly, in a genetically susceptible host it can be envisioned that the relationship between the IEC and the innate cells within the lamina propria is also abnormal. In this context, innate immune cells within the lamina propria are inappropriately responding to bacterial components such as individuals who have polymorphisms such as the *NOD2* gene. This abnormal innate immune signaling from dendritic cells would be predicted to result in the secretion of inflammatory cytokines (such as TNF and IL-6) as well as other important cytokines that modify the adaptive immune response leading in the genetically susceptible host to an exaggerated degree of adaptive immune T cells secreting highly proinflammatory cytokines as well as an inappropriately low number of T-regulatory cells or resistance of the effector T cells to the regulatory effects of the T-regulatory cells. In this model, cytokines such as IL-12 and IL-23 derived from aggressive innate immune cells within the lamina propria would be predicted to push T cells to secrete high quantities of TH1- and TH17-associated cytokines that have been recently appreciated to be associated with the development of CD. It can be predicted that blockade of IL-12p40 which is common to both IL-12 and IL-23 will lead to amelioration of this disease. Similarly, exaggerated innate immune signaling in an UC patient may lead to exaggerated production of inflammatory mediators that drive the development of aggressive TH2 cells although this pathway is not as well characterized to date. Thus, the insights provided by understanding the immunopathogenesis of IBD is increasingly providing opportunities for new therapeutic approaches in the treatment of patients with this very important immune mediated group of diseases.

Disclosure Statement

The author declares that no financial or other conflict of interest exists in relation to the content of this article.

References

1 Kaser A, et al: XBP1 links ER stress to intestinal inflammation and confers genetic risk for human inflammatory bowel disease. Cell 2008;134:743–756.
2 Hanauer SB, et al: Human anti-tumor necrosis factor monoclonal antibody (adalimumab) in Crohn's disease: the CLASSIC-I trial. Gastroenterology 2006;130:323–333.
3 Ito H, et al: A pilot randomized trial of a human anti-interleukin-6 receptor monoclonal antibody in active Crohn's disease. Gastroenterology 2004;126:989–996.
4 Present DH, et al: Infliximab for the treatment of fistulas in patients with Crohn's disease. N Engl J Med 1999;340:1398–1405.
5 Sandborn WJ, et al: Certolizumab pegol for the treatment of Crohn's disease. N Engl J Med 2007;357:228–238.
6 Targan SR, et al: A short-term study of chimeric monoclonal antibody cA2 to tumor necrosis factor α for Crohn's disease. N Engl J Med 1997;337:1029–1035.
7 Mannon PJ, et al: Anti-interleukin-12 antibody for active Crohn's disease. N Engl J Med 2004;351:2069–2079.
8 Hommes DW, et al: Fontulizumab, a humanized anti-interferon-γ antibody, demonstrates safety and clinical activity in patients with moderate to severe Crohn's disease. Gut 2006;55:1131–1137.

Targeted Therapies in Inflammatory Bowel Disease

Britta Siegmund

Charité, Campus Benjamin Franklin, Medizinische Klinik I, Berlin, Germany

Key Words

Inflammatory bowel disease, pathogenesis · Targeted therapies · Genome-wide association studies

Abstract

The pathogenesis of inflammatory bowel disease (IBD) is still not completely understood, however the ongoing research of the last decade is allowing the hypothesis that in genetically predisposed individuals distinct environmental factors result in a dysregulation of the mucosal immune system and thus IBD. Until today the majority of patients are being treated with rather unspecific medications exerting suppressive effects on the mucosal immune system. Nevertheless, these substances including azathioprine and steroids have proven excellent efficacy for defined subgroups of patients. However, the better understanding of the underlying pathogenesis resulted in the clinical development of novel therapeutic strategies with specific targets. The most prominent example being antibodies targeting tumor necrosis factor-α which are routinely administered in patients suffering from either Crohn's disease (CD) or ulcerative colitis. A second strategy is targeting the protein subunit p40 which heterodimerizes either with p35 resulting in the pro-inflammatory cytokine IL-12 or with p19 thus forming the pro-inflammatory IL-23. Experimental data suggest a crucial role for both cytokines in experimental colitis. Various antibodies against p40 are currently in clinical trials for patients with CD. In areas of inflammation, the blood vessel endothelial cells upregulate adhesion molecules resulting in the infiltration of leukocytes into the respective area. Natalizumab blocks these adhesion molecules. Treatment with natalizumab was associated with clinical improvement in patients with CD and has been approved in the USA. In summary, several therapeutic targets have already entered our clinical routine and have for some patients resulted in significant changes of the disease course.

Copyright © 2009 S. Karger AG, Basel

Introduction

The research of the last decade has contributed significantly to the understanding of the pathogenesis of inflammatory bowel disease (IBD) and consequently to the development of novel therapeutic strategies targeting single molecules. In particular the genome-wide association studies (GWAS) have and will reveal further novel molecules which may serve as future targets in the treatment of IBD.

With the present overview, selected targeted therapies and their suggested modes of action will be discussed. The mechanisms involved aim at maintaining the epithelial barrier, inhibiting pro-inflammatory innate cells as well as effector T cells within the lamina propria and prevent the infiltration of inflammatory cells through the vascular epithelium. An overview is provided in figure 1.

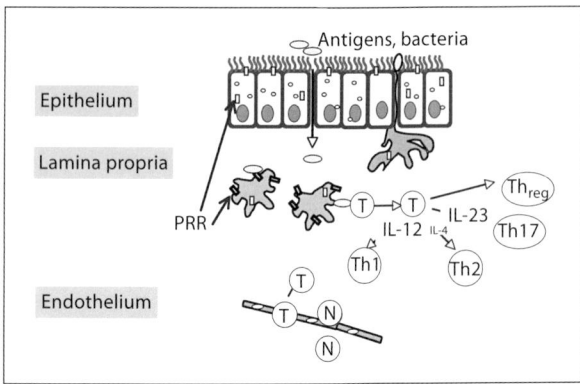

Fig. 1. Therapeutic targets in the mucosa.

Targeted Therapy – From Bench to Bedside

Anti-Tumor Necrosis Factor-α

Anti-tumor necrosis factor-α (TNF-α) strategies are established as anti-inflammatory therapy for a subgroup of patients with Crohn's disease (CD) as well as for patients suffering from ulcerative colitis [1, 2]. While a subgroup of patients show an impressive therapeutic efficacy, others do not respond at all. What is the mechanism behind this efficacy and are there experimental data providing an explanation for this discrepancy?

In 2001, the first experimental data from studies performed with peripheral blood mononuclear cells from patients treated with the chimeric anti-TNF-α antibody infliximab were examined. As early as 4 h after the infliximab infusion an increase in the apoptotic rate of peripheral blood mononuclear cells could be observed suggesting that apoptosis might play a role [3]. This idea was further expanded in a study published in 2007 investigating experimental colitis models as well as patients with CD [4]. The authors demonstrated in two independent animal models, the trinitrobenzene sulfonic acid-induced colitis model and the transfer model of colitis, that anti-TNF-α treatment resulted not only in an amelioration of disease but was also associated with an increase in apoptosis at the site of inflammation. Similarly, in patients with CD where infliximab treatment was followed by a decrease of the Crohn's Disease Activity Index, a paralleled increase of the apoptotic rate at the site of inflammation was observed. These results strongly suggest that anti-TNF-α exerts efficacy in patients when an increase of apoptosis can be observed. Similar mechanisms have been suggested for adalimumab. Perplexingly, no apoptosis induction could be proven for the certolizumab that has also been shown to exert clinical efficacy [5, 6].

For infliximab, a second, though related mechanism has been proposed. In this study, not the cells of the lamina propria or the peripheral blood built the endpoint but the intestinal epithelial cells. The initial hypothesis was based on the fact that in CD the barrier function is impaired, thus an efficacious treatment should be able to re-establish the intestinal barrier. Two parameters were evaluated in patients with CD before and 14 days after the infliximab infusion as well as in control patients: (1) the local epithelial apoptosis rate, and (2) the epithelial resistance was determined by alternating current impedance analysis in Ussing chambers. Before infliximab infusion, the apoptotic rate in epithelial cells was increased in CD patients when compared to healthy controls and vice versa, the epithelial resistance was decreased in CD patients. However, 14 days after infliximab infusion the apoptotic rate in intestinal epithelial cells from CD patients decreased, and in parallel, the epithelial resistance increased. Thus, infliximab treatment induced a normalization of the epithelial barrier function [7].

Thus, while induction of apoptosis provides one mechanism involved, other yet unidentified pathways might in addition contribute to the clinical efficacy.

Targeting p40 – IL-12 or IL-23?

Targeting key cytokines was an early-on approach to control effector T-cell function. One subpopulation of effector T cells, the so-called T-helper cells type 1 (Th1 cells), was already in the focus of therapeutic targets over 10 years ago, since cytokines secreted by this subpopulation could be shown to be increased locally in patients with CD. Functional data proving this concept were first provided in an animal model of intestinal inflammation. In this model system, anti-'IL-12' antibody treatment resulted in amelioration of disease when compared to mice receiving a control antibody [8]. This concept was then transferred to humans with CD and a first study, published in 2004, provided evidence that anti-'IL-12' exerts efficacy in a subgroup of patients [9].

However, GWAS caused some confusion about this concept. Thus, GWAS revealed a highly significant association between CD and the IL-23 receptor (IL-23R) gene on chromosome 1p31, which encodes a subunit of the receptor for the pro-inflammatory cytokine IL-23 [10, 11]. Why should this cause confusion? IL-23 as well as IL-12 belong to the IL-12 cytokine family. Both are heterodimers and share the common subunit p40. In the case of IL-12, p40 forms a heterodimer with the subunit p35, and

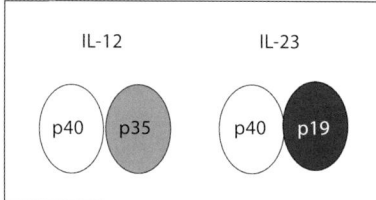

Fig. 2. p40 can either form a heterodimer with p35 resulting in IL-12 or form a heterodimer with p19 resulting in IL-23.

in the case of IL-23, p40 builds a heterodimer with the subunit p19 (fig. 2).

From these publications the obvious question arose whether or not IL-12 or rather IL-23 represents the key target. Remarkably, in the clinical study as well as in the animal model investigated initially, the antibody applied was targeting not p35 but p40, thus the neutralization of which cytokine resulted in the observed clinical benefit remains to be clarified [9]. This controversy was immediately picked up by the scientific community providing at least some insight to date. This research puts the spotlight on the pro-inflammatory cytokine IL-23 [12, 13] – prioritizing this molecule and associated signaling pathways as therapeutic target in IBD. IL-23 activates a subset of Th cells characterized by the production of the cytokine IL-17. These so-called Th17 cells express the master transcription factor RORγt and have been shown to mediate chronic inflammatory and autoimmune diseases in animal models [14]. Numerous animal data have been performed targeting specifically p35 for IL-12 or p19 for IL-23, respectively [13, 15–17].

The IL-23R is also expressed on the surface of macrophages and dendritic cells and may thereby control barrier function and immune response against the commensal microflora in the gut. Consistent with this hypothesis, IL-23 is required for gut inflammation via innate immune mechanisms in T-cell-deficient animals [15]. This finding clearly shows that IL-23 may cause gut inflammation in the absence of T lymphocytes, further highlighting a master control function of IL-23 in the gut [18].

From a mechanistic point of view, the results obtained by the transfer model of colitis offer a clear view. In this model, naive T cells are adoptively transferred into immunodeficient, RAG knockout mice causing chronic intestinal inflammation. The authors found that colitis was suppressed in recipient mice deficient in p19 and p40 – but not in p35, the subunit thought to be specific for IL-12 [16].

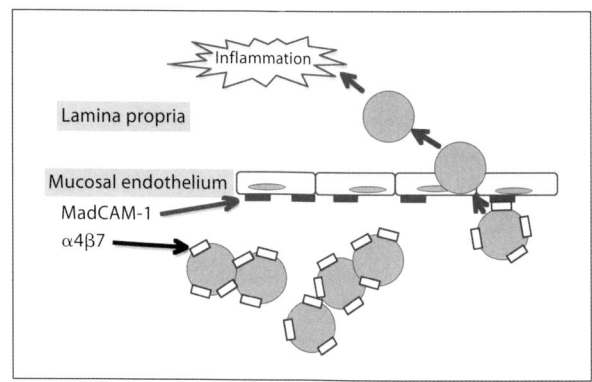

Fig. 3. Infiltration of activated cells by binding of α4β7 to MadCAM in gut endothelial cells.

Taken together, all these data indicate that IL-23 initiates and perpetuates both innate and T-cell-mediated intestinal inflammation. Thus, selective targeting of IL-23 is now emerging as an attractive concept – not only with new findings, but also because IL-12 mediates protective systemic antimicrobial immunity. Consequently, blockade of IL-23 may be as effective as blocking both cytokines – but may result in fewer infectious problems [18].

In the near future, we can expect to learn how IL-23 signaling affects gut inflammation in patients with CD, since clinical studies selectively targeting p19 are currently ongoing.

Blocking Adhesion Molecules – Preventing Infiltration of Inflammatory Cells

An upregulation of adhesion molecules on activated lymphocytes and monocytes as well as on the endothelial cells of the respective organs results in an increased infiltration of activated cells and consequently in an aggravation of the inflammatory process. Thus, selective inhibition of adhesion molecules represents a self-evident target when considering anti-inflammatory strategies. Animal models have shown that the adhesion molecule mucosal addressin cell adhesion molecule-1 (MadCAM-1) as well as the vascular adhesion molecule-1 (VCAM-1) is dramatically elevated in the chronically inflamed colonic vasculature. To address the role of MadCAM, it could be demonstrated that labeled T cells adhere to the vasculature while this can be prevented when MadCAM-1 is blocked by an antibody [19]. Functional data further underlining the role of MadCAM provided by a second study showed that experimental colitis can be ameliorated by treatment with blocking MadCAM antibodies [20]. The process of cell infiltration is illustrated in figure 3.

MadCAM is expressed at the endothelial cells and does bind to the integrin α4β7 expressed on lymphocytes and monocytes in the peripheral blood, thus allowing these cells to infiltrate the lamina propria. While α4β7 expression is required to transfer mucosal endothelium, the integrin α4β1 binds to the VCAM-1 which is expressed on various organs including the brain.

The strategy was transferred to humans by using an antibody targeting α4, thus preventing the binding to MadCAM-1 and VCAM-1, respectively. The antibody was named natalizumab and the clinical efficacy could be proven in clinical trials with CD patients [21, 22]. In addition, natalizumab exerted clinical efficacy in multiple sclerosis [23].

The enthusiasm about this targeted therapy was somewhat reduced by reports published in 2005 in the *New England Journal of Medicine* describing 3 patients in whom progressive multifocal leukencephalopathy developed during treatment with natalizumab [24–26]. These patients were among 3,000 whom had participated in clinical trials of natalizumab for the treatment of multiple sclerosis of CD. Progressive multifocal leukencephalopathy is a deadly opportunistic infection of the central nervous system for which there is no specific treatment. It is caused by reactivation of a clinically latent JC polyomavirus infection. The prevention of normal trafficking of lymphocytes led to unbridled JC virus replication in these patients. Consistent with this scenario, inflammatory infiltrates were conspicuously absent in the brain lesions [27]. Indeed, the cellular immune response, principally mediated by CD8+ cytotoxic T lymphocytes, has been shown to play a major role in the containment of JC virus [28, 29]. These were 3 patients out of 3,000 included in the clinical trials and receiving natalizumab. Natalizumab was withdrawn from the market but is still available in Europe. Due to the excellent efficacy in particular in multiple sclerosis, natalizumab has been approved again in the USA, however every patient has to be included in a treatment registry.

Novel approaches targeting specifically α4β7 and not α4β1 will have to prove comparable efficacy in CD with less severe side effects.

Future Perspective

These new discoveries have led mucosal immunology in IBD into a new era. The key questions are whether GWAS will reveal further target molecules or involved pathways and which subgroup of patients will respond to which therapy.

Disclosure Statement

B. Siegmund has received lecture fees from Abbott, Essex, Shire, Falk, and Merckle Recordati.

References

1 Hanauer SB, Feagan BG, Lichtenstein GR, Mayer LF, Schreiber S, Colombel JF, et al: Maintenance infliximab for Crohn's disease: the ACCENT I randomised trial. Lancet 2002;359:1541–1549.
2 Rutgeerts P, Sandborn WJ, Feagan BG, Reinisch W, Olson A, Johanns J, et al: Infliximab for induction and maintenance therapy for ulcerative colitis. N Engl J Med 2005; 353:2462–2476.
3 Lugering A, Schmidt M, Lugering N, Pauels HG, Domschke W, Kucharzik T: Infliximab induces apoptosis in monocytes from patients with chronic active Crohn's disease by using a caspase-dependent pathway. Gastroenterology 2001;121:1145–1157.
4 Van den Brande JM, Koehler TC, Zelinkova Z, Bennink RJ, te Velde AA, ten Cate FJ, et al: Prediction of antitumour necrosis factor clinical efficacy by real-time visualisation of apoptosis in patients with Crohn's disease. Gut 2007;56:509–517.
5 Schreiber S, Khaliq-Kareemi M, Lawrance IC, Thomsen OO, Hanauer SB, McColm J, et al: Maintenance therapy with certolizumab pegol for Crohn's disease. N Engl J Med 2007; 357:239–250.
6 Sandborn WJ, Feagan BG, Stoinov S, Honiball PJ, Rutgeerts P, Mason D, et al: Certolizumab pegol for the treatment of Crohn's disease. N Engl J Med 2007;357:228–238.
7 Zeissig S, Bojarski C, Buergel N, Mankertz J, Zeitz M, Fromm M, et al: Downregulation of epithelial apoptosis and barrier repair in active Crohn's disease by tumour necrosis factor-α antibody treatment. Gut 2004;53: 1295–1302.
8 Neurath MF, Fuss I, Kelsall BL, Stuber E, Strober W: Antibodies to interleukin-12 abrogate established experimental colitis in mice. J Exp Med 1995;182:1281–1290.
9 Mannon PJ, Fuss IJ, Mayer L, Elson CO, Sandborn WJ, Present D, et al: Anti-interleukin-12 antibody for active Crohn's disease. N Engl J Med 2004;351:2069–2079.
10 Duerr RH, Taylor KD, Brant SR, Rioux JD, Silverberg MS, Daly MJ, et al: A genome-wide association study identifies IL-23R as an inflammatory bowel disease gene. Science 2006;314:1461–1463.
11 Tremelling M, Cummings F, Fisher SA, Mansfield J, Gwilliam R, Keniry A, et al: IL-23R variation determines susceptibility but not disease phenotype in inflammatory bowel disease. Gastroenterology 2007;132: 1657–1664.

12 Oppmann B, Lesley R, Blom B, Timans JC, Xu Y, Hunte B, et al: Novel p19 protein engages IL-12p40 to form a cytokine, IL-23, with biological activities similar as well as distinct from IL-12. Immunity 2000;13:715–725.

13 Becker C, Wirtz S, Blessing M, Pirhonen J, Strand D, Bechthold O, et al: Constitutive p40 promoter activation and IL-23 production in the terminal ileum mediated by dendritic cells. J Clin Invest 2003;112:693–706.

14 Ivanov II, McKenzie BS, Zhou L, Tadokoro CE, Lepelley A, Lafaille JJ, et al: The orphan nuclear receptor RORγt directs the differentiation program of proinflammatory IL-17+ T-helper cells. Cell 2006;126:1121–1133.

15 Uhlig HH, McKenzie BS, Hue S, Thompson C, Joyce-Shaikh B, Stepankova R, et al: Differential activity of IL-12 and IL-23 in mucosal and systemic innate immune pathology. Immunity 2006;25:309–318.

16 Kullberg MC, Jankovic D, Feng CG, Hue S, Gorelick PL, McKenzie BS, et al: IL-23 plays a key role in *Helicobacter hepaticus*-induced T-cell-dependent colitis. J Exp Med 2006; 203:2485–2494.

17 Hue S, Ahern P, Buonocore S, Kullberg MC, Cua DJ, McKenzie BS, et al: Interleukin-23 drives innate and T-cell-mediated intestinal inflammation. J Exp Med 2006;203:2473–2483.

18 Neurath MF: IL-23: a master regulator in Crohn disease. Nat Med 2007;13:26–28.

19 Shigematsu T, Specian RD, Wolf RE, Grisham MB, Granger DN: MAdCAM mediates lymphocyte-endothelial cell adhesion in a murine model of chronic colitis. Am J Physiol 2001;281:G1309–G1315.

20 Kato S, Hokari R, Matsuzaki K, Iwai A, Kawaguchi A, Nagao S, et al: Amelioration of murine experimental colitis by inhibition of mucosal addressin cell adhesion molecule-1. J Pharmacol Exp Ther 2000;295:183–189.

21 Ghosh S, Goldin E, Gordon FH, Malchow HA, Rask-Madsen J, Rutgeerts P, et al: Natalizumab for active Crohn's disease. N Engl J Med 2003;348:24–32.

22 Targan SR, Feagan BG, Fedorak RN, Lashner BA, Panaccione R, Present DH, et al: Natalizumab for the treatment of active Crohn's disease: results of the ENCORE Trial. Gastroenterology 2007;132:1672–1683.

23 Tubridy N, Behan PO, Capildeo R, Chaudhuri A, Forbes R, Hawkins CP, et al: The effect of anti-α4 integrin antibody on brain lesion activity in MS. The UK Antegren Study Group. Neurology 1999;53:466–472.

24 Kleinschmidt-DeMasters BK, Tyler KL: Progressive multifocal leukoencephalopathy complicating treatment with natalizumab and interferon-$β_{1a}$ for multiple sclerosis. N Engl J Med 2005;353:369–374.

25 Langer-Gould A, Atlas SW, Green AJ, Bollen AW, Pelletier D: Progressive multifocal leukoencephalopathy in a patient treated with natalizumab. N Engl J Med 2005;353:375–381.

26 Van Assche G, Van Ranst M, Sciot R, Dubois B, Vermeire S, Noman M, et al: Progressive multifocal leukoencephalopathy after natalizumab therapy for Crohn's disease. N Engl J Med 2005;353:362–368.

27 Berger JR, Koralnik IJ: Progressive multifocal leukoencephalopathy and natalizumab – unforeseen consequences. N Engl J Med 2005;353:414–416.

28 Du Pasquier RA, Kuroda MJ, Zheng Y, Jean-Jacques J, Letvin NL, Koralnik IJ: A prospective study demonstrates an association between JC virus-specific cytotoxic T lymphocytes and the early control of progressive multifocal leukoencephalopathy. Brain 2004;127:1970–1978.

29 Du Pasquier RA, Schmitz JE, Jean-Jacques J, Zheng Y, Gordon J, Khalili K, et al: Detection of JC virus-specific cytotoxic T lymphocytes in healthy individuals. J Virol 2004;78: 10206–10210.

Mucosal Healing: Impact on the Natural Course or Therapeutic Strategies

Morten H. Vatn

University of Oslo, Institute of Clinical Epidemiology and Molecular Biology (EpiGen), Akershus University Hospital, Lørenskog, and Medical Clinic of Gastroenterology, Oslo University Hospital, Rikshospitalet, Oslo, Norway

Key Words
Inflammatory bowel disease, mucosal healing · Mucosal healing · Inflammatory bowel disease, natural course

Abstract
Background: The treatment with anti-TNF in inflammatory bowel disease (IBD) has shown a much higher rate of mucosal healing (MH) compared to previous treatments. As MH after treatment also seemed to predict a positive outcome of disease regarding long-term outcome and reduced economic burden on the healthcare system, the question was if MH would have an impact on both the natural course of disease and treatment strategy. *Areas of Experience:* Literature search includes population-based cohort studies, such as the Norwegian IBSEN study, and hospital-based studies, such as the GETAID study from France, both referring to MH in prospective follow-up studies of treatment prior to the introduction of biologics. Additionally, experience is based on short- and long-term efficacy studies with anti-TNF treatment, especially infliximab. From all studies, predictability of MH on long-term outcome of disease, including surgery and hospitalization, was assessed. *Results:* MH predicts a generally favorable outcome of disease based on all types of treatment strategies, except glucocorticosteroids, and is related to treatment efficacy-reduced frequency of surgery and hospitalizations. Scheduled treatment with anti-TNF is superior to episodic treatment and a top-down strategy has a favorable effect on healing. A limitation of MH as a universal marker is the fact that less than 50% of patients with a clinical effect of treatment acquire complete healing and MH appears in less than 30% of all patients on anti-TNF. *Conclusion:* MH has become a valuable marker of efficacy in IBD, predicting a favorable disease outcome. In the future, additional markers of healing are expected to be combined with today's endoscopic and histologic assessments.

Copyright © 2009 S. Karger AG, Basel

Introduction

Mucosal healing (MH) is an important treatment goal in various gastrointestinal disorders, such as peptic ulcer and other chronic diseases. After the introduction of biologic treatment in Crohn's disease (CD) [1, 2], MH was observed in a substantial number of patients, leading to the question if MH could be a general predictor of disease course or a main endpoint of efficacy in clinical trials [3]. The percentage of patients achieving complete MH on scheduled therapy in the ACCENT I study at week 54 was above 40% of those who had ulcers at baseline, which was more than twice the percentage of healing among patients on episodic treatment, a significant difference (fig. 1). From the same original studies of infliximab therapy, the sustained effect was also related to reduced hospitalizations and surgeries which also have attracted attention to the question if MH could be a valuable mark-

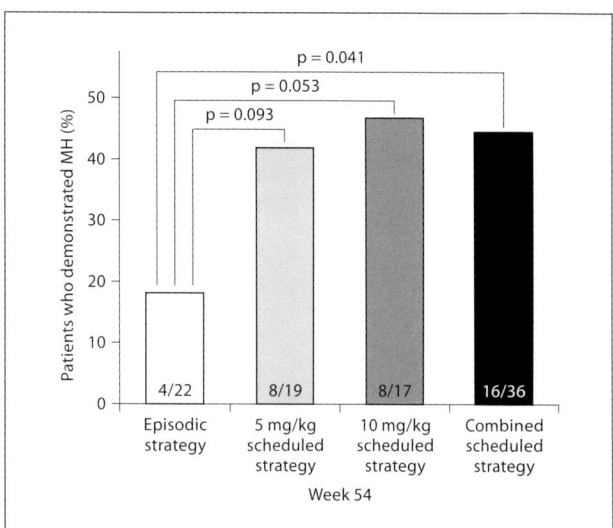

Fig. 1. Proportion of patients demonstrating MH at week 54 in the ACCENT 1 study [3]. Of 81 patients, 58 had baseline and follow-up endoscopy at week 54. MH was defined as the complete absence of mucosal ulcerations that were observed at baseline.

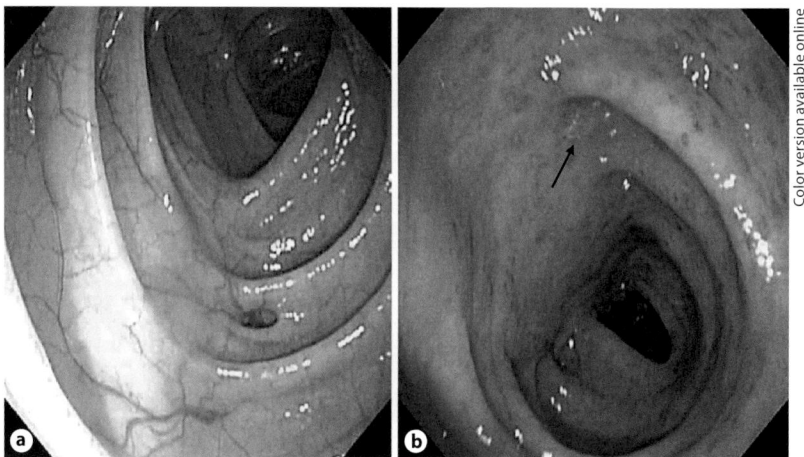

Fig. 2. Endoscopic picture of a normal colon (**a**) and colitis in IBD (**b**) with general inflammation, multiple erosions and an ulcer (↑).

er, even in fistulizing disease, for cost-benefit and utility questions in society [4].

In the following presentation, an attempt has been made to emphasize some important issues as a background for further discussion on the role of MH in the follow-up of patients with inflammatory bowel disease (IBD).

Theoretic Relevance of MH as a Predictive Factor

Before limiting the scope to direct answers to the questions in the title, it might be important to discuss the meaning of MH in general. A prerequisite for the use of MH as a reliable prognostic marker, either of severity or of response to treatment, would be, on the one hand that MH is connected to an individual patient's ability to heal, or, on the other hand, that the effect of a certain treatment is high enough to significantly affect the healing process. These factors might be partly connected in the sense that individual features, such as the ability to heal, might also include individual response to treatment or severity of disease. MH depends on the aggressiveness of a lesion as part of a continuous balance between epithelial damage and the healing process.

If we hypothesize that any chronic disease always has an organic lesion, one might indeed postulate that this lesion is a stimulus for healing and that any stage of the disease process would include the presence of this stimu-

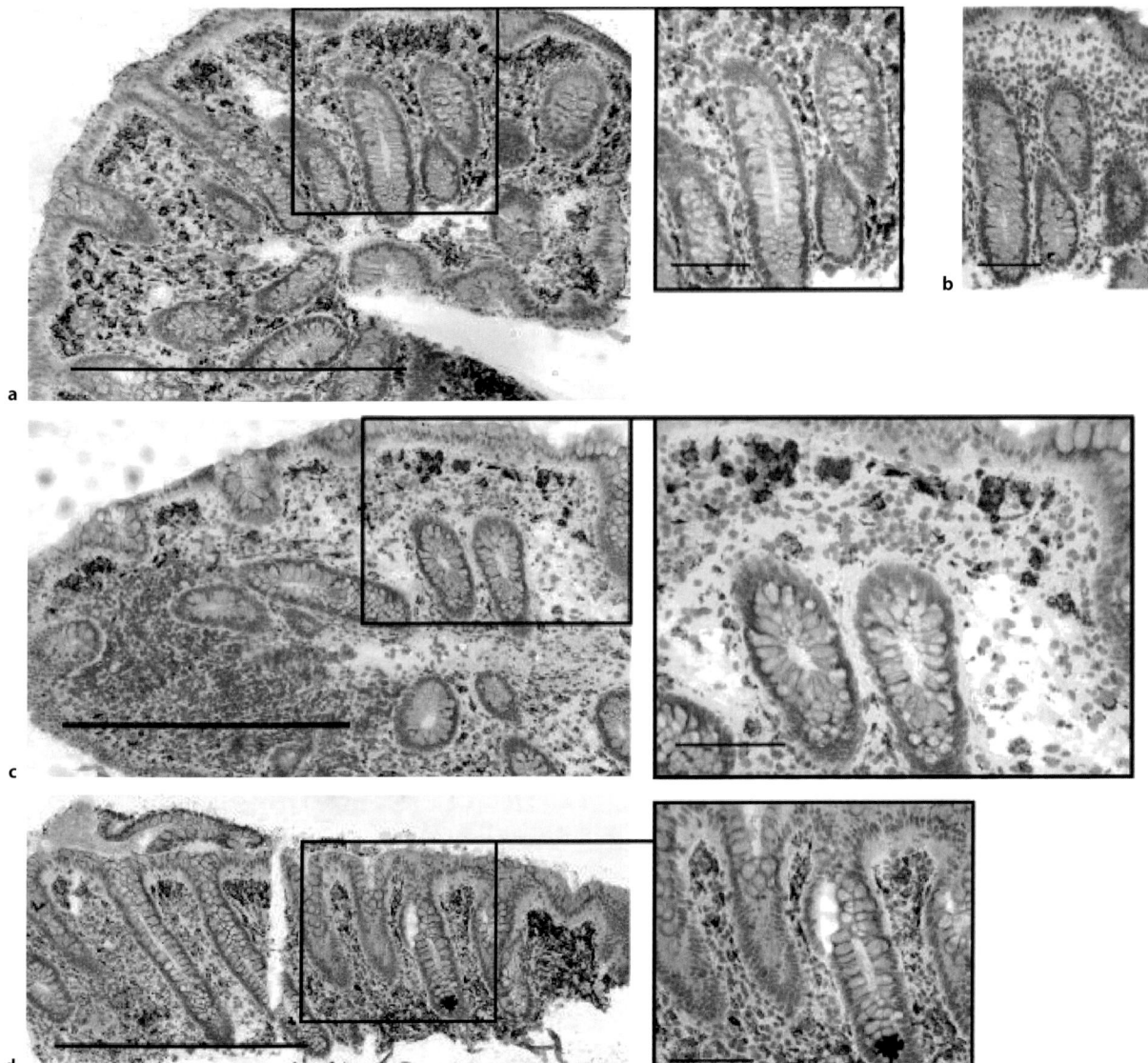

Fig. 3. Immunoperoxidase staining on cryosections of colonic biopsies from non-IBD controls and pediatric Crohn's disease showing the predominant pattern of subepithelial CD68 expression representing macrophages. **a** Adult non-IBD colon; scale bar = 500 μm (selected field, 100 μm). **b** Adult non-IBD negative control; scale bar = 100 μm. **c** Pediatric non-IBD colon; scale bar = 500 μm (selected field, 100 μm). **d** Pediatric Crohn's disease colon; scale bar = 500 μm (selected field, 100 μm) [4].

lation at any level of activity. The interesting part of the healing process for clinical aspects of IBD must be related to a certain clinical disease activity which is relevant to the patients' situation and if the recognition of MH might be relevant to management of treatment.

We then have to define the rational for observing a healing process (1) at a certain degree of severity, (2) at a certain localization, (3) at a certain point in time, and (4) with defined measures.

(1) The healing of an active process is a global goal in medicine. In IBD, much effort has been put on finding

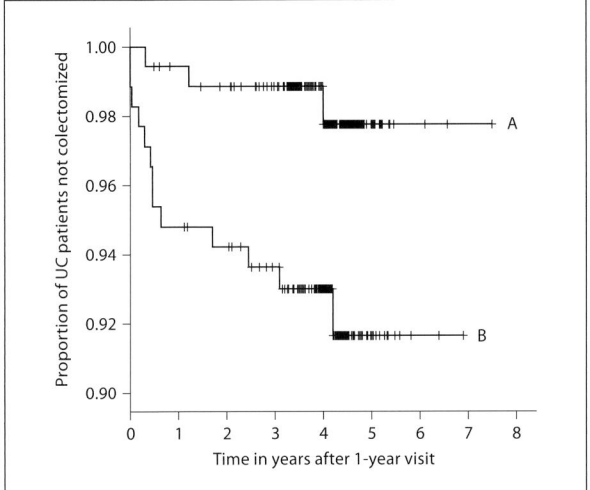
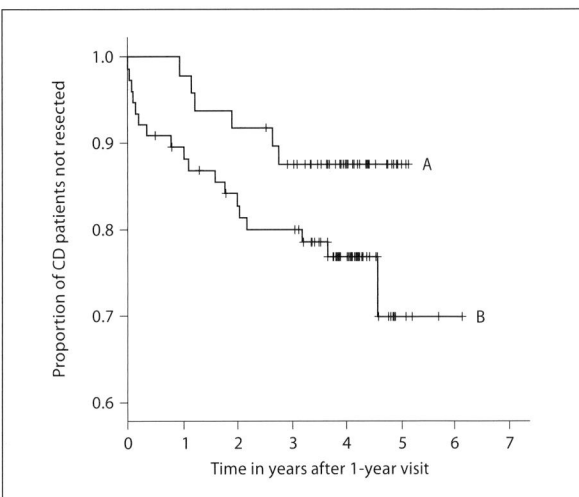

Fig. 4. Kaplan-Meier curves for colectomies in UC patients subsequent to 1-year follow-up after diagnosis. Line A represents the proportion of patients not undergoing subsequent colectomy among patients with established MH at the 1-year visit. Line B represents the proportion of patients not undergoing colectomy among patients without MH at the 1-year visit.

Fig. 5. Kaplan-Meier curves for resections in CD patients subsequent to 1-year follow-up after diagnosis. Line A represents the proportion of patients not undergoing subsequent resection among patients with established MH at the 1-year visit. Line B represents the proportion of patients not undergoing subsequent resection among patients without MH at the 1-year visit.

the most rational disease indices for measurement of disease activity. The combined indices have included both symptoms and signs in an effort to make close to linear or semiquantitative relationships to the characterization of disease activity. By applying the term MH, one may try to use macro- or microscopic indices for quantitative or semiquantitative measures, or simply land on qualitative measures like the presence or not of an ulcer. The latter has been used in recent literature, based on the rational that it represents a certain degree of severity and is easily observed by the endoscope (fig. 2).

(2) But how reliable are the observations of an ulcer over time, or how related is disease severity to the appearance and number of ulcerations? And maybe even more important, how representative is the superficial lesion to the active disease process? A recent study showed a significantly increased number of mucosal macrophages of colonic biopsies in areas with no apparent macroscopic lesions (fig. 3) [5].

(3) Another question is if the time points we are using for assessment of the mucosa are relevant for the understanding of the disease process. Is the observable ulcer a direct or indirect measure of the general disease process? If not directly related, what would be the 'window' for observation needed to adjust for this time span, alternatively to select the optimal length of time between active treatment and observation of effect.

(4) Then the next question is, of course, which instruments we are using to measure the rate of healing. As endoscopic healing is considered to be the most relevant object to observe today, the literature mostly refers to ulcer healing as a qualitative measure or changes in endoscopic scores as semiquantitative measures. In addition to the question if endoscopic activity is representative for the disease process, one is also faced with limitations of the instruments and observers. Fundamentally, the question is if new markers are emerging that might be more reliable for evaluation of the disease process [6].

Since IBD is a chronic relapsing disease, we must regard MH as part of a continuous process of mucosal balance/imbalance, which may be influenced by a combination of endogenous and exogenous processes, as a basis for the natural history of disease, or by specific therapeutic interventions, whereby MH is used as a target of efficacy. An interesting question is if MH is a predictor of outcome of disease, regardless of the disease activity before treatment or if the prognosis is related to a minimum of disease activity, as shown for the TNF-α blockers in trials for patients with moderate to severe disease.

For the evaluation of impact on the natural course of disease, one must focus on the predictive role of MH for future disease outcome. For the evaluation of impact on therapeutic strategies, one must focus on both efficacy of the specific treatment and the role of MH as a predictor for disease outcome with respect to the specific treatment. Increased understanding of the role of MH, both with regard to natural course of disease and the choice of treatment strategy, may seem highly relevant to important decisions in handling of the patients and for the society.

Impact on the Natural Course of IBD

In a prospectively followed incidence cohort [7] of CD (n = 160) and ulcerative colitis (UC) (n = 410) patients in Norway, MH after 1 year of individual treatment could be significantly associated with a subsequent low risk of colectomy in UC (fig. 4) and resections in CD (fig. 5) after 5 and 10 years. In both groups, less inflammation and decreased steroid treatment was observed at 5 years. These observations may provide evidence for the use of endoscopic evaluation of MH in clinical practice. Since this study was performed prior to the introduction of biologics, the results indicate that MH is obtained in a proportion of the patients even with conventional treatment, both in UC and CD. The results may further suggest that MH is a universal predictor of disease outcome in populations with IBD.

Impact on Therapeutic Strategies

Although studies with conventional treatment, including immunosuppressants, have shown MH in a proportion of patients [8], the lack of documentation of MH after treatment with systemic glucocorticosteroids has not given reason to use this parameter as a primary target for evaluation of response to acute treatment in IBD, in spite of an obvious clinical effect of steroids on global disease activity. This situation changed dramatically by the introduction of biologic treatment.

In the ACCENT I trial [1], a significantly higher number of patients showed MH after scheduled treatment compared with episodic treatment with infliximab [3], suggesting a role for MH as a monitoring parameter during follow-up. Moreover, patients with MH showed less demands for hospitalization and surgery after infliximab, which was the case also after conventional treatment in the population-based study [7].

Recent investigations seem to indicate that long-term healing of the bowel mucosa can be achieved with immunosuppressives [8] and anti-TNF treatment [9] even beyond 1 year of scheduled treatment. A significantly longer disease-free interval was shown for the patients with MH in addition to improved long-term outcome and a lesser need for major abdominal surgery among patients on long-term maintenance treatment with infliximab [9]. A comparison between anti-TNF treatments with a top-down and top-up strategy showed significantly more cases with MH in the former [10]. Some studies in children also seem to support the effect of infliximab on MH with association to the restoration of growth [11].

Conclusion

UC and CD are chronic intermittently active diseases, and although MH may seem to be an important sign of efficacy in the acute stage, long-term healing may be difficult to predict in each individual case. We do not completely know which additional factors besides drugs influence the healing process and which factors are responsible for the maintenance of healing over time, and also why in a substantial number of patients the mucosa does not heal. Nevertheless, our recent experience, based on follow-up of population-based cohorts and clinical trials, gives reason to suggest MH is a sign of early response to treatment, as well as an indication for sustained medical treatment, complicated cases with immunosuppressives or biologics. MH seems to be an important prognostic marker associated with reduced frequency of surgeries, hospitalizations and cost of healthcare in IBD, and implies an early top-down strategy with potent drugs for patients with serious and complicated disease.

Since in the majority of cases complete MH is not obtained by the present regimes, more studies will be needed to assess the impact of long-term treatment in the future.

Disclosure Statement

The author declares that no financial or other conflict of interest exists in relation to the content of this article.

References

1 Hanauer SB, Feagan BG, Lichtenstein GR, Mayer LF, Schreiber S, Colombel JF, Rachmilewitz D, Wolf DC, Olson A, Weihang B, Rutgeerts P, and the ACCENT I Study Group: Maintenance infliximab for Crohn's disease: the ACCENT I randomized trial. Lancet 2002;359:1541–1549.

2 Sands BE, Anderson FH, Bernstein CN, Chey WY, Feagan BG, Fedorak RN, Kamm MA, Korzenik JR, Lashner BA, Onken JE, Rachmilewitz D, Rutgeerts P, Wild G, Wolf DC, Marsters PA, Travers SB, Blank MA, van Deventer SJ: Infliximab maintenance therapy for fistulizing Crohn's disease. N Engl J Med 2004;350:876–885.

3 Rutgeerts P, Feagan BG, Lichtenstein GR, Mayer LF, Schreiber S, Colombel JF, Rachmilewitz, Wolf DC, Olson A, Weihang B, Hanauer SB: Comparison of scheduled and episodic treatment strategies of infliximab in Crohn's disease. Gastroenterology 2004; 126:402–413.

4 Lichtenstein GR, Songkay Y, Mohan B, Blank M, Sands BE: Infliximab maintenance treatment reduces hospitalizations, surgeries, and procedures in fistulizing Crohn's disease. Gastroenterology 2005;128:862–869.

5 Perminow G, Reikvam DH, Lyckander LG, Brandtzaeg P, Vatn MH, Carlsen HS: Increased number and activation of colononic macrophages in pediatric patients with untreated Crohn's disease. Inflamm Bowel Dis 2009 [Epub ahead of print].

6 Roseth AG, Aadland E, Grzyb K: Normalization of faecal calprotectin: a predictor of mucosal healing in patients with inflammatory bowel disease. Scand J Gastroenterol 2004; 39:1017–1020.

7 Froeslie KF, Jahnsen J, Moum BA, Vatn MH, and the IBSEN Study Group: Mucosal healing in inflammatory bowel disease: results from a Norwegian population-based cohort. Gastroenterology 2007;133:412–422.

8 Lemann M, Mary J-Y, Colombel JF, Duclos B, Soule JC, Lerebours E, Modigliani R, Bouhinik Y; GETAID: A randomized, double-blind, controlled withdrawal trial in Crohn's disease patients in long-term remission on azathioprine. Gastroenterology 2005;128:1812–1818.

9 Schnitzler F, Fidder H, Ferrante M, Noman M, Arijs I, Van Assche G, Hoffman L, Van Steen K, Vermeire S, Rutgeerts P: Mucosal healing predicts long-term outcome of maintenance therapy with infliximab in Crohn's disease. Inflamm Bowel Dis 2009 [Epub ahead of print].

10 D'Haens G: Anti-TNF therapy: top-up versus top-down strategy. Lancet 2008;371: 660–667.

11 Borrelli O, Bascietto C, Viola F, Bueno de Mesquita M, Barbato M, Mancini V, Bosco S, Cucchiara S: Infliximab heals intestinal inflammatory lesions and restores growth in children with Crohn's disease. Dig Liver Dis 2004;36:342–347.

Diagnostic Approach to Small Bowel Involvement in Inflammatory Bowel Disease: View of the Endoscopist

Konstantinos A. Papadakis

University of Crete, Faculty of Medicine, University Hospital of Heraklion, Heraklion, Greece

Key Words

Balloon-assisted enteroscopy · Double-balloon enteroscopy · Inflammatory bowel disease, small bowel involvement · Intraoperative enteroscopy · Push enteroscopy · Single-balloon enteroscopy · Wireless capsule endoscopy

Abstract

Recent advances in endoscopic small bowel (SB) techniques have revolutionalized the diagnostic approach of patients with suspected or known inflammatory bowel disease (IBD). Wireless capsule endoscopy (WCE) has become an important diagnostic tool for the evaluation of suspected CD of the SB or in patients with known IBD to rule out SB involvement. The greatest utility of WCE has been observed in cases of suspected CD, where the initial evaluation with traditional radiographic and endoscopic studies has failed to establish the diagnosis. WCE can detect early SB lesions that can be overlooked by traditional radiological studies. The sensitivity of diagnosing SB CD by WCE is superior to other endoscopic or radiological methods such as push enteroscopy, computed tomography or magnetic resonance enteroclysis. The utility of WCE in patients with known CD, IBD unclassified (IBDU) and a select group of patients with ulcerative colitis (UC) can better define the diagnosis and extent of the disease and may lead to reclassification of IBD from UC/IBDU to definitive CD. In addition, previously diagnosed patients with CD may be found to have more significant disease burden in the SB. This information may facilitate more targeted and effective therapies and potentially lead to better patient outcomes. A disadvantage of WCE is its low specificity and the risk of being retained in a strictured area of the SB. Balloon-assisted enteroscopy has essentially replaced push enteroscopy, and has been used to treat CD strictures, obtain biopsies from areas of SB involvement and even retrieving a retained capsule.

Copyright © 2009 S. Karger AG, Basel

Introduction

Inflammatory bowel disease (IBD) represents chronic recurrent intestinal inflammatory disorders traditionally classified into ulcerative colitis (UC) and Crohn's disease (CD) [1]. Whereas UC involves the superficial layers of the colon, CD is a transmural inflammatory process that may affect any part of the gastrointestinal (GI) tract [1, 2]. Most cases of CD affect the distal small bowel (SB) and right colon, whereas ~20–30% of patients may have disease limited to the SB. This holds true for younger patients with CD who seem to have more involvement of the proximal SB compared to adults [3]. It is, therefore, critical to evaluate the SB in all patients with suspected IBD. Historically, CD of the SB has been assessed with a barium meal showing typical radiographic features of the disease [4]. Subsequently, other radiographic techniques have been introduced such as SB enteroclysis [5], SB ultrasonography (with oral or intravenous enhancing agents) [6–8]. More recently, CT enterography and MR enteroclysis have greatly improved the delineation of SB involvement in patients with SB CD [9–12].

From the endoscopic point of view, the SB has remained the last 'frontier' of the GI tract to be explored. This stems from the length of the SB (360–600 cm in the adult) and its tortuous anatomy in the abdominal cavity. Until the end of the 20th century, push enteroscopy (PE) was the most commonly used method for the endoscopic investigation of the SB [13]. However, PE has been largely replaced by double-balloon enteroscopy (DBE) [13]. Traditionally, PE has been used to evaluate the proximal SB in cases of obscure GI bleeding but has not been extensively used for the evaluation of patients with suspected or known CD. Sonde enteroscopy has been of historic interest only since this technique has been used in select centers, was time-consuming and uncomfortable for the patient. Until recently, intraoperative enteroscopy has been the only diagnostic tool for the evaluation of the entire SB [14]. WCE and DBE or single-balloon enteroscopy (SBE) have been introduced in an attempt to evaluate the SB in its entirety without the need for surgery [15–17]. The first breakthrough in the evaluation of patients with suspected or known CD was the introduction of the wireless capsule endoscopy (WCE) [18]. WCE was mainly introduced to evaluate patients with GI bleeding of presumed SB origin and for the evaluation of different SB diseases including tumors, celiac disease, and CD [15, 18, 19]. The main disadvantage of the WCE is the inability to provide a tissue diagnosis and the risk of capsule retention [20]. Another advance in the SB exploration was the introduction of techniques that can provide the opportunity for tissue diagnosis and therapeutic capabilities. Such techniques included the DBE and SBE techniques [16, 21]. Although these techniques are still under investigation for their role in patients with IBD, they can certainly provide important diagnostic information and therapeutic applications in a select group of patients with CD.

Wireless Capsule Endoscopy

WCE was introduced in 2000 for the evaluation of patients with GI bleeding of suspected SB origin [18]. Naturally, WCE was introduced in the IBD arena to study patients with suspected or known IBD. The PillCam SB video capsule (Given Imaging Inc., Yoqneam, Israel) measures 11 × 26 mm and weighs <4 g. It contains a color video camera and wireless radiofrequency transmitter, 4 LED lights, and enough battery power to take 50,000 color images during an 8-hour journey through the digestive tract [22]. About the size of a large vitamin, the capsule is made of specially sealed biocompatible material that is resistant to stomach acid and powerful digestive enzymes. The EndoCapsule® system from Olympus Medical Instruments (Tokyo, Japan) with a real-time viewer is also available and received FDA clearance in 2007 [22].

The first study by Mow et al. [23] utilized the M2A capsule (Given Imaging Inc.) in 50 patients with known or suspected IBD and ongoing symptoms. Indications included: (1) evaluation for SB involvement in patients with IBD with isolated colitis (n = 22), (2) determination of the extent of SB disease in patients with CD (n = 20), and (3) workup of suspected IBD (n = 8). WCE findings were diagnostic for CD in 20 patients and suspicious for SB CD in 10 patients. This early experience with the WCE showed that it is a clinically useful method of directly visualizing and diagnosing SB lesions in patients with IBD that cannot be reached by traditional endoscopic procedures and be missed by radiological techniques [23].

Several studies subsequently showed that WCE is more sensitive in detecting lesions in the SB compared to radiographic studies such as SBFT or SB and MR enteroclysis [4, 24–33]. WCE has higher sensitivity in depicting SB lesions compared to MR enteroclysis, primarily by detecting more proximal SB lesions [33]. In a recent meta-analysis, the yield for CE versus barium radiography for all patients was 63 and 23%, respectively (incremental yield = 40%, $p < 0.001$, 95% CI = 28–51%). A subanalysis of patients with established diagnosis of CD and suspected SB recurrence revealed a statistically significant difference in yield in favor of CE compared with all other modalities (barium radiography ($p < 0.001$), colonoscopy with ileoscopy ($p = 0.002$), CT enterography ($p < 0.001$), and PE ($p < 0.001$).

One of the first indications that the WCE was tested was in patients with suspected CD. These included generally young patients with symptoms of diarrhea, abdominal pain or iron-deficiency anemia and elevated inflammatory markers but with negative traditional endoscopic and radiographic studies [19]. WCE diagnosed CD of the SB with a diagnostic yield of 71% [19].

In patients with an established diagnosis of CD, WCE can be performed in order to evaluate the extent of the disease burden, to identify the source of overt GI bleed-

Table 1. Potential indications for the use of WCE in patients with IBDs [22]

a	Suspected CD (i.e. abdominal pain, diarrhea, elevated CRP) with negative findings on upper GI endoscopy and colonoscopy
b	Evaluation of obscure (gastroscopy- and colonoscopy-negative) GI bleeding in patients with CD
c	Evaluation of disease extent in patients with CD[1]
d	Evaluation of postoperative recurrence[2]
e	Evaluation of patients with IBDU
f	Evaluation of response to anti-inflammatory therapy if indicated (i.e. in patients with persistent symptoms despite appropriate therapy)

[1] If information of disease extent in the SB is likely to change patient management.
[2] Mainly in patients unwilling to undergo ileocolonoscopy.

Table 2. Contraindications to WCE [22]

Contraindications to WCE
1. Clinical or radiographic evidence of bowel obstruction or pseudo-obstruction
2. Severe and extensive SB CD with or without stricture or fistula
3. Patients with cardiac pacemakers or other implanted electromedical devices
4. Patients with swallowing disorders
5. Extensive small intestinal diverticulosis (rare)

Warnings to performing WCE
1. Previous abdominal or pelvic surgery
2. Pregnancy
3. Young children (<10 years)

ing, to assess for SB or postoperative recurrence and, finally, document mucosal healing in a select group of patients [22]. In a recent study of patients with SB CD who underwent WCE before and after treatment, the number of large ulcers was the only endoscopic variable that showed significant improvement after treatment [34].

CD recurrence at the neo-ileum (Rutgeert's score) was assessed in 24 patients by colonoscopy and capsule endoscopy [35]. All patients were asymptomatic and did not receive any prophylactic treatment. Recurrence was visualized with colonoscopy in 6 patients and with capsule endoscopy in 5. Ten additional recurrences were visualized only with capsule endoscopy. Moreover, proximal involvement was detected in 13 patients. Therapeutic management was modified in 16 patients. All patients preferred capsule endoscopy. The authors concluded that capsule endoscopy is more effective in the evaluation of recurrence after surgery for CD and is better tolerated than colonoscopy [35]. In contrast, the study by Bourreille et al. [36] showed that the sensitivity of WCE in detecting recurrence in the neo-terminal ileum was inferior to that of ileocolonoscopy. WCE detected lesions outside the scope of ileocolonoscopy in more than two-thirds of patients. The authors argued that WCE cannot systematically replace ileocolonoscopy in the regular management of patients after surgery [36].

Patients with a diagnosis of UC and atypical features or IBD unclassified (IBDU) may have SB findings on capsule endoscopy that are consistent with CD [32, 37]. This is more common in patients with a history of colectomy [32].

In the pediatric IBD patient group, WCE may be valuable in evaluating children with growth retardation when traditional studies have been unrevealing and in children with UC and IBDU may be used to reclassify the disease [38, 39]. In a recent study, 4 of the 7 (57%) older children and adolescents with unexplained growth failure and normal SB series were found to have CD involving the small intestine [38]. In another pediatric study, 4 of 5 patients with UC and 1 of 2 patients with IBDU (total 5 of 7, 71% of UC/IC patients) had their disease reclassified to CD based upon newly diagnosed SB mucosal lesions following CE examination [40]. Moreover, 13 of 21 (62%) patients with CD were found at the time of CE examination to have more extensive SB disease with newly diagnosed jejunal disease found in 12 of 13 (92%) patients [40]. We see similar results in adults with UC/IBDU and CD [32, 35, 36]. Recently, Gralnek et al. [41] developed and validated a capsule endoscopy activity index. The final index includes three parameters: villous edema, ulcer and stenosis. A score of <135 is designated normal or clinically insignificant mucosal inflammatory change, a score between 135 and 790 is mild, and a score ≥790 is moderate to severe. This capsule endoscopy activity index will help researchers use a common language in quantifying SB inflammatory changes for clinical and research purposes.

The indications for performing WCE in patients with suspected or known IBD continue to evolve. Tables 1 and 2 summarize potential indications and contraindications for performing WCE in patients with IBD [22].

Push, Intraoperative and Balloon-Assisted Enteroscopy

PE was the most commonly used method for the endoscopic investigation of the SB [13]. Intraoperative enteroscopy has previously been used in patients with CD and showed a higher burden of SB involvement than evaluated by radiography only [14]. This old observation has been recently re-emphasized with the increasing use of WCE in patients with an established diagnosis of CD [35, 36, 42]. Fortunately, these 'residual' lesions do not seem to predict postoperative recurrence [43]. Push-and-pull enteroscopy is very useful for diagnosis and directing therapy in patients with CD-associated strictures within the SB [21, 44, 45]. Balloon dilation with the push-and-pull enteroscopy device appears safe and effective and can be considered as an alternative to surgery in selected patients with medically refractory strictures [46]. Recently, however, PE has been almost completely replaced by DBE. DBE was introduced in 2001 by Yamamoto et al. [17] as a new endoscopic modality for visualization of the entire SB, and last year, the SBE technique was introduced by Tsujikawa et al. [16]. The term balloon-assisted enteroscopy (BAE) was introduced later on as a unifying terminology referring to both techniques [13, 47]. BAE is now considered the standard endoscopic technique for visualization and endoscopic therapy of SB lesions [47].

BAE has for the first time enabled endoscopists to observe the entire small intestine, and has provided endoscopic interventions such as cauterization of bleeding lesions, polypectomy, placement of SB stents, dilation of SB strictures and foreign-body extraction [13]. In the cases of CD, BAE may be used to confirm the diagnosis of CD histologically in cases of suspected CD on WCE and dilation of SB strictures. In a recent meta-analysis that included 11 studies, the overall diagnostic yield for WCE (60%, n = 397) was comparable to that of DBE (57%, n = 360).

A small recent study evaluated DBE in patients with suspected SB CD. In 50% of the patients (5 out of 10) with suspected SB CD, DBE revealed pathological results. In 4 patients, CD was verified histologically, whereas 1 patient was diagnosed with a lymphoma [48]. Several studies have also reported on the successful dilation of CD SB strictures and avoidance of surgery at least in the short term [21, 44, 49, 50].

Tsujikawa et al. [16] reported on their experience with 78 SBE procedures performed in 41 patients for suspected SB disease (GI bleeding, CD, abdominal pain, and tumor). Observation of the deep small intestine by the oral route was possible in 27 out of 38 procedures, although complete enteroscopy was only possible in 25% of the cases. SBE revealed several abnormal lesions, including ulcerations or scars in 16 patients with CD. The presence of CD lesions in the SB was an impediment for complete SB evaluation. There are several cases of successful retrieval of retained capsule endoscopes using the oral or anal approach of BAE reported in the recent literature [45].

The main limitations of BAE include the risk of bleeding and perforation, the latter could be related to the repeated push-and-pull maneuvers with stretching of the SB or during insertion of the overtube [16]. At present, the role of BAE in the evaluation of CD should be limited to patients with short fibrotic SB strictures that are amenable to dilation who are at risk of short-bowel syndrome from repeated surgeries, in patients with suspected SB CD to confirm the diagnosis histologically and to retrieve retained capsule.

Conclusions

Over the last decade, advances in SB imaging have had a positive impact on the evaluation and management of patients with IBD. WCE combined with sophisticated radiographic techniques such as MR enteroclysis, US with enhancing agents and CT enterography have assisted physicians caring for IBD patients to accurately define the extent and severity of CD involving the small intestine. The newer endoscopic techniques such as the BAE may be used in a select group of patients for diagnostic and mainly therapeutic purposes such as stricture dilation and removal of retained capsule. The cost-effectiveness of these newer modalities and the impact that they may have in the natural history of CD await long-term, well-designed studies.

Disclosure Statement

The author declares that no financial or other conflict of interest exists in relation to the content of this article.

References

1 Papadakis KA, Tabibzadeh S: Diagnosis and misdiagnosis of inflammatory bowel disease. Gastrointest Endosc Clin N Am 2002; 12:433–449.
2 Podolsky DK: Inflammatory bowel disease. N Engl J Med 2002;347:417–429.
3 Weiss B, Shamir R, Bujanover Y, Waterman M, Hartman C, Fradkin A, Berkowitz D, Weintraub I, Eliakim R, Karban A: NOD2/CARD15 mutation analysis and genotype-phenotype correlation in Jewish pediatric patients compared with adults with Crohn's disease. J Pediatr 2004;145:208–212.
4 Costamagna G, Shah SK, Riccioni ME, Foschia F, Mutignani M, Perri V, Vecchioli A, Brizi MG, Picciocchi A, Marano P: A prospective trial comparing small bowel radiographs and video capsule endoscopy for suspected small bowel disease. Gastroenterology 2002;123:999–1005.
5 Gourtsoyiannis NC, Grammatikakis J, Papamastorakis G, Koutroumbakis J, Prassopoulos P, Rousomoustakaki M, Papanikolaou N: Imaging of small intestinal Crohn's disease: comparison between MR enteroclysis and conventional enteroclysis. Eur Radiol 2006;16:1915–1925.
6 Serra C, Menozzi G, Labate AM, Giangregorio F, Gionchetti P, Beltrami M, Robotti D, Fornari F, Cammarota T: Ultrasound assessment of vascularization of the thickened terminal ileum wall in Crohn's disease patients using a low-mechanical index real-time scanning technique with a second-generation ultrasound contrast agent. Eur J Radiol 2007;62:114–121.
7 Pallotta N, Tomei E, Viscido A, Calabrese E, Marcheggiano A, Caprilli R, Corazziari E: Small intestine contrast ultrasonography: an alternative to radiology in the assessment of small bowel disease. Inflamm Bowel Dis 2005;11:146–153.
8 Parente F, Greco S, Molteni M, Anderloni A, Sampietro GM, Danelli PG, Bianco R, Gallus S, Bianchi PG: Oral contrast enhanced bowel ultrasonography in the assessment of small intestine Crohn's disease. A prospective comparison with conventional ultrasound, x-ray studies, and ileocolonoscopy. Gut 2004;53:1652–1657.
9 Gourtsoyiannis NC, Papanikolaou N, Karantanas A: Magnetic resonance imaging evaluation of small intestinal Crohn's disease. Best Pract Res Clin Gastroenterol 2006; 20:137–156.
10 Kohli MD, Maglinte DD: CT enteroclysis in small bowel Crohn's disease. Eur J Radiol 2009;69:398–403.
11 Siddiki H, Fidler J: MR imaging of the small bowel in Crohn's disease. Eur J Radiol 2009; 69:409–417.
12 Wiarda BM, Kuipers EJ, Heitbrink MA, van OA, Stoker J: MR Enteroclysis of inflammatory small-bowel diseases. AJR Am J Roentgenol 2006;187:522–531.
13 Monkemuller K, Bellutti M, Fry LC, Malfertheiner P: Enteroscopy. Best Pract Res Clin Gastroenterol 2008;22:789–811.
14 Lescut D, Vanco D, Bonniere P, Lecomte-Houcke M, Quandalle P, Wurtz A, Colombel JF, Delmotte JS, Paris JC, Cortot A: Perioperative endoscopy of the whole small bowel in Crohn's disease. Gut 1993;34:647–649.
15 Melmed GY, Lo SK: Capsule endoscopy: practical applications. Clin Gastroenterol Hepatol 2005;3:411–422.
16 Tsujikawa T, Saitoh Y, Andoh A, Imaeda H, Hata K, Minematsu H, Senoh K, Hayafuji K, Ogawa A, Nakahara T, Sasaki M, Fujiyama Y: Novel single-balloon enteroscopy for diagnosis and treatment of the small intestine: preliminary experiences. Endoscopy 2008; 40:11–15.
17 Yamamoto H, Sekine Y, Sato Y, Higashizawa T, Miyata T, Iino S, Ido K, Sugano K: Total enteroscopy with a nonsurgical steerable double-balloon method. Gastrointest Endosc 2001;53:216–220.
18 Iddan G, Meron G, Glukhovsky A, Swain P: Wireless capsule endoscopy. Nature 2000; 405:417.
19 Fireman Z, Mahajna E, Broide E, Shapiro M, Fich L, Sternberg A, Kopelman Y, Scapa E: Diagnosing small bowel Crohn's disease with wireless capsule endoscopy. Gut 2003; 52:390–392.
20 Cheifetz AS, Kornbluth AA, Legnani P, Schmelkin I, Brown A, Lichtiger S, Lewis BS: The risk of retention of the capsule endoscope in patients with known or suspected Crohn's disease. Am J Gastroenterol 2006; 101:2218–2222.
21 Monkemuller K, Weigt J, Treiber G, Kolfenbach S, Kahl S, Rocken C, Ebert M, Fry LC, Malfertheiner P: Diagnostic and therapeutic impact of double-balloon enteroscopy. Endoscopy 2006;38:67–72.
22 Saruta M, Papadakis KA: Capsule endoscopy in the evaluation and management of inflammatory bowel disease: a future perspective. Expert Rev Mol Diagn 2009;9:31–36.
23 Mow WS, Lo SK, Targan SR, Dubinsky MC, Treyzon L, Breu-Martin MT, Papadakis KA, Vasiliauskas EA: Initial experience with wireless capsule enteroscopy in the diagnosis and management of inflammatory bowel disease. Clin Gastroenterol Hepatol 2004;2:31–40.
24 Albert JG, Martiny F, Krummenerl A, Stock K, Lesske J, Gobel CM, Lotterer E, Nietsch HH, Behrmann C, Fleig WE: Diagnosis of small bowel Crohn's disease: a prospective comparison of capsule endoscopy with magnetic resonance imaging and fluoroscopic enteroclysis. Gut 2005;54:1721–1727.
25 Buchman AL, Miller FH, Wallin A, Chowdhry AA, Ahn C: Videocapsule endoscopy versus barium contrast studies for the diagnosis of Crohn's disease recurrence involving the small intestine. Am J Gastroenterol 2004;99:2171–2177.
26 Chong AK, Taylor A, Miller A, Hennessy O, Connell W, Desmond P: Capsule endoscopy vs. push enteroscopy and enteroclysis in suspected small-bowel Crohn's disease. Gastrointest Endosc 2005;61:255–261.
27 Efthymiou A, Viazis N, Vlachogiannakos J, Georgiadis D, Kalogeropoulos I, Mantzaris G, Karamanolis DG: Wireless capsule endoscopy versus enteroclysis in the diagnosis of small-bowel Crohn's disease. Eur J Gastroenterol Hepatol 2009;21:866–871.
28 Eliakim R, Fischer D, Suissa A, Yassin K, Katz D, Guttman N, Migdal M: Wireless capsule video endoscopy is a superior diagnostic tool in comparison to barium follow-through and computerized tomography in patients with suspected Crohn's disease. Eur J Gastroenterol Hepatol 2003;15:363–367.
29 Golder SK, Schreyer AG, Endlicher E, Feuerbach S, Scholmerich J, Kullmann F, Seitz J, Rogler G, Herfarth H: Comparison of capsule endoscopy and magnetic resonance enteroclysis in suspected small bowel disease. Int J Colorectal Dis 2006;21:97–104.
30 Liangpunsakul S, Chadalawada V, Rex DK, Maglinte D, Lappas J: Wireless capsule endoscopy detects small bowel ulcers in patients with normal results from state of the art enteroclysis. Am J Gastroenterol 2003;98: 1295–1298.
31 Marmo R, Rotondano G, Piscopo R, Bianco MA, Siani A, Catalano O, Cipolletta L: Capsule endoscopy versus enteroclysis in the detection of small-bowel involvement in Crohn's disease: a prospective trial. Clin Gastroenterol Hepatol 2005;3:772–776.
32 Mehdizadeh S, Chen G, Enayati PJ, Cheng DW, Han NJ, Shaye OA, Ippoliti A, Vasiliauskas EA, Lo SK, Papadakis KA: Diagnostic yield of capsule endoscopy in ulcerative colitis and inflammatory bowel disease of unclassified type. Endoscopy 2008;40:30–35.
33 Voderholzer WA, Ortner M, Rogalla P, Beinholzl J, Lochs H: Diagnostic yield of wireless capsule enteroscopy in comparison with computed tomography enteroclysis. Endoscopy 2003;35:1009–1014.
34 Efthymiou A, Viazis N, Mantzaris G, Papadimitriou N, Tzourmakliotis D, Raptis S, Karamanolis DG: Does clinical response correlate with mucosal healing in patients with Crohn's disease of the small bowel? A prospective, case-series study using wireless capsule endoscopy. Inflamm Bowel Dis 2008;14:1542–1547.
35 Pons Beltrán V, Nos P, Bastida G, Beltrán B, Argüello L, Aguas M, Rubín A, Pertejo V, Sala T: Evaluation of postsurgical recurrence in Crohn's disease: a new indication for capsule endoscopy? Gastrointest Endosc 2007; 66:533–540.

36 Bourreille A, Jarry M, D'Halluin PN, Ben-Soussan E, Maunoury V, Bulois P, Sacher-Huvelin S, Vahedy K, Lerebours E, Heresbach D, Bretagne JF, Colombel JF, Galmiche JP: Wireless capsule endoscopy versus ileocolonoscopy for the diagnosis of postoperative recurrence of Crohn's disease: a prospective study. Gut 2006;55:978–983.

37 Maunoury V, Savoye G, Bourreille A, Bouhnik Y, Jarry M, Sacher-Huvelin S, Ben SE, Lerebours E, Galmiche JP, Colombel JF: Value of wireless capsule endoscopy in patients with indeterminate colitis (inflammatory bowel disease type unclassified). Inflamm Bowel Dis 2007;13:152–155.

38 Moy L, Levine J: Capsule endoscopy in the evaluation of patients with unexplained growth failure. J Pediatr Gastroenterol Nutr 2009;48:647–650.

39 Bousvaros A, Antonioli DA, Colletti RB, Dubinsky MC, Glickman JN, Gold BD, Griffiths AM, Jevon GP, Higuchi LM, Hyams JS, Kirschner BS, Kugathasan S, Baldassano RN, Russo PA: Differentiating ulcerative colitis from Crohn disease in children and young adults: report of a working group of the North American Society for Pediatric Gastroenterology, Hepatology, and Nutrition and the Crohn's and Colitis Foundation of America. J Pediatr Gastroenterol Nutr 2007;44:653–674.

40 Cohen SA, Gralnek IM, Ephrath H, Saripkin L, Meyers W, Sherrod O, Napier A, Gobin T: Capsule endoscopy may reclassify pediatric inflammatory bowel disease: a historical analysis. J Pediatr Gastroenterol Nutr 2008; 47:31–36.

41 Gralnek IM, Defranchis R, Seidman E, Leighton JA, Legnani P, Lewis BS: Development of a capsule endoscopy scoring index for small bowel mucosal inflammatory change. Aliment Pharmacol Ther 2008;27: 146–154.

42 Melmed GY, Fleshner PR, Papadakis KA: Proximal small intestinal CD detected by CE. Gastrointest Endosc 2008;68:202–203.

43 Klein O, Colombel JF, Lescut D, Gambiez L, Desreumaux P, Quandalle P, Cortot A: Remaining small bowel endoscopic lesions at surgery have no influence on early anastomotic recurrences in Crohn's disease. Am J Gastroenterol 1995;90:1949–1952.

44 Gay G, Delvaux M: Double balloon enteroscopy in Crohn's disease and related disorders: our experience. Gastrointest Endosc 2007;66:S82–S90.

45 Semrad CE: Role of double balloon enteroscopy in Crohn's disease. Gastrointest Endosc 2007;66:S94–S95.

46 Pohl J, May A, Nachbar L, Ell C: Diagnostic and therapeutic yield of push-and-pull enteroscopy for symptomatic small bowel Crohn's disease strictures. Eur J Gastroenterol Hepatol 2007;19:529–534.

47 Aktas H, Mensink PB: Therapeutic balloon-assisted enteroscopy. Dig Dis 2008;26:309–313.

48 Seiderer J, Herrmann K, Diepolder H, Schoenberg SO, Wagner AC, Goke B, Ochsenkuhn T, Schafer C: Double-balloon enteroscopy versus magnetic resonance enteroclysis in diagnosing suspected small-bowel Crohn's disease: results of a pilot study. Scand J Gastroenterol 2007;42:1376–1385.

49 Fukumoto A, Tanaka S, Yamamoto H, Yao T, Matsui T, Iida M, Goto H, Sakamoto C, Chiba T, Sugano K: Diagnosis and treatment of small-bowel stricture by double balloon endoscopy. Gastrointest Endosc 2007;66:S108–S112.

50 Oshitani N, Yukawa T, Yamagami H, Inagawa M, Kamata N, Watanabe K, Jinno Y, Fujiwara Y, Higuchi K, Arakawa T: Evaluation of deep small bowel involvement by double-balloon enteroscopy in Crohn's disease. Am J Gastroenterol 2006;101:1484–1489.

Significance of Abdominal Ultrasound in Inflammatory Bowel Disease

C.F. Dietrich

Medical Department 2, Caritas-Krankenhaus, Bad Mergentheim, Germany

Key Words
Abdominal ultrasound in inflammatory bowel disease · Antibiotic-associated colitis · Contrast-enhanced ultrasound · Neutropenic enterocolitis · Penicillin-induced segmental hemorrhagic colitis · Pseudomembranous colitis · Sonomorphology · Transabdominal ultrasound · Tuberculosis

Abstract

Transabdominal ultrasound is most commonly used to examine the liver, hepatobiliary-pancreatic and urogenital tract. Its use for imaging the intestinal tract is less well established and has been considered more difficult in the past. Improvements in technology and increasing experience with sonographic findings in a variety of intestinal diseases including inflammatory bowel disease (IBD), however, have contributed to firmly establishing the role of ultrasound as a clinically important, non-invasive and widely available imaging modality. In addition, newer techniques such as harmonic imaging and contrast-enhanced ultrasound have recently gained attention. Transabdominal ultrasound is clinically useful in the initial diagnosis of IBD by evaluating bowel wall thickness and surrounding structures including peri-intestinal inflammatory reaction, extent and localization of involved bowel segments and detection of extraluminal complications such as fistula, abscesses, carcinoma and ileus. Transabdominal ultrasound is currently accepted as a clinically important first-line tool in assessing patients with Crohn's disease irrespective of their clinical symptoms and/or disease activity. It helps to better characterize the course of the disease in individual patients and can guide therapeutic decisions. The topic of this review is to provide an updated overview of the role of transabdominal ultrasound in IBD including Crohn's disease, ulcerative colitis, tuberculosis and neutropenic colitis while summarizing the results of recent studies with special reference to sensitivity/specificity in detecting the disease and sonomorphologic features to evaluate disease activity and its luminal and extraluminal complications.

Copyright © 2009 S. Karger AG, Basel

Introduction

Transabdominal ultrasound is most commonly and traditionally used to examine the liver, hepatobiliary-pancreatic and urogenital tract. The use for imaging the intestinal tract is less well established and has been considered more difficult in the past. Improvements in technology and increasing experience with sonographic findings in a variety of intestinal diseases including inflammatory bowel disease (IBD), however, have contributed to firmly establishing the role of ultrasound as a clinically important, non-invasive and widely available imaging modality. In addition, techniques such as color Doppler imaging (CDI), harmonic imaging, 3D [1], panoramic imaging [2] and contrast-enhanced ultrasound (CEUS) have recently gained attention [3–5]. This review will provide an updated overview of the role of transabdominal ultrasound in IBD. A more detailed analysis of the IBD literature will soon be published by Allgayer and Dietrich.

Examination Technique

Imaging of the alimentary tract requires high-frequency (5–17 MHz), high-resolution linear or convex array transducers, a great deal of scanning experience, and patience. The standard evaluation should ideally take place preprandially since images from filled intestines can be difficult to interpret, particularly when motility is being evaluated. On the other hand, reliable diagnoses under emergency conditions, such as ileus (obstruction, incarcerated hernia or intussusception), appendicitis or diverticulitis can be performed postprandially.

Sonomorphology

The ileocecal region and the sigmoid colon can be identified by ultrasound imaging in most patients. Landmarks in the ileocecal region are the right iliac artery and vein, while landmarks in the sigmoid region are the left iliac artery and vein. The remaining colonic segments can also be adequately evaluated by continuous scanning in many patients. However, the rectum and distal parts of the colon cannot always be displayed satisfactorily by the transabdominal route. In contrast, perineal ultrasound has been useful in the evaluation of the perianal region and the distal rectum [6]. The small and large bowel can usually be distinguished by scanning the haustra of the colon and/or the circular folds of Kerckring in the small intestine. In unclear cases, scanning of the intestine during various stages of filling may be helpful.

A central problem of alimentary tract imaging is the correct estimation of wall thickness. More than 30 trials have been published within the last two decades measuring intestinal wall diameters, however, under a variety of conditions with greatly differing values defining normal from 1 up to 5 mm. Table 1 summarizes the results from studies in which data concerning the thickness of at least three distinct bowel segments (jejunum, ileum and colon) are presented and comparable techniques and frequencies have been used. In contrast, measurements from our ultrasound unit differ from several studies as we have found lower diameters for all segments (table 2).

The major reasons for this discrepancy may be different examination techniques, equipment and frequencies used,

Table 1. Bowel wall thickness at different intestinal sites in healthy controls (mm)

Jejunum	Ileum	Colon	Frequency, MHz	Reference
2.0	2.0	2.0–3.0	3.5; 5.0	7
<2.0	<2.0	2.0–5.0	5.0	8
<3.0	<3.0	<5.0	3.5; 5.0	9
<4.0	<4.0	<4.0	5.0	10
<4.0	<4.0	<4.0	3.5; 7.5	11
<5.0	<5.0	5.0	2.4–5.0	12
<5.0	<5.0	<5.0	NA	13
<5.0	<5.0	<5.0	3.5; 5.0	14

Table modified from Allgayer and Dietrich [unpublished data]. Studies using methods other than transabdominal ultrasound are not included in this table. For example, trials using endoscopic ultrasound, hydrocolon ultrasound, in vitro measurements or postmortem examination. < = Values below this level are considered normal; NA = not available.

Table 2. Determination of wall diameter at the ileum, ascending colon, hepatic flexure and sigmoid in healthy volunteers (n = 31; mean ± SD and range) [data compiled from 15]

Localization	Wall thickness, mm
Terminal ileum	1.1 ± 0.1 (1.0–1.2)
Ascending colon	1.1 ± 0.1 (0.9–1.3)
Right flexure	1.1 ± 0.1 (0.9–1.3)
Sigmoid	1.4 ± 0.1 (1.2–1.8)

Measurements were performed after having identified corresponding landmarks for each bowel segment (see text) using a high-resolution transducer (5.0 MHz) in the RES mode.

and particularly the presence or absence of externally exerted compression during the examination by the operator [15]. In our experience the normal intestinal tract thickness in the terminal ileum, cecum and right and left colon is generally <2 mm when examined with mild dose compression. It is important to mention that a contracted intestinal segment can be misinterpreted as a thickened wall and, on the other hand, that an inflamed ileal/cecal wall structure may appear normal. In addition to wall thickness, its overall echotexture and appearance within surrounding structures should always be carefully considered when interpreting data, as determination of wall thickness alone may be of very limited value clinically.

Table 3. Sonomorphology and intestinal wall structures from the lumen to serosa

Layer echogenicity	Anatomic structure
Lumen echo-poor (fluid), echo-rich	(air)
Echo-rich entrance echo	inner (luminal) layer transition lumen/mucosa
Echo-poor mucosa	inner layer
Echo-rich submucosa	layer
Echo-poor muscularis propria	outer layer
Echo-rich exit echoes	outer layer serosa/surrounding structures

Table 4. Sonographic findings in abdominal tuberculosis: review of the literature [17]

Authors	Year	n	LN	SM	HM	BWT	Ascites	Abscess	Mes. thick
Khan[a]	2007	110[a]	39[a]			28[a]			
Akgun	2005	80	11			10	19	20	
Uzunkoy	2004	11	2			2	11		3
Tarantino	2003	12	12	12	12	5	6	10	
Malik	2003	66	37			14	36		
Uygur-Bayramicli	2003	26	1	1	4	3	14		
Jain	1995	56	56				17		56
Lee	1995	46	6	9	11	3	46		10
Sheikh	1995	13	1	4	4	3	46		10
Kedar	1994	90	23			31	40	10	14
Lee	1993	41				38			

[a] This study summarized CT scan and ultrasound findings. n = Number of patients; LN = lymphadenopathy; SM = splenomegaly; HM = hepatomegaly; BWT = bowel wall thickening; Mes. thick. = mesenteric thickness.

High-resolution transducers usually permit visualization of five (up to nine) layers within the colonic and stomach wall, visualization being grossly enhanced in the presence of intraluminal fluid. Although the sonographic appearance cannot be completely assessed in terms of the exact anatomic wall structures, it can reasonably be assumed that these echolayers reflect approximately the structures as described in table 3.

Tuberculosis

Intestinal manifestation is a severe complication in the course of tuberculosis. Although these patients mostly suffer from general symptoms of abdominal disease such as abdominal pain or diarrhea, these symptoms remain too unspecific to prompt physicians towards a diagnosis of intestinal tuberculosis. The number of deaths per year from tuberculosis is steady at about 2 million. The widespread use of immunosuppressive therapy, the increasing population migration and the HIV epidemic have contributed to the return of the disease.

The most prominent ultrasonographic features suggestive for abdominal tuberculosis are mesenteric thickening of ≥15 mm with an increased echogenicity of the mesentery due to fat deposition and mesenteric lymphadenopathy. Furthermore, diffuse or focal hypoechoic bowel wall thickening of >5 mm and the presence of dilated small bowel loops have also been described to be significantly associated with the diagnosis of intestinal tuberculosis. Diffuse signs of intestinal disease such as ascites have also been found. In addition, the few available studies were mainly focused on just a few individual sonographic signs, but presentation of abdominal tuberculosis may vary widely. However, Khan et al. [16] have reported that in their investigation most cases presented with intestinal tuberculosis (103/209, 49%), followed by peritoneal tuberculosis in 42% (87/209). All segments of the gastrointestinal tract can be affected by tuberculosis, but predominantly the cecum (85–90%) and the ileocecal region are involved. This has been underlined by endoscopic investigation of proven intestinal tuberculosis. In descending order of frequency, tuberculosis is also observed in the ascending colon, jejunum, appendix, duodenum, stomach, esophagus, sigmoid and rectum. Intramural abscess, fistula and abscesses as well as mesenteric vein thrombosis and lymphatic infiltration are also typical signs of tuberculosis [17]. Sonographic findings in abdominal tuberculosis in the literature are summarized in table 4.

Neutropenic Enterocolitis

The incidence of neutropenic colitis in cytopenic patients ranges from 2.6 to 33% with a pooled incidence rate from 21 studies of 5.3%. With the use of more intensive chemotherapy regimens, especially after autologous and allogeneic stem-cell transplantations, the incidence of neutropenic colitis is rising. Various factors could play a role in the pathogenesis of neutropenic colitis. Apart from direct damage to the mucosa by leukemic of lymphatic infiltrates, toxic effects of chemotherapy agents contribute to the pathogenesis. Neutropenic colitis is mainly localized in the ileocecal region, although other parts of the bowel can be affected as well. The high concentration of lymphatic tissue in this area, the special anatomy of the terminal branches of the superior mesenteric artery with subsequent lower vascular perfusion, may contribute to ischemia. The cecum represents an area of relative stasis of bowel content and is easily distended, causing a high intramural pressure and insufficient blood supply (Laplace's law) [18].

The initial symptoms are not specific and usually occur during the nadir with rapid improvement after neutrophil regeneration. The symptoms very often consist of a combination of crampy abdominal pain (subileus symptoms), a palpable mass and tenderness in the right lower quadrant with rebound (as a sign of peritonism) and fever. Diarrhea, occasionally bloody diarrhea, may be present, but the leading symptom is abdominal pain in the right lower quadrant. Sepsis and signs of perforation with peritonism, as well as profuse bleeding are threatening complications.

Appendicitis is very often the main differential diagnosis. Because of the high perioperative mortality in these patients, the surgical approach should be avoided. A neoplastic (leukemic of lymphocytic) infiltration of the ileocecal region must be excluded especially in the case of a palpable mass in this area. In pancytopenic patients, one has also to think of an acute hemorrhage into the mucosal wall. Besides the routine laboratory and microbiological tests for bacteria (e.g. *Clostridium difficile* and toxin), viruses and parasites, one should perform the CMV PCR test and the CMV early (pp65) antigen test. The endoscopic approach during pancytopenia is usually contraindicated, although the definitive diagnosis of CMV colitis, leukemic or neoplastic infiltrates can only be definitively diagnosed by histological examination.

The characteristic sonographic features of neutropenic colitis are an echogenic, asymmetric thickening of the mucosal wall with transmural inflammatory reaction and areas of different echogenicity, caused by edema, necrosis and/or circumscript hemorrhages. Intramural air suggests an infection with anaerobic bacteria. Pericolic fluid is a sign of a (possible) perforation. Sonography may demonstrate free abdominal air, which is usually detected right-sided, e.g. perihepatic. In advanced disease with catastrophic prognosis, air bubbles in the vena porta may be demonstrated, as seen after application of contrast-enhancing agents. Another feature may be pneumatosis cystoides intestinalis, as seen in premature infants with necrotizing enterocolitis. It is worth mentioning that in these patients the hydrogen content of the expired air is massively increased. The macroscopic findings are dilated, edematous thickened bowel wall with areas of hemorrhage and necrosis. The characteristic histological lesions are mucosal ulceration without accompanying inflammatory response, which might progress to gangrene. Often, thrombosis of intestinal veins, in some cases extensive macroscopic thrombosis of adjacent mesenteric veins, is present, which probably is caused by endotoxins. The main histological features of neutropenic colitis are edema, hemorrhage and necrosis. Inflammatory, fungal, leukemic or neoplastic infiltrates, as well as frank perforation are only seen occasionally. The prognosis depends on the underlying disease and on the clinical condition of the patient. The mortality rate in patients with signs of perforation, sepsis and multiorgan failure is higher than 50% [18].

Antibiotic-Associated Colitis

Most patients with antibiotic-related diarrhea do not have colitis and thus have no detectable sonographic abnormalities of the bowel wall. On the other hand, patients who develop pseudomembranous colitis, or much less commonly, penicillin-induced colitis, may have sonographically detectable bowel wall changes [19].

Pseudomembranous Colitis

The most common finding in patients with pseudomembranous colitis caused by *C. difficile* is symmetric mucosal wall thickening, which is often most prominent in the left colon. However, sonographic findings are insufficiently specific to distinguish pseudomembranous colitis from other bacterial causes of colitis. In severe cases, the colonic wall thickening may resemble an intestinal lymphoma with asymmetric thickening of the bowel wall. Other sonographic features of severe infection include transmural inflammatory reactions, free pericolic fluid, and intramural gas echoes [20].

Penicillin-Induced Segmental Hemorrhagic Colitis

A characteristic sonographic feature of penicillin-induced segmental hemorrhagic colitis is the appearance of partially asymmetric wall thickening of the colon (typically in the right colon) with loss of intestinal wall layers due to edema and bleeding. Relative hypovascularization (and histologically ischemia) can be detected with color Doppler ultrasound examination. The surrounding colon may appear normal [20].

Crohn's Disease

Transabdominal ultrasound is clinically useful in the initial diagnosis of Crohn's disease (CD) by evaluating bowel wall thickness and surrounding structures including peri-intestinal inflammatory reaction, extent and localization of involved bowel segments and detection of extraluminal complications such as fistula, abscesses, carcinoma and ileus. In addition, several extraintestinal manifestations, particularly mesenteric and perihepatic lymph node involvement such as in sclerosing cholangitis, can also be reliably diagnosed [21, 22].

Initial Diagnosis by Ultrasound

Sensitivity and specificity in detecting IBD were reported generally in the range from 70 to 94 and 67 to 97%, respectively. When specific to CD alone, similar data were found as demonstrated by a series of additional studies comparing transabdominal ultrasound with other methods such as endoscopy and/or radiology. In these trials the sensitivity ranged generally from 73 to 96% and the specificity from 90 to 100%, respectively. The literature is summarized in table 5. Different values may be due to different reference methods (gold standard).

Although positive and negative predictive values would be clinically more relevant as they take prevalence and incidence of disease into account, only a minority of studies have reported such values and these are in the range from 79 to 100% and 57 to 95%, respectively.

Table 5. Sensitivity, specificity, positive and negative predictive value in the detection of CD

n	Sensitivity, %	Specificity, %	Positive predictive value, %	Negative predictive value, %	Ref.
296[a]	93	97	NA	NA	23
296[b]	79	98	95	NA	23
296[c]	90	100	100	NA	23
227 (69)	84	NA	98	76	24
142	91	100	NA	NA	25
175 (51)	84	91	80	93	26
115	89	94	NA	NA	29
181 (89)	81	80	79	81	27
127 (46)	78	91	NA	NA	14

Table modified from Allgayer and Dietrich [unpublished data]. NA = Not available; n = number of patients. Number of patients with proven CD in parentheses.
[a] Localization, disease spread. [b] Strictures, gold standard: endoscopy and radiological methods. [c] Gold standard: operation.

Assessment of Bowel Wall Thickness and Disease Activity

The assessment of bowel wall thickness and structures has been considered a particularly important issue. Attempts have been made to correlate wall thickness with disease activity, notably the Crohn's Disease Activity Index (CDAI). Although an association of wall thickness and disease activity generally is assumed, detailed data including correlation coefficients (e.g. Spearman rank coefficient) (R_s) with corresponding significance levels have only been reported rarely. In a large series of patients (n = 255) we have found that wall thickness is significantly higher than normal (4.9 ± 2.7 vs. <2.0 mm) and greater in active (CDAI >150) than in inactive disease (CDAI <150): 5.8 ± 2.9 vs. 4.3 ± 2.2 mm (p < 0.0001). In addition, in a second trial including 100 consecutive patients, we have found a weak, but significant correlation of wall thickness with the CDAI (R_s = 0.44, p < 0.00001).

In view of the conflicting results concerning the relationship between altered wall morphology such as a blurred aspect and/or transmural inflammatory reaction, with disease activity, we have investigated those characteristics and observed that a blurred wall layer morphology was significantly more frequent in active

Table 6. Sonomorphologic criteria and clinical activity in patients with CD (n = 100)

Criteria	Total, n	CDAI <150	CDAI >150	Significance[a], p
Wall thickness				
Normal	33/100 (33%)	26/71 (37%)	1/21 (5%)[b]	<0.05
Pathologic (>2 mm)	67/100 (67%)	45/71 (63%)	20/21 (95%)	<0.05
Mean ± SD (range)	5.0 ± 2.0 (3–12)	4.0 ± 1.0 (3–8)	6.0 ± 3.0 (3–12)	<0.05
Wall layer				
Accentuated	49/100	41/71 (58%)	7/21 (33%)	<0.05
Blurred	18/100	4/71 (5%)	1/21 (62%)	<0.05
Transmural inflammation	8/100 (8%)	4/8 (50%)	3/8 (38%)	0.1

[a] Comparison between CDAI >150 vs. CDAI <150.
[b] The sum of the number of patients with CDAI <150 and CDAI >150 does not yield n = 100, as 8 patients with ileostoma were excluded from calculations because the CDAI was not applicable.

than in inactive disease (62.0 vs. 5.0%, p < 0.05) and that conversely, accentuated wall layers were more frequent in inactive than active disease (table 6).

In contrast, transmural inflammatory reaction (definition, see above) was present only in 8% of the patients. The differences between active and inactive disease was not significant.

Assessment of Bowel Wall Involvement (Length and Extent) and Disease Activity

As CD often comprises more than one bowel segment, it may be important to estimate the overall length of the involved segments and to examine as many areas as possible. As this question has not been sufficiently addressed so far, we prospectively investigated 100 patients, of whom 67 had a bowel wall thickness >2.0 mm at initial presentation. 39 showed unisegmental and 28 multisegmental involvement. The majority of patients with unisegmental involvement (74.0%) had quiescent disease (CDAI <150) and a mean length of involved bowel segments of 16.0 ± 8.0 cm, the differences between patients with active and inactive disease, however, were not significant (p = 0.8). In patients with multiple segment disease, the exact determination of the total length of involved segments was not possible, but sonographic and clinical features including disease activity were not different from those with unisegmental involvement.

Detection of Complication

Besides morphologic evaluation of mural, transmural and adjacent structures, ultrasound is able to detect complications such as fistulae (and the early stage of fistula, transmural inflammation), abscesses, carcinoma and ileus/subileus with a high sensitivity and specificity (fig. 1, 2). Estimates of the sensitivity and specificity for detecting fistulae have ranged between 50–89 and 90–95%, respectively [28]. Estimates of the sensitivity and specificity for detecting abscesses have been reported in a somewhat higher range, i.e. between 71 and 100 for the sensitivity and between 77 and 94% for the specificity [27, 29–32].

Ultrasound as a Screening Procedure

A prospective study suggested that routine ultrasound in patients with CD can reveal unexpected pathological findings that have therapeutic implications [33]. The study included 255 patients with CD who underwent regular ultrasound irrespective of symptoms and disease activity. Patients with abnormal findings underwent further evaluation with additional radiological and/or endoscopic imaging and treatment as needed. Of 17 patients with inactive disease, ultrasound revealed 4 with an interenteric fistula, 7 with a mesenteric or perirectal fistula and 6 with transmural mesenteric inflammation without a fistula. Ultrasound of the remaining abdominal organs revealed pathological findings with further diagnostic implications in 25 of 255 (10%) patients and with therapeutic implications in 4%. In another series with 100 consecutive patients, we found 13 fistulae, 7 of which were not previously known, a percentage very close to our previous findings. The majority of the fistulae were again enteroenteric, 1 patient had an enterovesical and another an enterocutaneous fistula (table 7).

In a third trial comprising 46 consecutive patients, 19 cases with communicating fistulae were detected by ultrasound, 13 of which were enteroenteric with 9 patients having a CDAI >150 (median 222), thus further support-

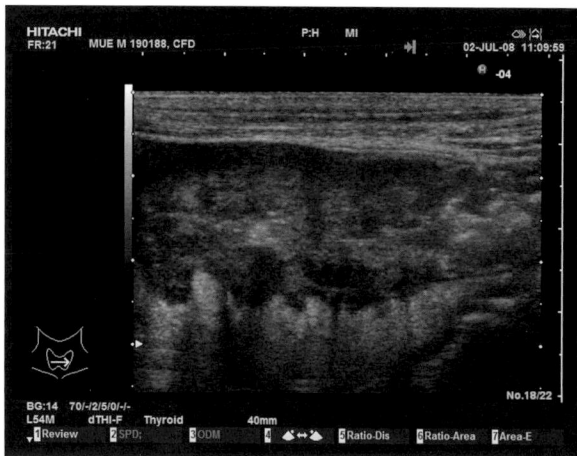

Fig. 1. CD with transmural inflammation (irregular wall delineation).

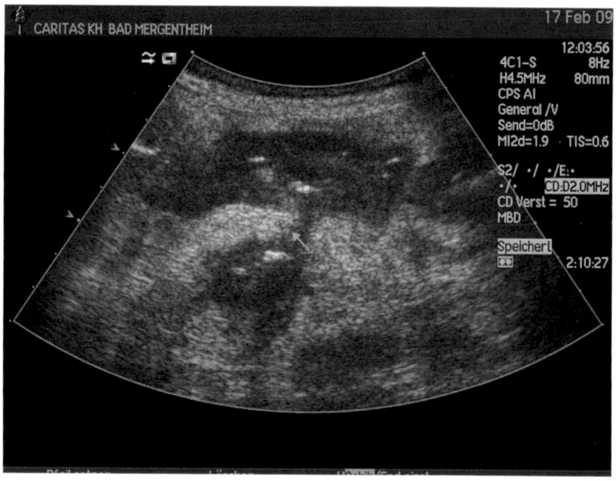

Fig. 2. CD with fistula (arrow) and abscess.

ing the view that fistula formation reflects a more active disease. Six of these had to be treated surgically, in 7 immunosuppressive therapy was started. In this context the question arose as to whether the presence of a fistula per se is associated with greater bowel wall thickness and/or otherwise altered morphology. In this same series, we found that the mean bowel wall thickness in patients with fistula formation was significantly greater than in those with no fistula: 8.0 ± 3.0 vs. 4.3 ± 1.2 mm ($p < 00002$). 8 out of 10 (80%) patients with a fistula showed a blurred wall structure compared to only 9 out of 54 without fistulas (17%, $p < 0.0002$). Signs of transmural inflammatory reaction were present in all patients with fistula formation. The median wall thickness in these patients was almost twofold higher than in those lacking these features (7.0 ± 2.0 vs. 4.0 ± 1.0 mm, $p < 3 \times 10^{-8}$). Mesenteric lymph nodes were detected in 42%, however no significant correlation to disease activity and/or sonographic/laboratory findings was found.

Extraluminal Findings (Ascites, Lymphadenopathy)

Transabdominal US findings of extraluminal phenomena such as free fluid collection and/or mesenteric lymph nodes may also reflect disease activity, but clinical data corroborating such a view is scanty. In the recent trial comprising 100 patients as mentioned above, we found free abdominal fluid in 13% of the patients; there was, however, no significant correlation with disease activity and/or laboratory parameters ($p = 0.236$). Although lymph node enlargement is a common sonographic finding in CD, it appears that US assessment of lymph nodes with regard to clinical parameters, particularly disease activity, is only of limited value and the clinical implications remain to be clarified further. Very early manifestation of CD in children might be mesenteric lymphadenopathy with or without bowel wall thickening [data not yet published]. Other acute and chronic intestinal diseases have to be excluded by appropriate stool and serological test.

Color Doppler Imaging

Intestinal Wall Vascularity. As in a variety of inflammatory intestinal disease states, vascularization is involved particularly in CD. Special ultrasound techniques to qualitatively assess perfusion and other flow parameters have been used for more than a decade. Although a number of authors have described the utility of color Doppler imaging in gastrointestinal disorders, particularly CD, celiac disease and mesenteric artery stenosis, its exact role in diagnosis and/or monitoring disease activity remains to be investigated further. In a trial with 22 patients with confirmed CD, a high concordance between a power Doppler ultrasound score (measuring vascularization) and the degree of local inflammation assessed with an endoscopic severity score was demonstrated with values from 0.83 to 0.98 [34]. A pilot study prospectively involving 20 patients demonstrated a highly significant correlation between the mean blood vessel density assessed by power Doppler sonography and the semiquantitative score tested by Limberg showing its potential application in routine clinical practice [35].

Table 7. Sonographic detection of fistulas in patients with CD [data compiled from 32]

Criteria	Total, n	CDAI <150	CDAI >150	Significance[a], p
Fistula	13/100 (13%)	3/17 (4%)	8/21 (38%)[b]	<0.05
Previously known	3/10 (30%)	1/71 (1%)	2/21 (5%)	
Newly detected	7/10 (70%)	5/71 (7%)	2/21 (10%)	
Enteroenteric	10/13 (77%)	3/71 (4%)	7/21 (33%)	
Enterovesical	1/13	0/71 (0%)	0/21 (0%)	

[a] Comparison between CDAI >150 vs. CDAI <150.
[b] The sum of the patients with CDAI <150 and CDAI >150 does not yield n = 100, as 8 patients with ileostoma were excluded from calculation because the CDAI is not applicable.

Intestinal Wall Vascularity Combined with Mesenteric Inflow Parameters. A newer promising approach is combining mesenteric inflow by duplex scanning such as systolic and diastolic peak velocities and resistance index with end-organ vascularity by CDI. Recent advances including harmonic imaging, power Doppler and CEUS have been added to improve sensitivity/accuracy further with regard to different disease aspects and potential therapeutic decisions, but their definitive clinical role still has to be more precisely defined.

Mesenterial Inflow and Prognosis. Investigations by Ludwig et al. [36, 37] indicate that the pulsatility index measured postprandially as well as in the fasting state allows calculation of the probability of a relapse in patients with active CD. Positive and negative predictive values range between 0.77 and 0.89. 52 patients were prospectively followed for 1 year. The major finding was that a decreased pulsatility index of the superior mesenteric artery was significantly associated with remission in CD, but not in ulcerative colitis [38]. This has led the authors to conclude that repeated Doppler ultrasound measurements may predict response to immunosuppressive therapy. In view of other studies that show a discrepancy to those findings [39], further research and experience in larger patient populations are clearly needed.

Contrast-Enhanced Ultrasound

Newer techniques such as power Doppler and the administration of echo-enhancing agents (Levovist® or SonoVue®) have further improved sensitivity and accuracy [40–44]. Although 2D and Doppler techniques have been grossly improved over the last decade, the performance of these techniques can still be limited by a variety of factors such as tissue motion artifacts (peristalsis) and/or transmural vessel perfusion below the detection threshold [44]. To circumvent such limitations, contrast harmonic imaging at a low mechanical index has been proposed [45–53], but its use in IBD is not yet currently widespread and is confined to a few specialized centers. Introduction into clinical routine use will depend on further developments and experience. Studies comparing new with more conventional approaches will help to clarify these issues. In a small pilot study including 15 patients with ileal CD, contrast-enhanced power Doppler and conventional power Doppler were compared with regard to clinical disease activity and laboratory tests. The results were promising when bowel wall perfusion was evaluated at the site of maximum bowel wall thickness. The prime result was that CEUS was found to be superior compared to conventional techniques with respect to those parameters [45–48]. In another study, 104 consecutive patients with CD were prospectively examined using CEUS with respect to the disease activity index [50]. It was found that the pattern of contrast enhancement and the ratio of enhanced to entire wall thickness had a positive predictive value of 63.0 and 58.6%, respectively, in distinguishing active from inactive disease [50]. It was therefore proposed that CEUS may be particularly able to more precisely characterize bowel wall thickness by differentiating fibrosis from edema and may, thereby, grade inflammation by assessing presence and distribution of vascularity within the intestinal layers, particularly the submucosa and/or the entire bowel wall [54]. Peri-intestinal inflammation can also be characterized in more detail [54], a view, however, which has to be confirmed in the near future. Some authors postulate that CEUS can also provide prognostic data concerning relapse and/or response to therapy.

In a preliminary trial with 20 patients, CEUS was suggested to be useful in the follow-up of infliximab treatment [47]. In addition, this technique has been helpful in surgical management, particularly in the decision of con-

Table 8. Sonomorphologic criteria and clinical activity in patients with ulcerative colitis (n = 36)

	Total	CAI <4	CAI >4	Significance
Patients	36	11	22	
Wall thickening	27/36 (75.0%)	11/11 (100.0%)	16/22 (73.0%)	NS
Wall thickness, mm	4.5 ± 1.3 (3.0–8.0)	4.6 ± 1.2 (3.0–7.0)	4.4 ± 1.3 (3.0–8.0)	NS
Symmetrical thickening	27/33 (82.0%)	11/12 (92.0%)	16/22 (73.0%)	NS
Accentuated mucosa	3/33 (9.0%)	1/11 (9.0%)	2/22 (9.0%)	NS
Thickened mucosa/submucosa	21/33 (64.0%)	9/11 (82.0%)	12/22 (55.0%)	NS
Transmural reaction	3/33 (9.0%)	1/11 (9.0%)	2/22 (9.0%)	NS
Pancolitis	17/33 (52.0%)	9/11 (82.0%)	8/22 (36.0%)	NS
Left-sided colitis	16/33 (48.0%)	2/11 (18.0%)	14/22 (64.0%)	NS
>2 mesenteric lymph nodes	4/36 (11.0%)	2/11 (18.0%)	2/22 (9.0%)	NS

Table modified from Allgayer and Dietrich [61]. NS = Not significant; CAI = Ulcerative Colitis Activity Index, for details see text. Wall thickness, symmetrical thickening, accentuated mucosa, thickened mucosa/submucosa, transmural reaction and lymph nodes were assessed in the same manner as in CD.

servative versus surgical treatment [52, 55]. Although results are promising, much more work is needed before CEUS can be considered a clinically useful tool in such decisions.

Differential Diagnosis of Inflammatory and Fibrotic Bowel Wall Changes

In patients with CD, the analysis of vascularity may facilitate the differentiation between inflammatory or cicatricial-fibroid stenosis, but the results are controversial. It has to be taken into account that cicatricial-fibroid stenoses are mostly in segments with wall thickening <20–30 mm, whereas inflammatory segments are >30 mm. This is more important for differential diagnosis of inflammatory and fibrotic bowel wall changes. Recently, 200 consecutive patients with CD have been examined, displaying hypervascularity in 180 patients with adequate visualization of the bowel wall [Siemens Elegra Advanced, 7 MHz] [54]. In 15 patients, hypervascularity could not be displayed due to reduced sensitivity in patients with a body mass index >30 (n = 14), or depth penetration >40 mm (n = 1) and, therefore, inadequate visualization and insensitivity of the method. In 3 patients the thickened bowel wall segment was <20 mm and hypovascularity was observed indicating cicatricial-fibroid stenosis. Hypovascularity was found in the remaining 2 patients. It was concluded that in patients with CD and thickened bowel wall with a segmental length of >30 mm, hypervascularity can virtually always be displayed. Lack of hypervascularity might be due to insensitivity of the equipment, poor optimization of Doppler parameters, depth penetration >40 mm with loss of sensitivity. In certain cases, contrast-enhanced sonography with a 2- to 5-MHz transducer can be helpful because there is less depth dependency than with Doppler techniques. Analysis of time intensity curves using contrast-enhanced techniques might be more promising than color Doppler imaging alone [54].

Ulcerative Colitis

The diagnosis of ulcerative colitis is usually based on the patient's history and typical endoscopic appearance of the mucosa and histology after exclusion of infectious agents by microscopic examination and stool cultures. As treatment is based in part upon the extent of the disease, it is useful at the initial presentation to document the extent of inflammation, which can be accomplished by combining flexible sigmoidoscopy and ultrasound, when complete colonoscopy is not possible and/or contraindicated. Early sonographic signs of active ulcerative colitis may include a thickened hypoechoic layer, reflecting endoscopic findings of congestion of the swollen mucosa with petechiae, exudates and friability. More severe cases may be associated with transmural bowel wall thickening and patients with fulminant disease may reveal also transmural inflammation similar to CD. However, it should be mentioned that none of these sonographic findings are specific and may be also seen in a number of other colonic disorders due to infectious agents and/or drugs. As a consequence, the value of transabdominal ultrasound in ulcerative colitis is less well established than in CD.

In order to address the role of ultrasound in ulcerative colitis in more detail, we evaluated sonomorphologic characteristics in a series of 36 consecutive patients, including wall thickness, symmetry of thickness, thickened mucosa/submucosa, transmural reaction and extraluminal signs (>2 lymph nodes) in a similar fashion as for CD [33]. Disease activity was assessed by the Ulcerative Colitis Index (CAI), a numerical index indicating active disease when >4 points, and inactive disease <4 points. Taken together, there were no significant correlations/associations between any of these sonographic features and the clinical disease activity and/or laboratory parameters (table 8). Based on the data from the literature and these findings, we consider the role of transabdominal ultrasound in ulcerative colitis less important than in CD, but helpful in evaluating the extent of the disease for treatment decisions.

Acute and Chronic Mesenteric Ischemia

Ultrasound, including color duplex imaging, can facilitate the identification of ischemic-hemorrhagic and secondary inflammatory or necrotic thickenings of the intestinal wall in patients with ischemic colitis and may also help predict patients at risk for complications. A slightly symmetrical hypoechoic wall thickening is often an indication of the non-obstructive form of ischemic colitis with chronic compensated changes. In contrast, asymmetric wall thickening with an ileus may be seen in patients with acute mesenteric ischemia. Duplex imaging reliably evaluates the velocity profile in the celiac trunk and the superior and inferior mesenteric arteries. Color duplex and, in some cases, additional echo-enhancing agents may be helpful in the evaluation of intestinal wall perfusion and in the identification of the mesenteric vessels. Systolic velocities of >250–300 cm/s are sensitive indicators of severe mesenteric arterial stenosis. However, the clinical significance of these findings is not always clear since US does not permit the evaluation of the compensatory collateral circulation (which often requires angiography) [54].

Acute Graft versus Host Disease
Acute graft versus host disease (aGvHD) of the gastrointestinal tract is one of the major complications after allogeneic hematopoietic cell transplantation. Conventional B-mode US and CDI were used in combination to assess the extent, severity, course and prognosis of aGvHD of the gastrointestinal tract in 12 patients with suspected intestinal and/or severe cutaneous aGvHD [56]. The structure and thickness of the bowel wall and blood flow pattern in the superior mesenteric artery and bowel wall were useful for detection of aGvHD even before symptoms developed. All patients had thickened bowel wall segments, particularly in the ileocecal region. Four patients had ischemic bowel wall lesions as evidenced by a high resistance flow pattern in the SMA; these patients did not respond to immunosuppressive therapy and ultimately died. These sonographic features can also be helpful for distinguishing aGvHD from other causes of bowel disturbance that occur in the transplant setting such as pseudomembranous or CMV colitis.

Ultrasound in Other Inflammatory and Non-Inflammatory Gastrointestinal Disease

Ultrasound has been established in other inflammatory and non-inflammatory gastrointestinal disease which is in IBD mainly of importance for differential diagnosis. Suggestions for the interested reader might be overviews [6, 15, 57–59], specific ultrasound signs in endemic sprue [60, 61], the so-called 'white bowel' [62], edema of the gastrointestinal wall [28], amyloidosis [63], cystic fibrosis [64] and other intestinal disease [65].

Conclusions

Transabdominal ultrasound is useful for the detection of bowel wall thickening and for determining the extent of involved segments in different kinds of IBD (CD, ulcerative colitis, intestinal tuberculosis and neutropenic enterocolitis). In CD, transabdominal ultrasound is able to detect complications and characterize disease activity. In ulcerative colitis, the sonographically assessed extent of disease can guide therapy decisions.

Disclosure Statement

The author declares that no financial or other conflict of interest exists in relation to the content of this article.

References

1 Dietrich CF: 3D real-time contrast-enhanced ultrasonography, a new technique (in German). Rofo 2002;174:160–163.
2 Dietrich CF, Caspary WF: SieScape – panorama imaging. Clinical value? (in German). Internist (Berl) 2000;41:24–28.
3 Ignee A, Jedrejczyk M, Schuessler G, Jakubowski W, Dietrich CF: Quantitative contrast-enhanced ultrasound of the liver for time intensity curves – reliability and potential sources of errors. Eur J Radiol 2009 [Epub ahead of print].
4 Dietrich CF, Ignee A, Seitz KH, Caspary WF: Duplex sonography of visceral arteries (in German). Ultraschall Med 2001;22:247–257.
5 Dietrich CF: Comments and illustrations regarding the guidelines and good clinical practice recommendations for contrast-enhanced ultrasound – update 2008. Ultraschall Med 2008;29(suppl 4):S188–S202.
6 Dietrich CF, Barreiros AP, Nuernberg D, Schreiber-Dietrich DG, Ignee A: Perianal ultrasound (in German). Z Gastroenterol 2008;46:625–630.
7 Worlicek H, Lutz H, Thoma B: Sonography of chronic inflammatory bowel diseases – a prospective study (in German). Ultraschall Med 1986;7:275–280.
8 Abu-Yousef MM, Bleicher JJ, Maher JW, Urdaneta LF, Franken EA Jr, Metcalf AM: High-resolution sonography of acute appendicitis. AJR Am J Roentgenol 1987;149:53–58.
9 Kedar RP, Shah PP, Shivde RS, Malde HM: Sonographic findings in gastrointestinal and peritoneal tuberculosis. Clin Radiol 1994;49:24–29.
10 Bozkurt T, Richter F, Lux G: Ultrasonography as a primary diagnostic tool in patients with inflammatory disease and tumors of the small intestine and large bowel. J Clin Ultrasound 1994;22:85–91.
11 Maconi G, Parente F, Bollani S, Cesana B, Bianchi PG: Abdominal ultrasound in the assessment of extent and activity of Crohn's disease: clinical significance and implication of bowel wall thickening. Am J Gastroenterol 1996;91:1604–1609.
12 DiCandio G, Mosca F, Campatelli A, Bianchini M, D'Elia F, Dellagiovampaola C: Sonographic detection of postsurgical recurrence of Crohn disease. AJR Am J Roentgenol 1986;146:523–526.
13 Dubbins PA: Ultrasound demonstration of bowel wall thickness in inflammatory bowel disease. Clin Radiol 1984;35:227–231.
14 Sheridan MB, Nicholson DA, Martin DF: Transabdominal ultrasonography as the primary investigation in patients with suspected Crohn's disease or recurrence: a prospective study. Clin Radiol 1993;48:402–404.
15 Dietrich CF, Brunner V, Lembcke B: Intestinal ultrasound in rare small and large intestinal diseases (in German). Z Gastroenterol 1998;36:955–970.
16 Khan R, Abid S, Jafri W, Abbas Z, Hameed K, Ahmad Z: Diagnostic dilemma of abdominal tuberculosis in non-HIV patients: an ongoing challenge for physicians. World J Gastroenterol 2006;12:6371–6375.
17 Barreiros AP, Braden B, Schieferstein-Knauer C, Ignee A, Dietrich CF: Characteristics of intestinal tuberculosis in ultrasonographic techniques. Scand J Gastroenterol 2008;43:1224–1231.
18 Dietrich CF, Hermann S, Klein S, Braden B: Sonographic signs of neutropenic enterocolitis. World J Gastroenterol 2006;12:1397–1402.
19 Dietrich CF: Ultrasonography of the small and large intestine; in UpToDate, Rose BD (ed), UpToDate, Wellesley, Mass., 2009.
20 Dietrich CF, Lembcke B, Seifert H, Caspary WF, Wehrmann T: Ultrasound diagnosis of penicillin-induced segmental hemorrhagic colitis (in German). Dtsch Med Wochenschr 2000;125:755–760.
21 Hirche TO, Russler J, Braden B, Schuessler G, Zeuzem S, Wehrmann T, et al: Sonographic detection of perihepatic lymphadenopathy is an indicator for primary sclerosing cholangitis in patients with inflammatory bowel disease. Int J Colorectal Dis 2004;19:586–594.
22 Dietrich CF, Zeuzem S, Caspary WF, Wehrmann T: Ultrasound lymph node imaging in the abdomen and retroperitoneum of healthy probands (in German). Ultraschall Med 1998;19:265–269.
23 Parente F, Maconi G, Bollani S, Anderloni A, Sampietro G, Cristaldi M, et al: Bowel ultrasound in assessment of Crohn's disease and detection of related small bowel strictures: a prospective comparative study versus X-ray and intraoperative findings. Gut 2002;50:490–495.
24 Hollerbach S, Geissler A, Schiegl H, Kullmann F, Lock G, Schmidt J, et al: The accuracy of abdominal ultrasound in the assessment of bowel disorders. Scand J Gastroenterol 1998;33:1201–1208.
25 Limberg B: Diagnosis of acute ulcerative colitis and colonic Crohn's disease by colonic sonography. J Clin Ultrasound 1989;17:25–31.
26 Sonnenberg A, Erckenbrecht J, Peter P, Niederau C: Detection of Crohn's disease by ultrasound. Gastroenterology 1982;83:430–434.
27 Pera A, Cammarota T, Comino E, Caldera D, Ponti V, Astegiano M, et al: Ultrasonography in the detection of Crohn's disease and in the differential diagnosis of inflammatory bowel disease. Digestion 1988;41:180–184.
28 Hollerweger A, Macheiner P, Dirks K, Dietrich CF: Differential diagnosis of severe hypoechoic oedema of the small bowel (in German). Ultraschall Med 2006;27:234–239.
29 Maconi G, Bollani S, Bianchi PG: Ultrasonographic detection of intestinal complications in Crohn's disease. Dig Dis Sci 1996;41:1643–1648.
30 Maconi G, Sampietro GM, Russo A, Bollani S, Cristaldi M, Parente F, et al: The vascularity of internal fistulae in Crohn's disease: an in vivo power Doppler ultrasonography assessment. Gut 2002;50:496–500.
31 Seitz K, Reuss J: Sonographic detection of fistulas in Crohn disease (in German). Ultraschall Med 1986;7:281–283.
32 Orsoni P, Barthet M, Portier F, Panuel M, Desjeux A, Grimaud JC: Prospective comparison of endosonography, magnetic resonance imaging and surgical findings in anorectal fistula and abscess complicating Crohn's disease. Br J Surg 1999;86:360–364.
33 Hirche TO, Russler J, Schroder O, Schuessler G, Kappeser P, Caspary WF, et al: The value of routinely performed ultrasonography in patients with Crohn disease. Scand J Gastroenterol 2002;37:1178–1183.
34 Neye H, Voderholzer W, Rickes S, Weber J, Wermke W, Lochs H: Evaluation of criteria for the activity of Crohn's disease by power Doppler sonography. Dig Dis 2004;22:67–72.
35 Kratzer W, Foeller T, Kaechele V, Reinshagen M, Tirpitz CV, Haenle MM: Intestinal wall vascularisation in Crohn's disease (in German). Z Gastroenterol 2004;42:973–978.
36 Ludwig D, Wiener S, Bruning A, Schwarting K, Jantschek G, Stange EF: Mesenteric blood flow is related to disease activity and risk of relapse in Crohn's disease: a prospective follow-up study. Am J Gastroenterol 1999;94:2942–2950.
37 Ludwig D: Doppler sonography in inflammatory bowel disease. Z Gastroenterol 2004;42:1059–1065.
38 Homann N, Klarmann U, Fellermann K, Bruning A, Klingenberg-Noftz R, Witthoft T, et al: Mesenteric pulsatility index analysis predicts response to azathioprine in patients with Crohn's disease. Inflamm Bowel Dis 2005;11:126–132.
39 Bremner AR, Griffiths M, Argent JD, Fairhurst JJ, Beattie RM: Sonographic evaluation of inflammatory bowel disease: a prospective, blinded, comparative study. Pediatr Radiol 2006;36:947–953.
40 Parente F, Greco S, Molteni M, Anderloni A, Sampietro GM, Danelli PG, et al: Oral contrast-enhanced bowel ultrasonography in the assessment of small intestine Crohn's disease. A prospective comparison with conventional ultrasound, x-ray studies, and ileocolonoscopy. Gut 2004;53:1652–1657.
41 Kratzer W, Schmidt SA, Mittrach C, Haenle MM, Mason RA, Von Tirpitz C, et al: Contrast-enhanced wideband harmonic imaging ultrasound (SonoVue): a new technique for quantifying bowel wall vascularity in Crohn's disease. Scand J Gastroenterol 2005;40:985–991.

42 Rapaccini GL, Pompili M, Orefice R, Covino M, Riccardi L, Cedrone A, et al: Contrast-enhanced power Doppler of the intestinal wall in the evaluation of patients with Crohn disease. Scand J Gastroenterol 2004;39:188–194.

43 Robotti D, Cammarota T, Debani P, Sarno A, Astegiano M: Activity of Crohn disease: value of color power Doppler and contrast-enhanced ultrasonography. Abdom Imaging 2004;29:648–652.

44 Schlottmann K, Kratzer W, Scholmerich J: Doppler ultrasound and intravenous contrast agents in gastrointestinal tract disorders: current role and future implications. Eur J Gastroenterol Hepatol 2005;17:263–275.

45 Plikat K, Klebl F, Buchner C, Scholmerich J, Schlottmann K: Evaluation of intestinal hyperaemia in inflamed bowel by high-resolution contrast harmonic imaging. Ultraschall Med 2004;25:257–262.

46 Schmidt T, Hohl C, Haage P, Honnef D, Mahnken AH, Krombach G, et al: Phase-inversion tissue harmonic imaging compared to fundamental B-mode ultrasound in the evaluation of the pathology of large and small bowel. Eur Radiol 2005;15:2021–2030.

47 Guidi L, De Franco A, De V, I, Armuzzi A, Semeraro S, Roberto I, et al: Contrast-enhanced ultrasonography with SonoVue after infliximab therapy in Crohn's disease. Eur Rev Med Pharmacol Sci 2006;10:23–26.

48 De Pascale A, Garofalo G, Perna M, Priola S, Fava C: Contrast-enhanced ultrasonography in Crohn's disease. Radiol Med 2006;111:539–550.

49 Pauls S, Gabelmann A, Schmidt SA, Rieber A, Mittrach C, Haenle MM, et al: Evaluating bowel wall vascularity in Crohn's disease: a comparison of dynamic MRI and wideband harmonic imaging contrast-enhanced low MI ultrasound. Eur Radiol 2006;16:2410–2417.

50 Serra C, Menozzi G, Labate AM, Giangregorio F, Gionchetti P, Beltrami M, et al: Ultrasound assessment of vascularization of the thickened terminal ileum wall in Crohn's disease patients using a low-mechanical index real-time scanning technique with a second-generation ultrasound contrast agent. Eur J Radiol 2007;62:114–121.

51 Migaleddu V, Quaia E, Scano D, Virgilio G: Inflammatory activity in Crohn disease: ultrasound findings. Abdom Imaging 2008;33:589–597.

52 Kunihiro K, Hata J, Manabe N, Mitsuoka Y, Tanaka S, Haruma K, et al: Predicting the need for surgery in Crohn's disease with contrast harmonic ultrasound. Scand J Gastroenterol 2007;42:577–585.

53 Martinez MJ, Ripolles T, Paredes JM, Blanc E, Marti-Bonmati L: Assessment of the extension and the inflammatory activity in Crohn's disease: comparison of ultrasound and MRI. Abdom Imaging 2009;34:141–148.

54 Dietrich CF, Jedrzejczyk M, Ignee A: Sonographic assessment of splanchnic arteries and the bowel wall. Eur J Radiol 2007;64:202–212.

55 Maconi G, Sampietro GM, Sartani A, Bianchi Porro G: Bowel ultrasound in Crohn's disease: surgical perspective. Int J Colorectal Dis 2008;23:339–347.

56 Klein SA, Martin H, Schreiber-Dietrich D, Hermann S, Caspary WF, Hoelzer D, et al: A new approach to evaluating intestinal acute graft-versus-host disease by transabdominal sonography and colour Doppler imaging. Br J Haematol 2001;115:929–934.

57 Nuernberg D, Ignee A, Dietrich CF: Current status of ultrasound in gastroenterology – Bowel and upper gastrointestinal tract. Part 1 (in German). Z Gastroenterol 2007;45:629–640.

58 Nuernberg D, Ignee A, Dietrich CF: Current status of ultrasound in gastroenterology – Bowel and upper gastrointestinal tract. Part 2 (in German). Z Gastroenterol 2008;46:355–366.

59 Nuernberg D, Braden B, Ignee A, Schreiber-Dietrich DG, Dietrich CF: Functional ultrasound in gastroenterology (in German). Z Gastroenterol 2008;46:883–896.

60 Dietrich CF, Brunner V, Seifert H, Schreiber-Dietrich D, Caspary WF, Lembcke B: Intestinal B-mode sonography in patients with endemic sprue. Intestinal sonography in endemic sprue (in German). Ultraschall Med 1999;20:242–247.

61 Allgayer H, Dietrich CF: Celiac sprue and malignancies: analysis of risks and prevention strategies (in German). Med Klin (Munich) 2008;103:561–568.

62 Hollerweger A, Dietrich CF: 'White bowel'. A sonographic sign of intestinal lymph edema? (in German). Ultraschall Med 2005;26:127–133.

63 Barreiros AP, Otto G, Ignee A, Galle P, Dietrich CF: Sonographic signs of amyloidosis. Z Gastroenterol 2009;47:731–739.

64 Bargon J, Stein J, Dietrich CF, Muller U, Caspary WF, Wagner TO: Gastrointestinal complications of adult patients with cystic fibrosis (in German). Z Gastroenterol 1999;37:739–749.

65 Dietrich CF, Caspary WF: What is collagen colitis and how is it treated? (in German). Internist (Berl) 1995;36:1016–1017.

New Insights into Whipple's Disease – A Rare Intestinal Inflammatory Disorder

Thomas Marth

Division of Internal Medicine, Krankenhaus Maria Hilf, Daun, Germany

Key Words

Whipple's disease · Whipple's disease, cardiac and neurologic involvement · Whipple's disease, clinical features · *Tropheryma whipplei*, characteristics

Abstract

Whipple's disease (WD) is a rare systemic infectious disorder caused by the actinomycete *Tropheryma whipplei*. This chronic disease, first described by Whipple as 'intestinal lipodystrophy', affects preferentially middle-aged white men who may present with weight loss, diarrhea, abdominal pain and arthralgia. Thus, it represents an important differential diagnosis of chronic diarrhea. A variety of other clinical patterns, such as involvement of the heart, lung, or central nervous system (CNS), are frequent. In addition, individuals with isolated heart valve involvement or asymptomatic carriers may be observed. The diagnosis often is established by small bowel biopsy, which is characterized by periodic acid-Schiff-positive inclusions representing the causative bacteria. *T. whipplei* can be detected by specific polymerase chain reaction, immunohistochemistry or electron microscopy and was cultured a few years ago. Several studies show that subtle defects of the cell-mediated immunity exist in active and inactive WD which may predispose individuals with a certain HLA type to a clinical manifestation of *T. whipplei* infection. As confirmed in a recent controlled trial, most patients respond well to a prolonged antibiotic treatment, but some patients with relapsing disease or CNS manifestation may have a poor prognosis. In the presentation, the relevance of WD in the differential diagnosis of chronic diarrhea and the new findings of this enigmatic rare disorder will be discussed.

Copyright © 2009 S. Karger AG, Basel

Introduction

Whipple's disease (WD) is caused by the rod-shaped bacterium *Tropheryma whipplei*. This rare chronic disease may occur in all ages, but most frequently affects middle-aged white males. Patients often present with symptoms of weight loss, diarrhea, arthralgia, and abdominal pain; involvement of the heart, lung and central nervous system (CNS) is also common. Therefore, WD should be considered primarily in the differential diagnosis of malabsorption syndromes and chronic diarrhea. The diagnosis is established by small-bowel biopsy which shows inclusions in macrophages of the lamina propria positive with the periodic acid-Schiff (PAS) stain. While untreated WD is chronic, progressive and fatal, many patients treated with antibiotics achieve rapid clinical improvement and maintain a long-lasting remission. Approximately 20% of patients do not respond sufficiently to antibiotic therapy and up to 40% have relapses afterwards.

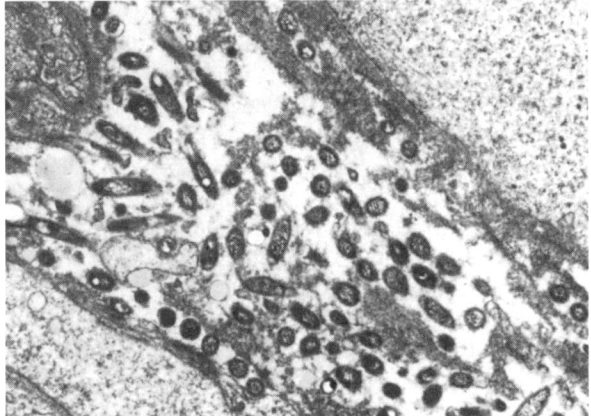

Fig. 1. Electron microscopic view of T. whipplei. The characteristic, rod-shaped (1–2.5 μm in size) organism can be observed in the extracellular space in florid disease or within cells in various stages of degradation. T. whipplei is characterized by a trilaminar plasma membrane, a surrounding homogeneous cell wall of 20 nm thickness, and an outer trilaminar membrane-like structure usually seen in Gram-negative bacteria. Other characteristics, including the central location of tubules and vesicles, are typical of Gram-positive organisms. ×20,000.

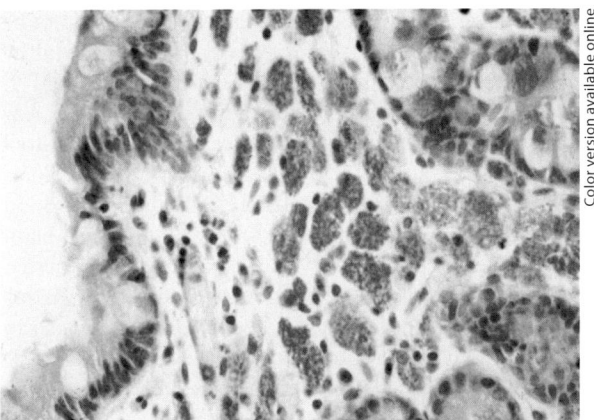

Fig. 2. PAS stain of a duodenal biopsy specimen in a patient with WD. Large numbers of stained macrophages in the lamina propria can be seen. ×40.

Characteristics of the Organism

T. whipplei is a rod-shaped bacterium and uniformly possesses a trilaminar plasma membrane, a surrounding homogenous cell wall of 20 nm thickness with two inner layers and an outer trilaminar membrane-like structure [1, 2] (fig. 1). Because of the frequent intestinal symptoms, an oral route of acquisition is generally assumed. It is probable that T. whipplei passes the stomach and enters the proximal small intestine where the bacteria invade the mucosa and then spread via the lymphatic system into the blood [2].

Typically, T. whipplei is found in macrophages of the lamina propria of the small bowel. In light microscopy the remnants of digested bacteria present as PAS-positive granular-foamy inclusions in large macrophages (fig. 2). In florid disease, undigested bacteria can also be seen in the extracellular space. Antibiotic treatment continuously decreases the number of PAS-positive macrophages and the organisms disappear usually slowly from the lamina propria resulting in clinical improvement [3].

The bacterium has an atypical morphology for a Gram-positive or a Gram-negative bacillus. Phylogenetic analysis of T. whipplei 16S rDNA sequence established that this bacterium is an actinomycete [4]. The organism is placed in an intermediate position between cellulomonads and a group of Actinomyces with group B peptidoglycan [5]. These bacteria are predominantly environmental bacteria and can be found in soil, water, and plants.

The bacillus was first propagated in peripheral blood mononuclear cells deactivated by interleukin-4, but then the growth of the bacillus was stably established in human fibroblast (HEL) cells [6]. T. whipplei is a slowly-growing organism with an estimated doubling time of 17 days; newer studies with cell-free media show a much faster replication rate [6, 7]. The site of multiplication in vivo is still controversial. Bacterial strains of T. whipplei show genetic heterogeneity and the genomic variants have been presumed to be associated with the geographic distribution. The natural habitat of T. whipplei is unknown, but polymerase chain reaction (PCR) studies suggest that the bacterium is ubiquitously present [8]. T. whipplei was found by PCR in 37% of influxes to sewage treatment plants around Vienna [9].

WD is approximately eight times more common in men than in women [1, 10]. There are several cases of familial clustering, but the majority of the analyzed cases do not exhibit familial components. Most of the cases stem from rural regions and farming is frequently documented occupation [1].

There is still some controversy regarding the prevalence of T. whipplei in healthy persons since T. whipplei DNA was found in the saliva from 19 to 35% of healthy subjects.

However, in other studies, *T. whipplei* DNA could not be identified in samples from duodenal biopsies in healthy persons, while 0.6 and 1.5% of healthy persons had *T. whipplei* DNA in saliva and stool, respectively [11, 12]. Another study reported the occurrence of *T. whipplei* in stool samples in 13 out of 208 (6%) healthy control individuals and in 5 out of 196 (2.5%) diseased control patients [13]. In a survey conducted in Austria, 25% of the sewage plant workers tested positive for *T. whipplei* in stool by nested PCR, whereas only 7% of controls (with different gastroenterological disorders) tested positive for *T. whipplei* in stool [9]. Thus, close contact to sewage water seems to increase the likelihood of excreting *T. whipplei* in stool.

Pathogenesis

Despite the presumed ubiquitous natural occurrence of *T. whipplei*, WD is extremely rare. The defective immune response in patients with WD would have to be quite specific since these patients are not generally predisposed to other infections. Martinetti et al. [14] recently found in the largest cohort examined so far an association with DRB1*13 and DQB1*06, but no HLA-B27 overexpression.

Changes in immunity have been identified. Populations of T cells are characterized by a low CD4/CD8 T-cell ratio, increased cell-activation markers, and shifts toward a mature T-cell subpopulation [15]. The reduced proliferative response of peripheral T cells occurs in response to lectins and to antibodies to CD2 [15, 16]. The small-bowel mucosa shows low numbers of IgA-positive B cells but an increased number of surface IgM-positive B cells [17]. Secretory IgA concentrations measured in intestinal aspirates and humoral immune responses to infectious agents in the periphery are normal. Serum concentrations of total IgG are normal, but IgM concentrations are low and those of IgA high in acute stages of the disease [15, 18].

In patients with WD, *T. whipplei* multiplies in both monocytes and macrophages [19], and the replication of *T. whipplei* in monocytes and macrophages correlates with interleukin-16 overexpression and thioredoxin downregulation. Recent studies have shown defective macrophage function in WD patients, and this could be of central importance in the development of the disease. It has been shown that intestinal macrophages of WD patients display in vivo the phenotype of M2/alternatively activated macrophages that favor the development of Th2 response and inhibit protective Th1 polarization [20a, 20b]. Macrophages from WD patients phagocytize bacteria normally but are unable to degrade bacterial antigens efficiently. This could be related to a reduced CD11b expression. CD11b serves as a facilitator of microbial phagocytosis, has a role in antigen processing, and mediates intracellular killing of ingested bacteria that is induced by IFN-γ [15]. Patients with inactive disease have a lower than normal number of circulating cells expressing CD11b, while during active disease intestinal macrophages do not express CD11b [20a].

Studies have also shown a reduced interleukin-12 production in macrophages [16, 21]. In addition, it was found that WD patients showed reduced or absent *T. whipplei*-specific Th1 response, whereas their capacity to react to other common antigens like tetanus toxoid, tuberculin, actinomycetes, *Giardia lamblia*, or cytomegalovirus (CMV) was not reduced compared with controls [22]. Even in successfully treated WD patients, the Th1 reactivity remains decreased.

In conclusion, the subtle defects of cellular immunity probably contribute to an important part to a disturbed phagocytosis, disturbed intracellular degradation and an impaired immunological clearance of *T. whipplei*. This may allow an invasion from the gastrointestinal mucosa to peripheral organs and result in a chronic infection and eventually in a fatal course of the disease.

Clinical Picture

WD is characterized in many patients by two stages – a prodromal stage and a progressive stage. The prodromal stage is characterized by protean symptoms, arthralgia, arthritis and non-specific findings. The progressive stage is characterized by weight loss, diarrhea and arthropathies in up to 75% of patients. The clinical presentation in the progressive stage may vary to a great extent, and even in the absence of gastrointestinal symptoms, cardiac or CNS symptoms may occur. The average time between the prodromal stage and the progressive stage is 6 years [23–25]. In patients already infected with *T. whipplei*, immunosuppression apparently accelerates the course of the infection and especially triggers the occurrence of intestinal manifestations [25]. Gastrointestinal symptoms usually lead to the diagnosis of WD.

Typical Clinical Features in Whipple's Disease

Common presenting clinical features of WD are weight loss, diarrhea, arthropathy, abdominal pain, low-grade fever and peripheral lymphadenopathy (table 1). Although WD has traditionally been regarded as a gas-

Table 1. Clinical characteristics of WD

Characteristic	Frequency, %
Major clinical characteristics	
Weight loss	90
Arthropathy	85
Diarrhea	75
Abdominal pain	60
Other signs and symptoms	
Fever	45
Lymphadenopathy	45
Hyperpigmentation	35
Hypotension	35
Peripheral edema	30
Cardiac murmurs	30
Occult bleeding	25
Myalgia	25
CNS involvement	15
Chronic cough	15
Splenomegaly	15
Hepatomegaly	10
Ascites	10

Table 2. Role of duodenal biopsy in the differential diagnosis of chronic diarrhea

Duodenal biopsies are
Diagnostic for:
    Whipple's disease (confirm by PCR or IH)
    Hypogammaglobulinemia
    Abetaproteinemia
Suggestive for:
    Celiac disease, collagenous celiac disease
    Intestinal lymphangiectasia
    Crohn's disease
    Lymphoma
    AIDS enteropathy
    Parasitic disorders
    Amyloidosis
    Eosinophilic enteritis
    Pharmacological causes
    Postradiation enteritis
    Deficiency in folic acid, vitamin B_{12}

trointestinal disease, the first symptom preceding the diagnosis by a mean of 8 years is often arthropathy. In one series, arthropathy as a prodromal symptom was found in 63% of patients [26]. The arthropathy consists of chronic migratory non-destructive and seronegative joint disease, involving predominantly the peripheral joints. Joint symptoms often diminish, for unknown reasons, with the occurrence of gastrointestinal symptoms. The joint symptomatology improves within 2–4 weeks after initiation of antibiotics [1, 10].

Weight loss is the major symptom by the time of diagnosis and is present in two thirds of the patients more than 4 years before diagnosis. Most patients respond well to antibiotic treatment and regain their initial weight after several months.

Watery diarrhea resulting from small intestine involvement is episodic and accompanied by colicky abdominal pain. Steatorrhea occurs rather rarely, and 20–30% of patients have evidence of occult blood in stool. These symptoms with concomitant anorexia can lead to a full malabsorption syndrome. The differential diagnosis of malabsorptive disorders includes celiac disease, Crohn's disease, lymphoma, AIDS enteropathy, parasitic disorders, amyloidosis as well as rare disorders such as hypogammaglobulinemia and abetaproteinemia (table 2).

Diarrhea responds well to antibiotic therapy and resolves within 1 or several weeks of therapy initiation. Endoscopic lesions disappear 6–9 months after antibiotics, and 12–18 months after the onset of antibiotic therapy most of the intestinal villi have a normal architecture.

Systemic symptoms occur in about one half of the WD patients. Frequent features are intermittent low-grade fever, night sweats and a peripheral and abdominal lymphadenopathy [1, 24].

Cardiac Involvement

Common clinical presentations of cardiac WD are cardiac murmurs and insufficiency of the valves necessitating valve replacement. Clinically apparent endocarditis is less frequent, and congestive heart failure and fever are not frequently observed in patients with Whipple's endocarditis [27]. Recent studies have described a syndrome of 'blood culture-negative endocarditis' in patients with T. whipplei infection but no other evidence of WD. In these cases, PCR is useful to confirm T. whipplei endocarditis which then should lead to an effective treatment regimen. Pathologic valve alterations in WD patients are most frequently found on the mitral valve, while the most significant clinical symptoms are caused by affection of the aortic valve [1, 27, 28].

Neurologic Involvement

Neurologic manifestations can resemble any neurologic disease. Therefore, some cases of WD with CNS involvement are not diagnosed until postmortem. Neurologic manifestations may occur in three situations: neurologic involvement in classic WD, isolated neurologic symptoms due to *T. whipplei* infection without evidence of intestinal involvement, and neurologic relapse of WD [1, 29].

Neurologic symptoms have been reported in series in 6–63% (mean ca. 15–20%) of patients with intestinal WD [1, 29]. Typical symptoms include cognitive changes which are associated with various psychiatric alterations. Other clinical signs are ophthalmoplegia, nystagmus and myoclonia, which are frequently noted in combination with disturbed sleep pattern, ataxia, seizures or symptoms of cerebral compression [29, 30]. In addition, cranial nerve symptoms such as hearing loss and blurred vision have been reported. A specific infrequent oculomasticatory myorhythmia and oculofacial skeletal myorhythmia have been considered to be characteristic for CNS WD and are accompanied by supranuclear vertical gaze palsy (supranuclear ophthalmoplegia) [31].

Neurological manifestations of cerebral WD rarely include stroke-like symptoms. The pathogenesis of cerebral infarction may be due to cerebral vasculitis, arterial fibrosis, thrombosis and thickening associated with the inflammation of adjacent brain parenchyma and leptomeninges, caused by the hematogenous spread of *T. whipplei* to the brain.

Isolated neurologic symptoms have been described in 32 patients, 19 of whom had systemic symptoms such as fever, weight loss, articular pain and peripheral lymphadenopathy, but no diarrhea. Of the 30 patients for whom follow-up data were available, 60% improved after treatment and 33% died [23]. Patients with CNS involvement carry a high risk for disease recurrence [24], and a neurologic recurrence has a poor prognosis. Therefore, neurologic manifestation is a major cause of deaths in WD. Computer tomography or magnetic resonance imaging in CNS show abnormalities like mild to moderate brain atrophy or focal lesions without a predilection for a specific site. Results of cerebrospinal fluid examination are normal or show a mild pleocytosis. PAS-positive sickleform particle-containing cells may be found at cerebrospinal fluid cytology and PCR is positive for *T. whipplei* in up to 50% even in neurologically asymptomatic patients [29].

Other Manifestations

Skin hyperpigmentation, particularly affecting light-exposed areas of the body (commonly misinterpreted as Addison's disease), has been observed in one third of the patients with WD. The skin changes usually regress after treatment [1, 32]. Hepato- or splenomegaly can be present in some patients with this disorder. Quite rare involvement has been reported for the kidney, the genitourinary and endocrine system. Chronic non-productive cough or chest pain indicating lung involvement or pleuritis, polyserositis, ascites, hypotension and edema are also among frequent signs and symptoms, but patients only rarely have persistent symptoms [1, 10].

Association of Whipple's Disease to Other Disorders

The inflammatory reaction in WD may be granulomatous in approximately 9% of the patients. Sarcoid-like epithelioid non-caseating granulomas have been described most frequently [1, 33]. These epithelioid cell granulomas are speculated to be a result of partially digested antigen, although no products of bacterial degradation have been observed. Especially when WD affects the lung, sarcoidosis may be confused with WD [34]. In a recent series of 40 patients in a randomized trial testing antibiotic treatment, 2 patients had sarcoid-like lesions [Feurle et al., in preparation]. In several patients with WD, amyloidosis has been reported, but it is unclear whether the amyloid deposits result from chronic inflammatory responses.

An association of WD with malignancies has not been described frequently. There are reports of non-Hodgkin's lymphoma occurring after treatment of WD [35] and clonal expansions simulating B-cell lymphoma have been found in patients blood or bone marrow [36]. There are 3 patients out of 40 in the randomized trial [Feurle et al., in preparation] who experienced a non-Hodgkin's or Hodgkin's lymphoma.

Infections with non-tuberculous mycobacteria (mostly *Mycobacterium avium intracellulare*) in AIDS patients can mimic histologically WD [37] and has been named 'pseudo Whipple's disease'. WD can be associated in rare cases with a number of opportunistic infections [38]. In addition, the intestinal symptoms may occur shortly after the onset of immunosuppressive therapy (which is started in some patients due to unclear arthropathies) [25]. The association of WD with giardiasis has been reported in more than 15 cases [39]. In the recent series of mostly German patients, 4 out of 40 (10%) had had a giardiasis [Feurle et al., in preparation].

Laboratory Features

Laboratory abnormalities can show evidence of malabsorption and protein-losing enteropathy such as low β-carotene, vitamin deficiencies (B_{12}, D, K, and folic acid), low albumin and cholesterol concentration, raised stool fat excretion and low D-xylose absorption. Some patients show pronounced eosinophilia and serum immunoglobulin abnormalities. Other laboratory abnormalities are increased C-reactive protein, lymphocytopenia, thrombocytosis and hypochromic anemia [25].

Diagnosis

The initial diagnostic procedure to a patient with clinical suspicion of WD is upper endoscopy with small-bowel mucosal biopsy. Histological appearance of the biopsy samples may reveal the diagnosis with PAS-positive cells (fig. 2). Duodenal biopsy has quite an important role in the diagnosis of WD as it is often the diagnostic procedure while duodenal biopsies are only suggestive for a number of other disorders in the differential diagnosis of chronic diarrhea (table 2). Biopsies should be taken from both the proximal and distal duodenum or jejunum. Infiltration of the bowel wall is associated with a widening and flattening of the villi and with dilated lacteals containing yellow lipid deposits [1]. PAS staining is not completely specific since patients with infection caused by *M. avium intracellulare*, *Rhodococcus equi*, *Bacillus cereus*, *Corynebacterium*, *Histoplasma* or fungi also have PAS-positive macrophages [23].

The lesions of WD are commonly described endoscopically as pale yellow shaggy mucosa alternating with an erythematous, erosive or mildly friable mucosa in the postbulbar region of the duodenum or jejunum. Whitish-yellow plaques can be seen in a patchy distribution [40].

Bacteria can also be visualized by electron microscopy, a technique which is nowadays used less frequently (fig. 1). Culture is currently not yet a method of diagnosis and is carried out only in highly specialized laboratories. Immunohistochemical staining for antibodies against *T. whipplei* can detect the organism in various tissues, body fluids and monocytes (fig. 3). This method provides direct visualization of the bacillus, has a great sensitivity and specificity and even can be used retrospectively on fixed samples. PCR can be used to detect *T. whipplei* in samples from various tissue types and fluids [23].

The proposed strategy for diagnosing WD is histologic examination of a small-bowel biopsy and routinely a PCR. In the absence of extraintestinal symptoms, a normal intestinal histology practically rules out the diagnosis. Routine PCR testing of cerebrospinal fluid in patients with diagnosed intestinal WD is obligatory since around 50% have a positive PCR in the cerebrospinal fluid even without neurologic or psychiatric symptoms [41]. Depending on the clinical manifestations, it is helpful to perform PCR testing on extraintestinal samples (such as cardiac valves, lymph nodes and synovia).

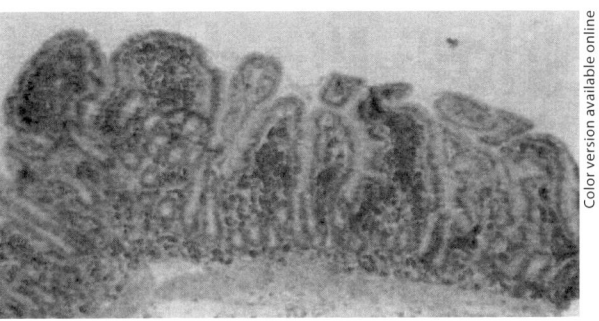

Fig. 3. Specific immunohistochemistry for *T. whipplei*. ×20.

Table 3. Recommended treatment in WD

Initial parenteral therapy (i.v.) 2 weeks of ceftriaxone (2 g daily) (alternatively: meropenem or penicillin + streptomycin)
Long-term therapy (oral) At least 1 year of trimethoprim-sulfamethoxazole (160/800 mg twice daily) (alternatively doxycycline [+ hydroxychloroquine] or cephalosporin)
Individual therapeutic approach Primary CNS manifestation Relapse with CNS manifestation Endocarditis Antibiotic resistance or refractory to antimicrobials (≥2 relapses)

Treatment

Up to the 1980s, many patients were treated with penicillin, streptomycin or tetracycline. Since tetracycline seems to be associated with a higher frequency of relapse, trimethoprim-sulfamethoxazole (160/800 mg orally twice daily) for 1–2 years is now recommended [10, 24]. Oral treatment should be preceded by a 2-week course of parenteral therapy with ceftriaxone (2 g daily), or alternatively by meropenem (table 3). This issue was clarified in a randomized controlled trial (SIMW) with 40 WD patients [Feurle et al., in preparation]. Another alternative, e.g. in cases of allergies, is a combination of streptomycin (1 g daily) together with penicillin G (1.2 million U daily).

The susceptibility of *T. whipplei* to various antimicrobial agents has been tested after its sequencing in vitro with the use of both cell and cell-free cultures. Doxycycline and sulfamethoxazole are active in vitro but not trimethoprim [41–43]. Cell culture cephalosporins including ceftriaxone and fluoroqinolones do not exhibit activity, whereas in axenic medium ceftriaxone and levofloxacin are active. Alkalizing agents like hydrochloroquine may increase the bactericidal effect of the antibiotics. The combination of doxycycline (200 mg daily) plus hydrochloroquine (200 mg three times daily) is a successful approach in vitro and was also successful in 4 patients [23].

In response to treatment, diarrhea and fever resolve within 1 week. Other symptoms improve in many cases after a few weeks [24]. Follow-up duodenal biopsies should be taken after 6 and 12 months. If by then no PAS-positive material is identified, antibiotic treatment can be stopped. In some patients, bacterial material persists, and few have an antibiotic refractory disease.

Disclosure Statement

The author declares that no financial or other conflict of interest exists in relation to the content of this article.

References

1 Dobbins WO III: Whipple's Disease. Springfield, Thomas, 1987.
2 Dobbins WO III, Ruffin JM: A light- and electron-microscopic study of bacterial invasion in Whipple's disease. Am J Pathol 1967;51:225–242.
3 Trier JS, Phelps PC, Eidelmann S, Rubin CE: Whipple's disease: light and electron microscope correlation of jejunal mucosal histology with antibiotic treatment and clinical status. Gastroenterology 1965;48:684–707.
4 Relman DA, Schmidt TM, MacDermot RP, Falkow S: Identification of the uncultured bacillus of Whipple's disease. N Engl J Med 1992;30:293–301.
5 Maiwald M, Ditton HJ, von Herbay A, Rainey FA, Stackerbrandt E: Reassessment of the phylogenetic position of the bacterium associated with Whipple's disease and determination of the 16S-23S ribosomal intergenic spacer sequence. Int J Syst Bacteriol 1996;46:1078–1082.
6 Raoult D, Birg ML, La Scola B, Fournier PE, Enea M, Lepidi H, Roux V, Piette JC, Vandenesch F, Vital Durand D, Marrie TJ: Cultivation of the bacillus of Whipple's disease. N Engl J Med 2000;342:620–625.
7 Renesto P, Crapoulet N, Ogata H, La Scola B, Vestris G, Claverie JM, Raoult D: Genome-based design of a cell-free culture medium for *Tropheryma whipplei*. Lancet 2003;362:447–449.
8 Maiwald M, Ditton HJ, von Herbay A, Rainey FA, Stackerbrandt E: Environmental occurrence of the Whipple's disease bacterium (*Tropheryma whippelii*). Appl Environ Microbiol 1999;64:760–762.
9 Schöniger-Hekele M, Petermann D, Weber B, Müller CT: Whipplei in the environment: survey of sewage plant influxes and sewage plant workers. Appl Environ Microbiol 2007;73:2033–2035.
10 Marth T, Raoult D: Whipple's disease. Lancet 2003;361:239–246.
11 Fenollar F, Fournier PE, Raoult D, Gérolami R, Lepidi H, Poyart C: Quantitative detection of *Tropheryma whipplei* DNA by real-time PCR. J Clin Microbiol 2002;3:1119–1120.
12 Maiwald M, von Herbay A, Persing DH, Mitchell PP, Abdelmalek MF, Thorvilson JN, Fredricks DN, Relman DA: *Tropheryma whippelii* DNA is rare in the intestinal mucosa of patients without other evidence of Whipple disease. Ann Intern Med 2001;2:115–119.
13 Amsler L, Bauernfeind P, Nigg C, Maibach RC, Steffen R, Altwegg M: Prevalence of *T. whipplei* DNA in patients with various gastrointestinal diseases and in healthy controls. Infection 2003;31:81–85.
14 Martinetti M, Biagi F, Badulli C, Feurle GE, Müller C, Moos V, Schneider T, Marth T, Marchese A, Trotta L, Sachetto S, Pasi A, De Silvestri A, Salvaneschi L, Corazza GR: The HLA alleles DRB1*13 and DQB1*06 are associated to Whipple's disease. Gastroenterology 2009;136:2289–2294.
15 Marth T, Roux M, von Herbay A, Meuer SC, Feurle GE: Persistent reduction of complement receptor-3 α-chain expressing mononuclear blood cells and transient inhibitory serum factors in Whipple's disease. Clin Immunol Immunopathol 1994;72:217–226.
16 Marth T, Neurath M, Cuccherini BA, Strober M: Defects of monocyte interleukin-12 production and humoral immunity in Whipple's disease. Gastroenterology 1997;113:442–448.
17 Eck M, Kreipe H, Harmsen D, Müller-Hermelink HK: Invasion and destruction of mucosal plasma cells by *Tropheryma whippelii*. Hum Pathol 1997;28:1424–1428.
18 Dobbins WO III: Is there a immune deficit in Whipple's disease? Dig Dis Sci 1981;26:247–252.
19 Desnues B, Raoult D, Mege JL: IL-16 is critical for *T. whipplei* replication in Whipple's disease. J Immunol 2005;175:4575–4582.
20a Desnues B, Lepidi H, Raoult D, Mege JL: Whipple disease: intestinal infiltrating cells exhibit a transcriptional pattern of M2/alternatively activated macrophages. J Infect Dis 2005;9:1642–1646.
20b Moos V, Schmidt C, Geelhaar A, Kunkel D, Allers K, Schinnerling K, Loddenkemper C, Fenollar F, Moter A, Raoult D, Ignatius R, Schneider T: Impaired immune functions of monocytes and macrophages in Whipple's disease. Gastroenterology 2009, Aug 4 [Epub ahead of print].
21 Marth T, Kleen N, Stallmach A, Ring S, Aziz S, Schmidt C, Strober W, Zeitz M, Schneider T: Dysregulated peripheral and mucosal Th1/Th2 response in Whipple's disease. Gastroenterology 2002;123:1468–1477.
22 Moos V, Kunkel D, Marth T, Feurle GE, La-Scola B, Ignatius R, Zeitz M, Schneider T: Reduced peripheral and mucosal *T. whipplei*-specific Th1 response in patients with Whipple's disease. J Immunol 2006;177:2015–2022.

23 Fenollar F, Puechal X, Raoult D: Whipple's disease N Engl J Med 2007;356:55–66.
24 Feurle GE, Marth T: An evaluation of antimicrobial treatment for Whipple's disease: Tetracycline versus trimethoprim-sulfomethoxazole. Dig Dis Sci 1994;39:1642–1648.
25 Mahnel R, Kalt A, Ring S, Stallmach A, Strober W, Marth T: Immunosuppressive therapy in Whipple's disease patients is associated with the appearance of gastrointestinal manifestations. Am J Gastroenterol 2005;100:1167–1173.
26 Marth T, Strober W: Whipple's disease. Semin Gastrointest Dis 1996;7:41–48.
27 Fenollar F, Lepidi H, Raoult D: Whipple's endocarditis: review of the literature and comparisons with Q fever, *Bartonella* infection, and blood culture-positive endocarditis. Clin Infect Dis 2001;33:1309–1316.
28 Geissdörfer W, Wittmann I, Seitz G, Cesnjevar R, Röllinghoff M, Schoerner C, Bogdan C: A case of aortic valve disease associated with *Tropheryma whippelii* infection in the absence of other signs of Whipple's disease. Infection 2001;29:44–47.
29 Gerard A, Sarrot-Reynauld F, Liozon E: Neurologic presentation of Whipple disease: report of 12 cases and review of the literature. Medicine (Baltimore) 2002;81:443–457.
30 Schneider T, Moos V, Loddenkemper C, Marth T, Fenollar F, Raoult D: Whipple's disease: new aspects of pathogenesis and treatment. Lancet Infect Dis 2008;8:179–190.

31 Louis ED, Lynch T, Kaufmann P, Fahn S, Odel J: Diagnostic guidelines in central nervous system Whipple's disease. Ann Neurol 1996;40:561–568.
32 Marth T: Whipple's disease; in Mandell GL, Dolin JE, Bennett R (eds): Principles and Practice of Infectious Disease, ed 6. Philadelphia, Churchill Livingstone, 2005, pp 1306–1310.
33 Rodarte JR, Garrison CO, Holley KE, Fontana RS: Whipple's disease simulating sarcoidosis. Arch Intern Med 1972;129:479–482.
34 Dzirlo L, Hubner M, Mueller C, Blaha B, Formann E, Dellinger C, Petzelbauer P, Muellauer L, Huber K, Kneussl M, Gschwantler M: A mimic of sarcoidosis. Lancet 2007;369: 1832.
35 Gillen CD, Coddington R, Monteith PG, Taylor RH: Extraintestinal lymphoma in association with Whipple's disease. Gut 1993; 11:1627–1629.
36 Fest T, Pron B, Lefranc MP, Pierre C, Angonin R, de Wazières B, Soua Z, Dupond JL: Detection of a clonal BCL2 gene rearrangement in tissues from a patient with Whipple disease. Ann Intern Med 1996;8:738–740.

37 Autran B, Gorin I, Leibowitch M, Laroche L, Escande JP, Hewitt J, Marche C: AIDS in a Haitian woman with cardiac Kaposi's sarcoma and Whipple's disease. Lancet 1983;8327: 767–768.
38 Meier-Willersen HJ, Maiwald M, von Herbay A: Whipple's disease associated with opportunistic infections. Dtsch Med Wochenschr 1993;23:854–860.
39 Fenollar F, Lepidi H, Gérolami R, Drancourt H, Raoult D: Whipple disease associated with giardiasis. J Infect Dis 2003;188:828–834.
40 Geboes, K, Ectors N, Heidbuchel H, Rutgeerts P, Desmet V, Vantrappen G: Whipple's disease: the value of upper gastrointestinal endoscopy for the diagnosis and follow-up. Acta Gastroenterol Belg 1992;2:209–219.
41 Von Herbay A, Ditton HJ, Schuhmacher F, Maiwald M: Whipple's disease: staging and monitoring by cytology and polymerase chain reaction analysis of cerebrospinal fluid. Gastroenterology 1997;113:434–441.
42 Boulos A, Rolain JM, Raoult D: Antibiotic susceptibility of *Tropheryma whipplei* in MRC5 cells. Antimicrob Agents Chemother 2004;48:747–752.
43 Raoult D, Ogata H, Audic S, Robert C, Suhre K, Drancourt M: *Tropheryma whipplei* Twist: a human pathogenic Actinobacteria with a reduced genome. Genome Res 2003;13: 1800–1809.

Joint Extraintestinal Manifestations in Ulcerative Colitis

A.E. Dorofeyev I.V. Vasilenko O.A. Rassokhina

National Medical University, Donetsk, Ukraine

Key Words

Colon mucosal barrier · Cytokine disturbances · Extraintestinal manifestations · Extraintestinal manifestations, pathogenic mechanisms · Joint manifestations · Ulcerative colitis, joint manifestations

Abstract

An extraintestinal manifestation (EIM) very often occurs in ulcerative colitis (UC) patients. EIM modifies the natural course of UC and decreases the quality of life in these patients. The aim of this study was to analyze clinical and laboratory findings in UC patients with joint EIM. 319 UC patients were examined. Among them were 131 (41.1%) patients with distal UC, 102 (32.0%) suffered from left-sided UC and 86 (26.9%) had pancolitis. 95 (29.8%) UC patients had joint EIM. Arthritis correlated with extensive forms of UC and was more often determined in patients with left-sided UC and pancolitis. Arthralgia was a prevalent symptom of joint EIM in patients with distal UC. Colon microbiocenosis and the mucosal barrier in UC patients were analyzed. The cytokine status with privileged cytokine profile changes was investigated. In all UC patients, dysbiosis with a decreasing quantity of bifidobacteria, lactobacilli and *Escherichia coli* was found, but an increase of facultative flora was also found. At the same time, an association of facultative flora in UC patients with arthritis was observed. In these patients, *Staphylococcus*, *Klebsiella* and *Proteus* were found more often in stool cultures. These associations correlated with a modification of the colonocytes' cell receptor maturity of mucus, a condition with a decreased staining intensity by lectins. A cytokine imbalance with an increase of proinflammatory and a decrease of anti-inflammatory cytokines was found in all UC patients. The privileged cytokine profile changes in UC patients with joint EIM were analyzed. Maximal increases of IL-1 and TNF with decreases of IL-10 in plasma in patients with joint EIM were observed.

Copyright © 2009 S. Karger AG, Basel

Introduction

Ulcerative colitis (UC) is one of the main pathologies of inflammatory bowel diseases. In most cases, UC induces systemic disorders and involves not only the inflammatory process but also the gastrointestinal tract [1–3]. Extraintestinal manifestations (EIM) include involvement of different organs and systems induced by UC or related to it. They have different pathogenic mechanisms, a different clinical picture and often an influence on the quality of life and long-term prognosis of UC [4, 5]. Joint manifestations are the most common EIM in UC patients. Involvement of joints was observed in 20–35% of UC patients [1, 4, 6]. Clinical features of joint EIM in UC vary from reactive arthritis to arthropathies and arthralgia, and from peripheral joint lesions to axial arthropathies, sacroiliitis and ankylosing spondylitis [3, 7].

The aim of this work was to analyze the frequency and clinical forms of joint EIM in UC patients and to investigate the pathogenic mechanisms of EIM evaluations, i.e. the colon mucosal barrier and cytokine profile modifications in these patients.

Materials and Methods

319 patients with distal, left-sided UC and pancolitis were examined for dynamics including period of acute phase with clinical symptoms. The patients included 172 women and 147 men. Average age was 43.2 ± 3.3 years. 131 (41.1%) patients had distal UC, 102 (32.0%) suffered from left-sided UC, and 86 (26.9%) had pancolitis. Diagnosis of UC was based on clinical symptoms, endoscopic picture, X-ray examination and histological investigation.

The colon mucosal barrier consists of several parts – colonic flora, mucus and bowel cells [8, 9]. To investigate colon flora, mucus production and intensity of inflammation in the large bowel were analyzed. The qualitative and quantitative composition of the colonic flora with the obligate and facultative flora was analyzed.

Feces were placed into a sterile box, transported to the laboratory, and divided into 1.0-gram samples and diluted by isotonic solution to 10^{-1}, 10^{-3}, 10^{-5}, 10^{-7}, 10^{-8}, and 10^{-9}. For pathogenic enterobacteria examination, feces diluted 10^{-1} were disseminated on Endo's, Ploscirev's culture medium, bismuth-sulfite agar and 1–2 ml on enriched magnesium and selenitic culture medium. Feces diluted 10^{-3} were disseminated on Sabourand's culture medium and penicillin and streptomycin added for *Candida* detection, and for staphylococci detection the feces in this dilution were disseminated on GSA culture medium. Feces diluted 10^{-5} were disseminated on Endo's culture medium and on 5% blood agar for *Enterobacter*, cocci and hemolytic bacteria detection. Feces diluted 10^{-7}, 10^{-8} and 10^{-9} were disseminated on Blaurock culture medium for *Bifidobacteria* detection, and for studying lactobacilli feces in this dilution disseminated on MRS-2 culture medium. Culture media were cultivated in a thermostat at 37°C for 24–48 h, and Sabourand's culture medium was cultivated for 48 h in thermostat at 37°C and 3 days at room temperature. Using Gram stain to estimate the quantity of bacteria, we microscopically determined the number of evolved microorganisms in 1 g of feces [10].

Before biopsies were taken, endoscopic examinations were carried out by examining the colon mucosa visually. Bioptates of colon mucosa were stained with hematoxylin and eosin, Alcian blue at pH 1.0 and 2.5 for determination of sulfated and non-sulfated glucosaminoglycans and glycoproteins, and for goblet cells and colon mucus. To characterize the mucus production, the PAS reaction was performed. Histochemical lectin tests using peroxidase-marked lectins were done. The following lectins were used: WGA affinity to NANA, PNA affinity to β-D-Gal, LAL affinity to α-L-Fuc, ML-1 affinity to α-D-Gal, SBA affinity to α-D-GalNAc, LCA affinity to α-D-Man, and HPA affinity to α-GlcNAc [11].

Bioptates were immersed in 5% formalin solution and passed on to the laboratory. Afterwards, successive processing was carried out using ethanol in increasing concentrations of 50, 60, 70, 80, 96% and absolute for 5 min in each solution. The bioptates were placed in an ortho-xylol solution for 20 min, then immersed in paraffin and put in a thermostat at 55°C. Paraffin blocks were then prepared. Two- to 3-μm-thick slices were prepared on a rotational microcutter. The slices were processed using ortho-xylol and ethanol with decreasing concentrations of water and stained with hematoxylin and eosin or Schiff's solution. The stains were prepared on a buffer solution of acetic acid pH 2.6 and 0.1 N solution of hydrochloric acid pH 1.0 for staining by Alcian blue. The slices were processed using 0.3% hydrogen peroxide solution before lectin staining. The peroxidase-marked lectins used were supplied by Lectinotest Laboratories (Lvov, Ukraine). Before staining, the lectins were diluted 1:15 in buffer solutions of NaCl, KCl, and $Na_2HPO_4 12H_2O$. Afterwards, the lectins were stained. The slices were processed using 3,3′-diaminobenzidine. The stain intensity of lectins was estimated using score points.

By carrying out the histological examinations, the number and maturity of goblet cells were determined as well as the content of mucus contained in them and the maturity of mucus. Furthermore, the intensity of cell infiltrations and their character were determined. The cytokine status with privileged cytokine profile changes was investigated in 150 patients. Finally, the interleukin levels in plasma were analyzed: IL-1, -2, -4, -6, -8, -10 and TNF. Analysis was performed using ELISA kits.

Results

All patients had suffered from UC for 1–20 years. Among the patients who had suffered from UC <5 years, those with distal UC and pancolitis predominated. However, in the patients who had suffered UC >5–10 years, left-sided UC was more predominant (table 1). Predisposing factors for UC were found in 285 patients. A genetic predisposition (UC or colon cancer or autoimmune diseases in relatives) was more commonly found in patients with pancolitis and left-sided UC ($p < 0.05$). Episodes of chemical and/or medicine damage were found more often in patients with left-sided UC, but nutrition disturbances were mostly observed in distal UC patients.

Among UC patients, persons with mild severity of disease [153 (47.9%) persons] predominated. 102 (32.0%) patients suffered from moderate UC, but 64 (20.1%) patients had severe UC. The severity of UC correlated with extensive inflammation of the colon. The activity of UC according to the Rachmilewitz activity index (CAI) was analyzed in all patients. The CAI score in all UC patient groups was 8.6 ± 0.9 points. In 95 (29.8%) UC patients, joint EIM were found. Among them, more than one half of the subjects (48, 50.5%) had arthritis. Arthropathies were observed in 23 (24.2%) patients and arthralgia in 24 (25.3%) UC patients.

Joint EIM in pancolitis (39.8%) and left-sided (35.1%) UC patients were found more often, but only in those patients (19.1%) with distal UC joint EIM, which could be

Table 1. Anamnestic data in patients with UC

Sign	Total number (n = 319)		Distal UC (n = 131)		Left-sided UC (n = 102)		Pancolitis (n = 86)	
	n	%	n	%	n	%	n	%
Duration of UC								
<5 years	156	48.9	68	51.9	24	23.5*	43	50.0
5–10 years	79	24.8	38	29.0	49	48.0*	31	36.0
>10 years	84	26.3	25	19.1	29	28.5	12	14.0
Predisposing factors								
Genetic predisposition	66	20.7	17	13.0	22	21.6*	27	31.4*
Allergy	70	21.9	24	18.3	22	21.6	24	27.9*
Chemical and medicines damages	36	11.3	10	7.6	15	14.7*	11	12.8
Stress	54	16.9	24	18.3	15	14.7	15	17.4
Nutrition disturbances	59	18.5	34	25.9	13	12.7*	12	13.9*

* Significant difference ($p < 0.05$) observed in left-sided UC and pancolitis patients as compared to distal UC patients.

related to more aggressive immunopathological and metabolic disturbances in patients with extensive forms of UC [3, 12]. Severe and extensive forms of UC correlated with more complicated joint involvement (table 2). In UC patients with pancolitis, arthritis and polyarthritis were observed significantly more often ($p < 0.05$). Arthropathies predominated in left-sided UC patients, but in patients with distal UC, arthralgia was significantly more common. Arthralgia predominated in patients with mild severity of UC, but in moderate and severe UC arthritis a prevalence was observed ($p < 0.05$). Arthropathies in patients with moderate and severe UC occurred with the same frequency. The severity of UC reflects inflammation; however, immune and metabolic changes in colon joint EIM directly depend of inflammation of UC severity.

The clinical activity of UC calculated by the CAI score shows the grade of inflammation intensity at an exact period of observation. The CAI score correlated with frequency and types of joint EIM. Among patients with joint EIM, those with a CAI score of 7–12 points predominated, but in UC patients with a CAI score of <6 points joint EIM were rarely found ($p < 0.05$). The clinical picture of joint lesions depends on the CAI score. In patients with a CAI score of >12 points, arthritis predominated (80.6%), but in persons with a CAI score of <6 points, arthralgia was observed significantly more often ($p < 0.05$). The frequency of arthropathies decreased from 35.0% in patients with a minimal CAI score to 16.1% in those with a high CAI score.

UC duration has less influence on joint EIM frequency. Among UC patients with joint EIM, persons with an UC duration of <5 years were observed more often. However, this prevalence was influenced by the absence of arthropathies in patients with an UC duration of <5 years, but arthralgia was found more often in these patients. The frequency of arthritis in patients with a different UC duration was almost the same (52.5, 52.0 and 46.7%, respectively) ($p < 1.0$).

Genetic predispositions and allergy have an influence on joint EIM in UC patients. Predisposing factors were found in 65 (68.4%) patients with joint EIM. 38 (40.0%) patients had genetic predisposition and 31 (32.6%) suffered from an allergy. In patients with a genetic predisposition, severe joint manifestations predominated, e.g. polyarthritis, arthropathies. None of the patients in this group had minimal joint lesion, i.e. arthralgia. At the same time, one half of the patients were observed to have allergy arthralgia, 14 (45.2%) suffered from arthritis, and only 1 patient had arthropathy. Thus, a genetic predisposition to UC leads to more aggressive and severe joint manifestations in such patients.

In UC patients, vertebral to peripheral hand and leg joints can be involved in the inflammatory process [3, 4, 13]. In the UC patients evaluated, arthritis of the large joints was found twice as often as in small and vertebral joints. Patients who had extensive UC oligo- and polyarthritis with or without vertebral involvement predominated. Large joint manifestations in patients with left-sided UC and pancolitis with moderate severity and high

Table 2. Joints lesion in different forms of UC

Sign	Total joint EIM		Type of joint lesion							
			arthritis		arthropathy		p <	arthralgia		p <
	n	%	n	%	n	%		n	%	
Total	95	100	48	50.5	23	24.2	0.05	24	25.3	0.05
Distal UC	25	26.34	6	24.0	3	12.0	0.05	16	64.0	0.05
Left-sided UC	36	37.9	19	52.8	14	38.9	0.5	3	8.3	0.05
p1<		0.05		0.05		0.05			0.01	
Pancolitis	34	35.8	23	67.6	6	17.6	0.05	5	14.8	0.05
p1<		1.0		0.05		0.5			0.05	
UC severity										
Mild	19	20.0	5	26.3	3	15.8	0.05	11	57.9	0.05
Moderate	43	45.3	24	55.8	12	27.9	0.1	7	16.3	0.05
p2<		0.05		0.05		0.05			0.05	
Severe	33	34.7	19	57.6	8	24.2	0.05	6	18.2	0.05
p2<		0.05		0.05		0.1			0.05	
CAI										
Less than 6 s.p.	20	21.0	3	15.0	7	35.0	0.05	10	50.0	0.05
7–12 s.p.	44	46.3	20	45.5	11	25.0	0.05	13	29.5	0.05
p3<		0.05		0.05		0.05			0.05	
More than 12 s.p.	31	32.7	25	80.6	5	16.1	0.01	1	3.3	0.01
p3<		0.1		0.05		0.01			0.01	
Duration of UC										
Less than 5 years	40	42.1	21	52.5	2	5.0	0.01	17	42.5	0.5
5–10 years	25	26.3	13	52.0	9	36.0	0.5	3	12.0	0.05
p4<		0.05		1.0		0.01			0.05	
More than 10 years	30	31.6	14	46.7	12	40.0	0.5	4	13.3	0.05
p4<		0.2		1.0		1.0			0.05	

p = Compared to patients with arthritis, p1 = compared to distal UC patients, p2 = compared to UC patients with mild severity, p3 = compared to UC patients with CAI score <6 points, p4 = compared to patients with duration of UC less than 5 years.

activity were found more often. Large joint lesions are characterized by migrative, reversible non-symmetrical arthritis of the knees, shoulders, and elbows. Arthritis activity is strongly correlated with UC acuteness. Sometimes, arthritis preceded UC relapse and was the initial symptom of UC acuteness. The duration of arthritis was longer than the UC relapses, but no more than 5–7 weeks. One quarter of patients with maximal UC activity had a reduction of arthritis syndrome. Sacroiliitis in UC patients was symmetric and combined with a vertebral lesion. Pathogenic mechanisms of large and small joint lesions were different. Large joint arthritis is mostly reactive and strongly corresponds to UC acuteness, severity and activity of disease. Probably as in other types of reactive arthritis, crossover antibodies play the main role in induction of this EIM [4, 12].

Small joint affections involving five or more joints as a symmetric polyarthritis were observed slightly more often in left-sided UC patients. These joint manifestations are rarely combined with large joints and vertebral involvement. Small joint affection is characterized by persistent hand and foot arthritis, which is symmetric in most cases. Morning stiffness, joint pain, swelling, limitations of movement, redness and formation of stable joint deformations were typical. The activity of joint manifestations usually did not correlate with UC acuteness. More than one half of these patients had moderate or severe UC with a CAI score of up to 7 points. The duration of small joint arthritis was much longer than UC relapses (from 3 to 8 months) and joint deformation was retained. In pathogenesis of small joint manifestations, immunopathogenic modifications with direct autoim-

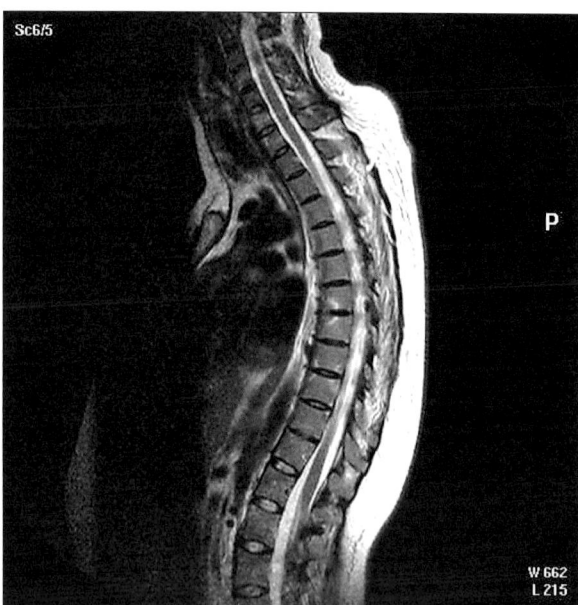

Fig. 1. Ankylosing spondylitis in a patient with UC.

mune aggression against cartilage tissue are probably more important [14, 15].

In patients with a vertebral lesion, more than one half suffered from left-sided UC. These patients had severe and moderate UC with a high clinical activity. In 52.1%, the duration of UC was <5 years and the frequency of vertebral manifestations decreased instead of increased the duration of UC. Patients suffered from vertebral and sacroiliac joint symmetric pain in combination with movement limitation which decreased after physical loads. Vertebral damages were persistent and torpid, but had a clear tendency to progression. Progressions of vertebral lesions were usually observed after UC relapses. These abnormalities in UC patients were similar to ankylosing spondylitis (Bechterew's disease) and were diagnosed in 8 UC patients (fig. 1). The pathogenesis of vertebral manifestations is mostly linked to autoimmune disease association [3, 16].

Arthropathies were found more often in moderate left-sided UC with a CAI score of 7–12 points. Patients with these manifestations complained of pain with limitation of joint movement. Large joints were mostly involved and correlated with UC acuteness. Arthropathies are probably one stage where metabolic modifications of cartilage are more important than immune changes [15].

Arthralgia was revealed mostly in patients with distal UC and mild severity. The CAI score in these patients was <12 points and UC duration <5 years. In 3 patients with distal UC and arthralgia, long-term isolation induced an aggressive severe course of UC with pancolitis and modification of arthralgia to polyarthritis of large joints. Arthralgia was observed which was strongly correlated with UC relapse and maximal intensity of joint pain at a higher level of UC. In arthralgia, pathogenesis probably presents the same mechanisms as in arthritis, but the absence of genetic predispositivity or lower antigen loading does not lead to arthritis.

Thus, joint manifestations were found in every third UC patient. Joint lesions varied from arthralgia to severe polyarthritis which was limited according to the patient's functional abilities. More often, joint EIM in moderate and severe UC with extensive forms (left-sided and pancolitis) and high clinical activity were found. Arthritis of large joints in left-sided UC and pancolitis with a high clinical activity were commonly observed and joint EIM correlated with UC relapse. Polyarthritis of small joints in left-sided UC patients with a moderate CAI score were found, but these joint manifestations did not depend of UC acuteness. Arthropathies were observed in patients with moderate, left-sided UC disease duration of >5 years. However, in mild, distal UC with a disease duration of <5 years, arthralgia occurred.

The mucosal colon barrier is one of the important factors in the UC [9, 17]. The condition of mucus-producing cells in the colon mucosa and the degree of mucus maturity have an influence on the severity of UC, EIM presence and the prognosis of this disease [1, 3, 12]. Inflammation of the mucosa initiates abnormalities in the colon flora and cause dysbiosis [4], in which modified antigen loads and induces EIM.

All of the UC patients had different degrees of dysbiosis. The microflora was characterized by an increase of the facultative flora and a decrease of number of obligate bacteria (table 3). The total number of *E. coli* was decreased, but levels of *E. coli* with reduced fermentative ability, lactose-negative *E. coli* and hemolytic *E. coli* were increased. The number of bifidobacteria and lactobacilli were decreased. The increase of facultative flora was characterized by high levels of *Staphylococcus* and *Enterococcus* of different species, e.g. *Klebsiella* and *Proteus*. The frequency of identification in stool and the number of facultative bacteria in patients with UC was significantly higher than in the normal population. In UC patients with joint EIM, *Enterobacter, Staphylococcus, Klebsiella* and *Proteus* were identified more often than in

Table 3. Colonic bacterial flora in patients with UC

Type of bacteria		Healthy persons	All groups of UC patients	UC patients without EIM	UC patients with joint EIM
Escherichia	Frequency, %	100.0	98.7	100.0	100.0
	Number l g CFU/g	7.82 ± 0.24	6.75 ± 0.61*	6.75 ± 0.65*	6.44 ± 0.64*
Bifidobacterium	Frequency, %	100.0	97.4	100.0	100.0
	Number l g CFU/g	8.72 ± 0.25	7.29 ± 0.71*	7.92 ± 0.76	7.56 ± 0.75*
Lactobacillus	Frequency, %	100.0	96.1	100.0	100.0
	Number l g CFU/g	6.60 ± 0.14	5.77 ± 0.51*	6.33 ± 0.63	6.55 ± 0.65
Enterococcus	Frequency, %	100.0	42.1*	43.0*	33.1*
	Number l g CFU/g	7.37 ± 0.33	7.33 ± 0.63	7.05 ± 0.59	7.12 ± 0.61
Enterobacter	Frequency, %	24.0	40.8*	28.6	46.1*, #
	Number l g CFU/g	1.11 ± 0.32	2.81 ± 0.21*	1.51 ± 0.14	3.09 ± 0.31*, #
Staphylococcus	Frequency, %	46.0	52.6*	30.0	61.5*, #
	Number l g CFU/g	4.05 ± 0.35	4.41 ± 0.43	4.11 ± 0.41	4.13 ± 0.41
Klebsiella	Frequency, %	32.0	46.1*	0.0*	66.1*, #
	Number l g CFU/g	0.99 ± 0.27	3.46 ± 0.32*	0.0*	5.49 ± 0.34*, #
Proteus	Frequency, %	16.0	36.8*	0.0*	46.1*, #
	Number l g CFU/g	0.4 ± 0.1	2.52 ± 0.25*	0.0	2.85 ± 0.28*, #
Cytobacter	Frequency, %	56.0	31.6*	39.3	15.4*, #
	Number l g CFU/g	1.79 ± 0.32	2.28 ± 0.22*	1.13 ± 0.12	2.23 ± 0.22*, #
Candida	Frequency, %	32.0	31.6	32.1	32.3
	Number l g CFU/g	3.36 ± 0.41	3.50 ± 0.35	3.01 ± 0.31	3.11 ± 0.31

* Significant difference ($p < 0.05$) observed in UC patients as compared to norm.
# Significant difference ($p < 0.05$) observed in UC patients with joint EIM as compared to UC patients without EIM.

healthy persons and UC patients without EIM. The number of these bacteria in UC patients with joint EIM was significantly higher than in the normal population and UC patients without EIM. Moreover, stable facultative bacterial combinations were found in patients with joint EIM. In 90 (94.7%) UC patients with joint EIM, two or more types of facultative bacteria occurred. In patients with arthritis, bacterial associations such as Staphylococcus-Klebsiella, Staphylococcus-Proteus or Staphylococcus-Klebsiella-Proteus were observed more often. In all patients with joint manifestations, these facultative flora quantities were significantly higher than in the healthy population and UC patients without EIM. Changes of colonic facultative bacteria could modify the mucosal barrier with an increase of antigen loads with immune response stimulation. This was caused by EIM inductions, especially joint manifestations [3, 4, 12].

The histological examination of biopsies demonstrated an increase of infiltrated cells in all patients, while the number of goblet cells was decreased. However, in 34 patients with distal UC (25.9%) and 13 (12.7%) patients with left-sided UC, the decrease of goblet cell number was moderate at the expense of immature goblet cells with small vacuoles and a lower content of mucus. In other patients, the decrease of goblet cells was severe. The severity of the goblet cell reduction correlated with the intensity of the mucosa injury. The severity of goblet cell reduction did not correlate with EIM presence and was similar in patients with and without EIM. At the same time, severe qualitative mucus modification was observed in UC patients with joint EIM. The PAS reduction showed a moderate level of PAS-positive substances in 111 (34.7%) patients, while the intensity of the PAS reaction was decreased in 102 (31.9%) patients, which indicates a defect of mucus production and decrease of glycoprotein level which fulfils a protective function. In 81 (85.2%) UC patients with joint EIM, a reduction of the PAS reaction was found. Active leukocytes containing glycogen were found in all patients. The number of active leukocytes was correlated with clearer endoscopic changes. Using an Alcian blue technique at pH 1.0, moderate staining was found in 259 (81.2%) patients, while weak staining was discovered in 60 (18.8%) patients – one half of these were patients with joint EIM. However, at pH 2.5,

Table 4. Lectin staining of UC patients compared to healthy persons

Type of lectins	Norm	All groups of UC patients	UC patients without EIM	UC patients with joint EIM
WGA	3.8 ± 0.2	1.7 ± 0.4	2.0 ± 0.3	1.2 ± 0.1*
PNA	3.8 ± 0.2	1.9 ± 0.4	2.0 ± 0.4	1.5 ± 0.1*
LAL	3.8 ± 0.2	1.8 ± 0.3	2.1 ± 0.2	2.0 ± 0.3
ML-1	3.7 ± 0.2	0.9 ± 0.1	1.4 ± 0.2	1.0 ± 0.2
SBA	3.6 ± 0.3	0.7 ± 0.1	1.5 ± 0.4	0.8 ± 0.4*
LCA	3.4 ± 0.3	0.6 ± 0.1	1.3 ± 0.3	0.8 ± 0.4
HPA	3.3 ± 0.3	0.3 ± 0.05	0.9 ± 0.2	0.6 ± 0.3

Values indicate score points.
* Significant difference ($p < 0.05$) observed in UC patients with joint EIM as compared to UC patients without EIM.

Table 5. Cytokine levels in plasma of patients with UC

Type of cytokines	Norm	All groups of UC patients	UC patients without EIM	UC patients with joint EIM
IL-1, pg/ml	49.7 ± 4.9	178.7 ± 17.1*	56.7 ± 5.4	211.9 ± 21.1*, #
IL-6, pg/ml	15.2 ± 1.5	26.3 ± 3.4*	18.6 ± 0.9	24.0 ± 2.4*
IL-8, pg/ml	15.1 ± 1.5	118.9 ± 27.0*	56.8 ± 2.2*	79.3 ± 17.9*
TNF-α, pg/ml	48.9 ± 2.0	93.4 ± 9.3*	54.1 ± 1.2	107.5 ± 4.7*, #
IL-2, MU/ml	0.18 ± 0.02	1.21 ± 0.22*	0.42 ± 0.04*	0.99 ± 0.47*
IL-4, pg/ml	124.0 ± 12.4	63.3 ± 6.2*	100.7 ± 10.0	87.0 ± 7.9*
IL-10, pg/ml	32.4 ± 3.2	22.9 ± 2.2*	25.2 ± 2.5*	17.2 ± 2.0*, #

* Significant difference ($p < 0.05$) observed in UC patients as compared to norm.
# Significant difference ($p < 0.05$) observed in UC patients with joint EIM as compared to UC patients without EIM.

moderate and intensive staining was found in 206 (64.6%) patients. In 113 (35.4%) patients, however, a weak staining was observed which indicates a change of the ratio between sulfated and unsulfated glucosaminoglycans and therefore a change of the mucus properties in patients with UC. These changes in UC patients with joint EIM were found significantly more often than in patients without EIM.

Lectin staining was performed in order to study the composition of the different glycoprotein receptors. Staining by WGA gave 1.7 ± 0.4 points, by PNA 1.9 ± 0.4 points, and by LAL 1.8 ± 0.3 points ($p < 0.05$ in comparison to the normal healthy population; see table 4). Stainings by ML-1, SBA, and LCA were decreased by <1.0 point, but HPA staining was practically absent. However, a decrease of the staining intensity by WGA was correlated with a decrease of the total *E. coli* level and/or an increase of *E. coli* with modified fermentative abilities. In patients with joint EIM, a decrease of staining of the lectins PNA, SBA and WGA was observed which indicates a decrease of the quantity of β-D-Gal, α-D-GalNAc and NANA in cell receptors and in colon mucus (fig. 2). These changes induce a modification of the mucosal barrier by decreasing the number of bacterial receptor adhesions and the flora's colonial matrix modifications.

Thus, in UC patients with joint EIM, severe dysbiosis with a facultative bacteria association were found. *Staphylococcus*, *Klebsiella* and *Proteus* were more commonly identified in patients with arthritis. At the same time, modification of mucus compositions in UC patients with joint EIM was observed. In these patients, there was a reduction of PAS reaction, changes of the ratio between sulfated and unsulfated glucosaminoglycans, a decrease of the quantity of β-D-Gal, α-D-GalNAc and NANA in mucus, and therefore changes of the mucus properties occurred (table 5).

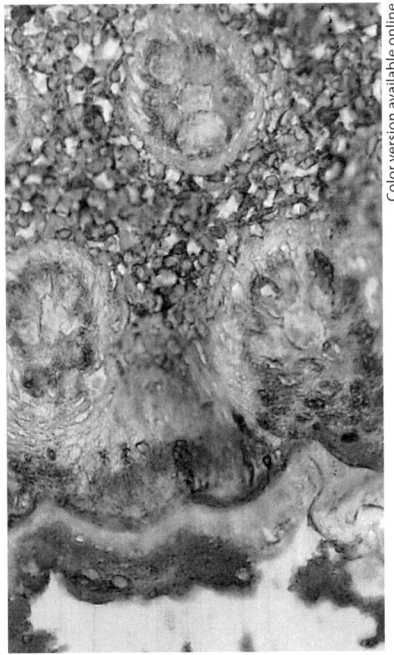

Fig. 2. Colon mucosa biopsy staining by SBA lectin affined to α-GalNAc in a patient with UC compared with normal mucosa.

In UC pathogenesis, immunopathological disturbances with an autoimmune component play the main role [4, 18]. Systemic damage and EIM are linked with these chances [3], which are realized by modifications of the cytokine profile [1, 12, 18]. In UC patients, cytokine cascade abnormalities were found with an increase of proinflammatory cytokines levels and a decrease of anti-inflammatory interleukins. There were also maximally increased levels of IL-1, -6, -8 and tumor necrosis factor (TNF) with a decrease of IL-4 and IL-10. These cytokines change according to extensity, severity and activity of UC. Cytokine abnormalities were minimal in patients with distal UC with mild activity, but in severe left-sided UC or pancolitis with a high clinical activity the maximal level of proinflammatory cytokines with a significant decrease of anti-inflammatory IL occurred. An increase of proinflammatory cytokines was seen in patients with joint EIM ($p < 0.05$). However, significant differences between UC patients with joint EIM and UC patients without EIM for IL-1 and TNF only were observed ($p < 0.05$). In these patients, a significant decrease of the IL-10 level occurred. Thus, in UC patients with joint EIM, we observed a cytokine imbalance with an increase of IL-1 and in TNF with a decrease of IL-10. Among patients with joint manifestations, these disturbances were more severe in patients with arthritis. Cytokine profile changes in UC patients with EIM could reflect not only the intensity of immune changes and severity of systemic manifestations, but could also be the basis of a rational therapeutic strategy.

Conclusions

UC is a systemic disease. Joint manifestations are one of the most common EIM which occur in 29.8% of patients with UC. Joint EIM varies from arthritis to arthropathies and arthralgia, and can involve small, large and vertebral joints with heterogeneous clinical features. Joint manifestations have different pathogenic mechanisms which depend of modifications of colonic flora, the mucosal barrier and cytokine disturbances.

Disclosure Statement

The authors declare that no financial or other conflict of interest exists in relation to the content of this article.

References

1. De Vos M: Joint involvement in inflammatory bowel disease. Aliment Pharmacol Ther 2004;20:36–42.
2. Salvarani C, Fornaciari G, Beltrami M, Macchioni PL: Musculoskeletal manifestations in inflammatory bowel disease. Eur J Intern Med 2000;11:210–214.
3. Danese S, Semeraro S, Papa A, Roberto I, Scaldaferri F, Fedeli G, Gasbarrini G, Gasbarrini A: Extraintestinal manifestations in inflammatory bowel disease. World J Gastroenterol 2005;11:7227–7236.
4. Rothfuss KS, Stange EF, Herrlinger KR: Extraintestinal manifestations and complications in inflammatory bowel diseases. World J Gastroenterol 2006;12:4819–4831.
5. Bernstein CN, Blanchard JF, Rawsthorne P, Yu N: The prevalence of extraintestinal diseases in inflammatory bowel disease: a population-based study. Am J Gastroenterol 2001;96:1116–1122.
6. Ricart E, Panaccione R, Loftus EV Jr, Tremaine WJ, Harmsen WS, Zinsmeister AR, Sandborn WJ: Autoimmune disorders and extraintestinal manifestations in first-degree familial and sporadic inflammatory bowel disease: a case-control study. Inflamm Bowel Dis 2004;10:207–214.

7 Mendoza JL, Lana R, Taxonera C, Alba C, Izquierdo S, Diaz-Rubio M: Extraintestinal manifestations in inflammatory bowel disease: differences between Crohn's disease and ulcerative colitis. Med Clin (Barc) 2005; 125:297–300.
8 Van Staa TP, Cooper C, Brusse LS, Leufkens H, Javaid MK, Arden NK: Inflammatory bowel disease and the risk of fracture. Gastroenterology 2003;125:1591–1597.
9 Loginov AS, Parfenov AI: Intestinal Diseases. Moscow, Meditsina, 2000, pp 137–211.
10 Nesvizhsky YuV, Dorofeyev AE: Normal and pathological microbiocenosis and immune status in human. Arch Clin Exp Med 1995, v.4, N2, pp 175–179.
11 Lutsyk MD, Panasjuk EN, Lutsyk AD: The Lectins/Vishcha shkola. Lvov, Lvov University, 1981, pp 114–118.
12 Oshitani N, Watanabe K, Nakamura S, Higuchi K, Arakawa T: Extraintestinal complications in patients with ulcerative colitis. Nippon Rinsho 2005;63:874–878.
13 Kruithof E, De Rycke L, Roth J, Mielants H, Van den Bosch F, De Keyser F, Veys EM, Baeten D: Immunomodulatory effects of etanercept on peripheral joint synovitis in the spondylarthropathies. Arthritis Rheum 2005;52:3898–3909.
14 Orchard TR, Dhar A, Simmons JD, Vaughan R, Welsh KI, Jewell DP: MHC class I chain-like gene A and its associations with inflammatory bowel disease and peripheral arthropathy. Clin Exp Immunol 2001;126: 437–440.
15 Orchard TR, Wordsworth BP, Jewell DP: Peripheral arthropathies in inflammatory bowel disease: their articular distribution and natural history. Gut 1998;42:387–391.
16 De Vlam K, Mielants H, Cuvelier C, De Keyser F, Veys EM, De Vos M: Spondyloarthropathy is underestimated in inflammatory bowel disease: prevalence and HLA association. J Rheumatol 2000;27:2860–2865.
17 Rogler G, Daig R, Aschenbrenner E, Vogl D, Falk W, Scholmerich J, Gross V, Andus T: Epithelial cells in inflammatory bowel disease; in Inflammatory Bowel Diseases – From Bench to Bedside. Dordrecht, Kluwer Academic, 1997 pp 103–116.
18 Bernstein CN, Wajda A, Blanchard JF: The clustering of other chronic inflammatory diseases in inflammatory bowel disease: a population-based study. Gastroenterology 2005;129:827–883.

Joint Involvement Associated with Inflammatory Bowel Disease

M. De Vos

Ghent University, Ghent, Belgium

Key Words

Inflammatory bowel disease · Spondylarthropathy · Arthritis · Genetics · Angiogenesis · Therapy

Abstract

Joint involvement associated with inflammatory bowel disease (IBD) belongs to the concept of spondyloarthritis (SpA) and includes two types of arthritis: a peripheral arthritis characterized by the presence of pauciarticular asymmetrical arthritis affecting preferentially joints of lower extremities and an axial arthropathy including inflammatory back pain, sacroiliitis and ankylosing spondylitis (AS). Treatment of arthritis includes a short-term use of NSAIDs associated with optimized treatment of gut inflammation. Safety concerns mean that long-term treatment with NSAIDs is best avoided if possible. Salazopyrine can be recommended for treatment of peripheral arthritis. Methotrexate and azathioprine are generally ineffective. Finally, efficacy of anti-TNF therapy (infliximab and adalimumab) is well established. However, use of etanercept is not recommended because of the increased risk for intestinal disease relapse. Pathogenesis of gut-joint iteropathy is not elucidated. Both inflammations are tightly related as suggested by human evidence of gut inflammation in patients with other forms of SpA and animal evidence of gut and joint inflammation in HLA-B27/human β_2-microglobulin transgenic rat model and $TNF^{\Delta ARE}$ mice. Several clues for the linkage between gut and joint inflammation have been put forward including an altered recognition and handling of bacterial antigens, an aberrant trafficking of CD8+ T cells with an impaired T-helper type 1 cytokine profile and expression of aEb7 integrin, an altered trafficking of macrophages expressing CD163 and evidence of an increased angiogenesis. A transcriptome analysis of mucosal biopsies identified a set of 95 genes that are differentially expressed in both CD and SpA as compared with healthy controls suggesting common pathways. TNF plays a key role in the pathogenesis of various arthritic diseases and IBD. Mesenchymal/myofibroblast-like cells may represent the local primary targets of TNF in the induction of gut and joint pathology. Selective expression of TNFRI on these cells seems to be sufficient to orchestrate the complete development of SpA-related pathologies at least in $TNF^{\Delta ARE}$ mice. Finally, genetic susceptibility is probably required to develop these pathologies. Genotyping of AS patients provided evidence for an important overlap between determinants of inherited predisposition to CD and AS. The best documented common association is with an IL-23R polymorphism, although the exact role remains unexplored. In addition, evidence suggests that a number of recently identified CD-susceptibility loci are associated with AS. Clinical, genetical, immunological and therapeutic evidence support the tight junction between gut and joint inflammation in two linked diseases, IBD and SpA, belonging to the 'immune-mediated inflammatory diseases'.

Copyright © 2009 S. Karger AG, Basel

Clinical Evidence

Joint involvement associated with inflammatory bowel disease (IBD) belongs to the concept of spondyloarthritis (SpA), a cluster of interrelated rheumatologic diseases with similar clinical and genetic features. The *peripheral arthritis* preferentially affects the joints of the upper or lower limbs in an asymmetrical pattern. The clinical inflammation is transient, migratory and mostly non-deforming. It occurs in 10–20% of patients, preferentially during a relapse of the intestinal disease [1]. The difference between this type 1 arthritis and a rarer type 2 polyarticular disease unrelated to activity of intestinal disease (in 2–4% of patients) was retained in the study of Orchard et al. [2] by retrospective analysis of case notes of 1,459 IBD (976 UC + 483 CD) and validation by a questionnaire in outpatients. *Enthesitis* or inflammation of insertion of tendon to bone occurs in about 7% of patients. The *axial arthropathy* includes inflammatory back pain present in 20–30% of patients, radiologic evidence of sacroiliitis in 20–25% of patients and full diagnosis of ankylosing spondylitis (AS) according to Rome criteria in 2–10% of patients [1–3]. Sacroiliitis and AS are diagnosed on conventional rheumatological grounds supported by characteristic radiologic changes, magnetic resonance imaging being the most sensitive. Arthralgia (pain without evidence of inflammation) is not recognized as extraintestinal manifestation but frequently reported by the patients and associated with a significant impact on quality of life. In a population-based cohort, 16% of patients reported this problem [4].

SpA includes not only IBD-related arthritis, but also AS, reactive arthritis, psoriatic arthritis, juvenile-onset SpA and a group of undifferentiated arthritis. In European countries, the general incidence is estimated at 0.1–0.5% of the total population. In all various forms of SpA, subclinical gut inflammation was described in about 60% of patients with a higher risk for evolution to overt Crohn's disease (CD) than expected in a general population. Predominantly the presence of chronic gut inflammation associated with blunted fused villi and distorted crypts, an infiltration with a mixed cell population with predominance of lymphoid cells, represents a high risk for CD development [5, 6].

Genetic Crossroads

Several candidate genes possibly involved in the coincidence of gut and joint pathology have recently been put forward.

The first candidate gene is HLA-B27 that is tightly associated with AS. 75–95% of those patients carry HLA-B27. However, this frequency lowers to 25–78% in the IBD population with AS and remains normal in IBD patients without evidence of AS. The presence of asymptomatic sacroiliitis is not related with HLA-B27 [3]. The possible mechanisms by which HLA-B27 exerts its pathogenic role were reviewed by Reveille [7]. In an HLA-B27/human β_2-microglobulin transgenic rat model, genetically predisposed strains (Lewis or Fisher rats) with a high copy number of the transgene developed an inflammatory syndrome consisting of sacroiliitis, peripheral arthritis, enterocolitis and psoriariform skin lesions. The absence of flora prohibited this clinical syndrome as observed in germ-free animals. Animals with lower transgene copy numbers remain healthy. A most recent hypothesis suggests that misfold of heavy chain leads to an accumulation in endoplasmatic reticulum with forming of disulfide-linked homodimers triggering a stress response and changes in cellular metabolism. Additional human β_2-microglobulin reduced the misfold of the heavy chain of HLA-B27 and the following response, and led to an aggravation of the arthritis and an abolishment of colitis [8]. This supports the evidence that HLA-B27 misfolding may play a role in the development of intestinal inflammation, at least in this animal model, by producing conditions favorable for intracellular persistence of intestinal bacteria. However, the clinical observation that gut inflammation was rarer in HLA-B27-negative AS patients and the observation that neither B27 misfolding nor intestinal inflammation are critical to the development of B27-associated arthropathy in animals deny the central role of B27 and suggest that other genes are implicated.

A second candidate gene is CARD15 since three polymorphisms have been associated with development of CD in many studies. These variants increase the risk for CD 3-fold for heterozygous individuals and 33- to 44-fold for homozygous and compound heterozygous individuals. Although the presence of these polymorphisms is associated with some specific clinical features as ileal involvement and stricturing disease, no association could be found with development of arthropathy. Moreover, the prevalence is not altered in the general SpA population (20%) compared with a healthy population (17%) [9–11]. However, a detailed analysis of SpA patients demonstrated that the presence of CARD15 mutations in SpA patients was associated with a high risk for the development of chronic gut inflammation [9].

Table 1. Coding variants in the population studied

IL-23R	Controls, % (n = 789)	Crohn's, % (n = 1,086)	Ankylosing spondylitis, % (n = 182)
rs11209026 Non-synonymous*	G 87.5 A 12.5	G 94.9 A 5.1	G 93.0 A 7.0
rs11465804 Intron**	A 93.8 C 6.2	A 96.7 C 3.3	G 96.3 C 3.7

Protective allele: * CD vs. controls: p < 0.001; AS vs. controls: p = 0.043. ** CD vs. controls: p = 0.014; AS vs. controls: p = 0.051.

The third candidate gene is IL-23 receptor gene present on chromosome 1p31. An uncommon coding variant (rs11209026, Arg381Gln) has been shown to confer protection against CD, AS and psoriasis. In our population, it has been confirmed that IL-23R polymorphisms protect against CD and AS (table 1). However, the presence of a polymorphism does not seem to influence the risk for AS in CD and CD in AS, although the number of patients was too small to be conclusive [pers. unpubl. data].

We recently analyzed the overlap between the susceptibility loci in CD and AS by genotyping a cohort of 182 AS patients for SNP markers corresponding to 39 of the 40 CD risk loci (not including CARD15) described in Barrett et al. [12]. For genotyping, an Illumina GoldenGate Assay was used (genotyping success rate: 97%) and marker allele frequencies were compared between AS cases and 789 previously described Belgian replication controls using a one-sided Fisher's exact test. A significant association was found with rs3763313 corresponding to the well-established major effect of the MHC. Another significant association was found with rs2872507 mapping to a locus closely linked to ORMDL3. ORMDL3 encodes a transmembrane protein domain anchored in the endoplasmatic reticulum and probably involved in protein folding. This gene has been associated with risk for asthma [13]. A nominally significant association was found with NKX2-3, PTPN2, ICOSLG and IL-23R but was not retained after Bonferroni correction. However, the distribution of p values for the remaining 36 SNPs was significantly skewed towards low p values unless the top 5 SNPs were removed from the analysis, hence supporting at least 5 novel associations with AS [14].

Finally, we analyzed the mucosal gene expression profile in CD and SpA patients and found 95 differentially expressed genes clustering CD and SpA with chronic gut inflammation [15].

Immunological Evidence

Adaptive Immunity

Circulation of T cells and/or macrophages has been put forward in recent years as a link between gut and joint inflammation. Evidence includes [reviewed in 16]:
- Aberrant trafficking of CD8+ T cells with impaired Th1 cytokine profile primed in intestine, circulating and homing to synovium.
- Enrichment of T cells carrying α4β7 and αEβ7 integrins in inflamed synovial tissue of SpA patients suggesting an intestinal origin. However, this altered expression may be only circumstantial and influenced by other cytokines such as TGF-β.
- Identification in reactive arthritis of identical clonally expanded T cells in intestine and joint. However, only a few expanded T-cell clones were shared by both compartments.
- Identification of macrophage subpopulation expressing scavenger receptor CD163 simultaneously upregulated in joint and intestine.

Innate Immunity

Using the $TNF^{\Delta ARE}$ mutant mice model it has been demonstrated that in the presence of chronic TNF overexposure, mesenchymal cells, such as fibroblasts/myofibroblasts of the joint and the intestine, are primary responder cells sufficient for full pathogenic TNF/TNFRI signaling in arthritis, sacroiliitis and CD-like IBD [17]. Mesenchymal cell replacement by stem cell or bone marrow transplantation may offer therapeutic approaches for the resolution of chronic inflammatory processes. The attenuation of the TNFRI pathway in these cells or their precursors may hold promise for therapeutic interventions [17].

Immune-Driven Angiogenesis

Mucosal microvasculature is a non-immune component crucially involved in intestinal inflammation. Several mechanisms are involved:
- Inflammatory cells stimulate angiogenesis: (a) *directly* by secretion of VEGF, FGF, HGF, PDGF, TNF-α and TGF-β, or (b) *indirectly* via stimulation of secretion of angiogenic factors by endothelial cells and fibroblasts [18].
- Extravasation of plasma fibrinogen induces neovascularization [19].
- Hypoxia with induction of HIF upregulates proangiogenic factors [20].
- Increased blood flow in inflammatory foci induces shear stress and stimulates angiogenesis [21].

Angiogenesis is the growth of new capillary blood vessels from existing ones, whereas microvascular remodeling involves structural alterations. Angiogenesis in inflammation has a dual role:
- It is a fundamental component of growth, development and repair of tissue and promotes tissue homeostasis by the regulation of the type and number of infiltrating leukocytes.
- It perpetuates inflammation by several mechanisms including: (a) endothelial activation and expression of adhesion molecules (leukocyte adhesion and infiltration); (b) increased vascular permeability (edema); (c) remodeling of the vascular bed (influx inflammatory cells), and (d) microvascular dysfunction by vasodilatation (ischemia and ulcerations).

Simplified, it can be stated that chronic inflammation upregulates pro-angiogenic factors via inflammatory mediators and that angiogenesis perpetuates inflammation via continuous supply of inflammatory cells [22].

The best characterized positive regulators of angiogenesis are vascular endothelial growth factors (VEGF) interacting with three receptors: VEGFR-1 (flt-1), VEGFR-2 (flk-1/KDR), and VEGFR-3 (flt-4). VEGF-A also binds to non-tyrosine kinase receptors inducing a switch for the endothelial cell to an angiogenetic phenotype with induction of uPA, MMP-1, MMP-3, MMP-9 and integrin $β_3$. Besides their role in angiogenesis, VEGFs have shown to exert potent proinflammatory activities by: (a) induction of adhesion molecules VCAM-1 and ICAM-1 on the surface of endothelial cells; (b) promotion of cytokine production, and (c) induction of expression of protease involved in matrix degradation [23].

As previously described by Danese et al. [18], we were able to demonstrate an increased vascular density and expression of VEGF in active inflamed intestinal mucosa of CD patients. Moreover, we found similar evidence for angiogenesis in intestinal mucosa of SpA patients, predominantly in the subgroup of patients with associated active or quiescent inflammation, supporting the evidence that this immune-driven intestinal angiogenesis is also important in this population. No differences were found for serum VEGF concentrations [manuscript in preparation].

Therapeutic Evidence

Treatment of IBD-related arthropathy is based almost entirely on extrapolation from treatment of other forms of SpA [24]. In the case of peripheral arthritis there is general support for use of short-term treatment with nonsteroidal anti-inflammatory agents, local corticosteroid injections and physiotherapy (EL4, RG D). The emphasis should be on treatment of underlying CD (EL2c, RG C). Sulfasalazine has a role in persistent peripheral arthritis (EL1a, RG B).

In axial arthropathy, arguments in favor of intensive physiotherapy (EL1b, RG B) associated with NSAIDs are stronger, but safety concerns mean that long-term treatment with NSAIDs is best avoided if possible (EL1b, RG C). Sulfasalazine (EL1a), methotrexate (EL1b) or azathioprine (EL4) are generally ineffective, or only marginally effective. The efficacy of anti-TNF therapy for patients with AS and CD intolerant or refractory to NSAIDs is well established (EL1b, RG B) (ECCO Consensus 2009).

The relative safety of NSAIDs is based on a recent study demonstrating that the use of low-dose NSAIDs was not associated with an increased risk. However, use of high-dose NSAIDs was associated with higher disease activity among CD patients with colonic involvement, but this was not reflected by an increase in significant disease flares [25]. Use of selective COX-2 inhibitors is an alternative [26, 27].

The efficacy of infliximab and adalimumab has been demonstrated in several placebo-controlled trials and is well established [24]. Although etanercept is efficacious in AS, its use in IBD is not recommended. In 2007, Braun et al. [28] published a synthesis of the incidence of new cases or relapses of IBD in studies performed in patients with AS and treated with anti-TNF: infliximab (n = 366–618 patient-years), adalimumab (n = 295–132 patient-years) or etanercept (419–625 patient-years) versus placebo (434–150 patient-years). The diagnosis of IBD was reported in 76 of 1,130 patients (6.7%) before treatment. One new case was reported in patients treated with placebo, 0 cases in infliximab or adalimumab, and 5 new cases in the etanercept group. In parallel, 1 relapse was reported in the placebo group, 1 relapse in infliximab, 3 relapses in adalimumab, and 9 relapses in etanercept. These data demonstrate a 10-fold increased risk for active IBD in the etanercept group as compared to the control group (p = 0.001), although the absolute risk remains low. The incidence of IBD was 1.3 cases per 100 patient-years for placebo, 0.2 cases per 100 patient-years for infliximab, 2.2 cases for etanercept, and 2.3 cases for adalimumab (NS).

In conclusion, these data provide evidence for common genetic, etiopathogenic and clinical overlap between 'immune-mediated inflammatory diseases'.

Disclosure Statement

The author declares that no financial or other conflict of interest exists in relation to the content of this article.

References

1 De Vlam K, Mielants H, Cuvelier C, et al: Spondyloarthropathy is underestimated in inflammatory bowel disease: prevalence and HLA association. J Rheumatol 2000;27: 2860–2865.
2 Orchard TR, Wordsworth BP, Jewell DP: Peripheral arthropathies in inflammatory bowel disease: their articular distribution and natural history. Gut 1998;42:387–391.
3 Peeters H, Vander Cruyssen B, Mielants H, et al: Clinical and genetic factors associated with sacroiliitis in Crohn's disease. J Gastroenterol Hepatol 2008;23:132–137.
4 Palm O, Bernklev T, Moum B, Gran JT: Non-inflammatory joint pain in patients with inflammatory bowel disease is prevalent and has a significant impact on health-related quality of life. J Rheumatol 2005;32:1755–1759.
5 De Vos M, Cuvelier C, Mielants H, et al: Ileocolonoscopy in seronegative spondylarthropathy. Gastroenterology 1989;96:339–344.
6 De Vos M, Mielants H, Cuvelier C, et al: Long-term evolution of gut inflammation in patients with spondylarthropathy. Gastroenterology 1996;110:1696–1703.
7 Reveille JD: Major histocompatibility genes and ankylosing spondylitis. Best Pract Res Clin Rheumatol 2006;20:601–609.
8 Tran TM, Dorris ML, Satumtira N, et al: Additional human β_2-microglobulin curbs HLA-B27 misfolding and promotes arthritis and spondylitis without colitis in male HL-B27 transgenic rats. Arthritis Rheum 2006; 54:1317–1365.
9 Laukens D, Peeters H, Marichal D, et al: CARD15 gene polymorphisms in patients with spondyloarthorpathies identify a specific phenotype previously related to Crohn's disease. Ann Rheum Dis 2005;64:930–935.
10 Micelli-Richard C, Zouali H, Lesage S, et al: CARD15/NOD2 analyses in spondyloarthropathy. Arthritis Rheum 2002;46:1405–1406.
11 Craene AM, Bradbury L, Van Heel DA, et al: Role of NOD2 variants in spondyloarthritis. Arthritis Rheum 2002;46:1629–1633.
12 Barrett JC, Hansoul S, Nicolae DL, et al; NIDDK IBD Genetics Consortium, Belgian-French IBD Consortium, and Wellcome Trust Case-Control Consortium: Genome-wide association defines more than 30 distinct susceptibility loci for Crohn's disease. Nat Genet 2008;40:955–962.
13 Moffatt MF, Kabesch M, Liang L, et al: Genetic variants regulating ORMDL3 expression contribute to the risk of childhood asthma. Nature 2007;448:470–473.
14 Georges M, Laukens D, Libioulle C, et al: Evidence for significant overlap between common risk variants for Crohn's disease and ankylosing spondylitis. Acta Gastroenterol Belg 2009;72:I03.
15 Laukens D, Peeters H, Cruyssen BV, et al: Altered gut transcriptome in spondyloarthropathy. Ann Rheum Dis 2006;65:1293–1300.
16 Jacques P, Mielants H, Coppieters K, et al: The intimate relationship between gut and joint in spondyloarthropathies. Curr Opin Rheumatol 2007;19:353–357.
17 Armaka M, Apostolaki M, Jacques P, et al: Mesenchymal cell targeting by TNF as a common pathogenic principle in chronic inflammatory joint and intestinal diseases. J Exp Med 2008;205:331–337.
18 Danese S, Sans M, De la Motte C, et al: Angiogenesis as a novel component of inflammatory bowel disease pathogenesis. Gastroenterology 2006;130:2060–2073.
19 Hatton MW, Southward SM, et al: Fibrinogen catabolism within the procoagulant VX-2 tumor of rabbit in lung in vivo: effluxing fibrin(ogen) fragments contain antiangiogenic activity. J Lab Clin Med 2004;143:241–254.
20 Robinson A, Keely S, Karhausen J, et al: Mucosal protection by hypoxia-inducible factor prolyl hydroxylase inhibition. Gastroenterology 2008;134:145–155.
21 Deban L, Correale C, Vetrano S, et al: Multiple pathogenic roles of microvasculature in inflammatory bowel disease: a jack of all trades. Am J Pathol 2008;172:1457–1466.
22 Costa C, Incio J, Soares R: Angiogenesis and chronic inflammation: cause or consequence? Angiogenesis 2007;10:149–166.
23 Danese S: VEGF in inflammatory bowel disease: a master regulator of mucosal immune-driven angiogenesis. Dig Liver Dis 2008;40: 680–683.
24 Zochling J, Van der Heijde D, Dougados M, Braun J: Current evidence for the management of ankylosing spondylitis: a systematic literature review for the ASAS/EULAR management recommendations in ankylosing spondylitis. Ann Rheum Dis 2006;65:423–432.
25 Bonner GF, Fakhri A, Vennamanen SR: A long-term cohort study of non-steroidal anti-inflammatory drug use and disease activity in outpatients with inflammatory bowel diseases. Inflamm Bowel Dis 2004;10: 751–757.
26 Sandborn WJ, Stenson WF, Brynskov J, Lorenze RG, et al: Safety of celecoxib in patients with ulcerative colitis in remission: a randomised placebo-controlled pilot study. Clin Gastroenterol Hepatol 2006;4:203–211.
27 El Miedany Y, Youssef S, Ahmed I, El Gaafary M: The gastrointestinal safety and effect on disease activity of etoricoxib, a selective COX-2 Inhibitor in inflammatory bowel diseases. Am J Gastroenterol 2006;101:311–317.
28 Braun J, Baraliakos X, Listing J, et al: Differences in the incidence of flares or new onset of inflammatory bowel disease in patients with ankylosing spondylitis exposed to therapy with anti-TNF agents. Arthritis Rheum 2007;57:639–647.

Can We Modulate the Clinical Course of Inflammatory Bowel Diseases by Our Current Treatment Strategies?

Jacques Cosnes

Service de Gastroentérologie et Nutrition, Hôpital St-Antoine et Université Pierre-et-Marie Curie (Paris VI), Paris, France

Key Words

Inflammatory bowel disease, clinical course · Inflammatory bowel disease, natural history · Thiopurines, efficacy · Anti-TNF

Abstract

Ulcerative colitis and Crohn's disease are chronic disabling lifelong diseases which may be disturbed by severe flares and anatomical complications requiring surgery. Until the very last years there was no clear indication that treatment was able to modify the long-term natural history of the disease. In particular, there are no data demonstrating a clear improvement through the period 1950–2003 in disease activity, occurrence of complications and need for surgery, in spite of an increased use of immunosuppressants since the 1990s. However, in inflammatory bowel disease, both thiopurines and methotrexate are very efficient in about one half of the patients, and in responders, may heal the mucosa and decrease the need for surgery. The early use of immunosuppressants in selected patients may have an impact on occurrence of severe flares and complications, and need for surgery. Moreover, anti-TNF now used for 10 years in Crohn's disease and for 5 years in ulcerative colitis demonstrated in two thirds of the patients a remarkable anatomic effect, healing the mucosa, closing fistulae and preventing strictures. Infliximab does prevent endoscopic recurrence following ileal resection for Crohn's disease. Actually, because irreversible anatomical damage may develop during the first years of disease, there is a need to classify early in the course of the disease patients who will benefit from anti-TNF and classical immunosuppressants, respectively. There is the need in the next few years to better define these subgroups and to compare different strategies within each group through randomized interventional studies.

Copyright © 2009 S. Karger AG, Basel

Ulcerative colitis (UC) and Crohn's disease (CD) are chronic disabling lifelong diseases, disconcerting in their evolution, which may be deranged by severe flares and complications requiring surgery. Their evolution has remained poorly predictable, and until recently there was no clear indication that treatment was able to modify the long-term natural history of the disease. However, new biological therapies and changing therapeutic strategies are emerging [1], and there are some signals of modifications of the clinical course of inflammatory bowel diseases (IBD).

Natural History of Inflammatory Bowel Diseases

Crohn's Disease
CD is a chronic disease, with usual onset in young adulthood, which continues lifelong without clear burn-

ing out. CD may involve any part of the gastrointestinal tract, from mouth to anus; however, ileal and colonic localization are the more prevalent [2]. Although the extent of involvement present at the time of diagnosis may progress, or regress, during follow-up, initial localization usually determines cumulative localization [3]. Perianal location is another important problem in CD [4]. At presentation, about 30% of patients share perianal lesions and 20% have or have had a fistula [5]. During the disease course, the cumulative risk of developing a perianal fistula increases to 45% after 20 years [5]. The risk of perianal fistula is twice more important in patients with colonic disease than in patients with ileal disease [6, 7].

The natural history of CD is marked by the occurrence of complications: perforation (abscess, fistula, or peritonitis) and strictures. The occurrence of complications, nearly constant in such a lifelong disease with progressive and irreversible anatomical damage, is highly related to disease location. Small bowel involvement may be complicated at diagnosis or during the very first years by an abscess/fistula or by a stricture followed by a fistula formation [8], whereas a colonic disease may remain 'uncomplicated', inflammatory, for many years. Perianal disease should be considered in particular because of the anatomy of the anal verge and the potential of these lesions to create fistulae and abscesses [7].

Most of these complications are inaccessible to medical therapy and require surgery. Less commonly, medicines fail to control disease activity and removal of the diseased segment is the only alternative. In the Copenhagen cohort, the 20-year cumulative risk of intestinal resection was 82% [9]. Other series from 1970 to 2000 showed very similar rates [10, 11].

Another fear of CD patients is the risk of permanent stoma. Proctocolectomy for Crohn's colitis is less often performed, as segmental colonic resection gives somewhat similar results to total colectomy [12]. Among patients with perianal disease, it was estimated that roughly one half of the patients required permanent fecal diversion, which was even more frequently true for patients with colonic CD and anal stenosis. This represents 12% of the total CD population in a recent surgical series from the USA [13].

Mortality in CD is slightly elevated when compared to the general population. A recent meta-analysis using a random-effects model showed the pooled estimate for standardized mortality ratio in CD was 1.52 (95% confidence interval 1.32–1.74) [14]. In other terms, being diagnosed with CD increases the risk of death by 50% in a given period of time.

Ulcerative Colitis

UC usually starts during the third decade of life; however, it may be diagnosed later in life, particularly in men who quit smoking. UC involves only the colon, from the anus, and flare after flare extends proximally from the rectum. The cumulative involvement includes the rectum in the great majority of cases, left colon in two thirds of the cases, and the right colon in one third to one half of the cases [15].

Colectomy is necessary in fulminant flares or chronic active disease refractory to therapy and in case of advanced neoplasia. The cumulative risk of colectomy is highly variable from one series to another, usually about 20–30% after 25 years, sometimes more in series from referral centers [16], or less in population-based studies and in series from Southern Europe [17]. This risk is particularly elevated during the year following diagnosis, then reaches a plateau at an annual rate of 1%. Disease extension and severity at presentation are the best predictors of the risk of colectomy.

Mortality is not significantly different from that of the general population [18], although there is an increased risk during the first attack [19].

Effect of Treatments before 2003

In CD, a systematic review published in 2004 which analyzed population-based studies with a complete follow-up failed to demonstrate a significant improvement of disease outcome during the last four decades [20]. Of note, disease activity, occurrence of complications and need for surgery did not change significantly during that period. For example, curves of first intestinal surgery were very similar [21, 22]. Rates of second surgery for postoperative recurrence did not change through the years 1950–1990, and about 35% of the patients had to be re-operated on 10 years after the first intestinal resection in most series [20]. Similarly, the mortality ratio has slightly decreased over the past 30 years, but this decrease has not reached the level of significance [14]. Finally, the larger use of immunosuppressants in CD patients from the end of the 1990s was not shown to be associated with fewer complications and a decreased surgical rate [22].

In UC, the main progress has been the standardization of management of fulminant colitis with intensive intravenous treatment according to the Oxford guidelines [23, 24]. Cyclosporine was introduced in the early 1990s [25] and was demonstrated to control the acute phase in two thirds of non-responders to intravenous steroids; however, in many patients it recurred during the follow-up.

To conclude, before 2003 there were no signs of a real impact of treatment on the disease course, both in CD and in UC.

New Data

Better Knowledge of the Efficacy of Thiopurines

Thiopurines (azathioprine and 6-mercaptopurine) have proven to be an effective and relatively safe treatment for IBD and are now widely used in the management of these patients. In the most recent years, about 60 and 30% of patients with CD and UC, respectively, are placed under thiopurines within the first 10 years of the disease. Thiopurines and methotrexate have a potent action on disease damage and are able to heal the mucosa after 2 years [26]; however, they may be poorly tolerated in some patients and their onset of action is slow. If started relatively late in the disease course, at a time when the anatomical damage has become irreversible, they will not prevent the occurrence of complications. Conversely, the classical study of Markowitz et al. [27] showed that 6-mercaptopurine was able to modify the disease course when given early in children with CD. A too late prescription may explain why their increased use over time was not associated in our patients with a decrease of annual rates of intestinal resection [22]. In contrast to our results in adult patients with CD, a large prospective study from the Lille group in pediatric CD found that early prescription of azathioprine was associated with lower rates of surgery. After adjustment on propensity scores, azathioprine was found to divide by a factor 2 the risk of surgery [28]. Further indirect evidence for the efficacy of immunosuppressants may be the recent decrease of the surgical rate in Danish patients diagnosed in 2003–2004 when compared to previous cohorts [21].

Taken together, these data (slow mode of action, impact on need for surgery only in case of an early prescription) favor a more rapid use of thiopurines in selected patients. However, there is no demonstration by a randomized controlled trial of the superiority of an early prescription. This study is an ongoing trial currently being performed by the GETAID.

Effect of Anti-TNF

Anti-TNF drugs are very potent agents in the treatment of IBD and have revolutionized the management of these patients. Up to two thirds of patients, even those who failed on classical immunosuppressants, are clinical responders. There is also some evidence from randomized control trials that anti-TNF may decrease the need for surgery in CD. In the ACCENT I study, scheduled treatment strategies resulted in fewer surgeries when compared to an episodic treatment strategy [29]. In the ACCENT II study, among patients randomized as responders, those who received infliximab maintenance therapy (5 mg/kg every 8 weeks) had significantly fewer mean numbers of hospitalizations, all surgeries and procedures, and major surgeries, compared with those who received placebo maintenance [30]. Similarly, patients undergoing maintenance therapy with adalimumab had a decreased probability of requiring surgery in the CHARM trial [31].

However, two recent still unpublished studies, one in the USA, the other in Spain, compared calendar cohorts of patients who started their disease before or after 2000 and showed that the availability of infliximab had little impact on the initial course of CD. In particular, the occurrence of stricturing and penetrating complications and the need for surgery were similar from one cohort to another. This does not mean that infliximab has no effect on the natural history of CD, but means that it has no effect when used in the setting of a step-up therapeutic program. Actually there is a large difference when considering patients from prospective randomized control trials and selecting responders to a given drug, and a large cohort of unselected patients.

We believe, however, that, over time, with a more accurate prescription of immunosuppressants and anti-TNF, respectively, patients will do better. Immunosuppressants in patients who respond to these treatments (about half the patients) do change the disease course, decreasing year-by-year activity (fig. 1) and the annual surgical rate from 4 to 2% (fig. 2). The effect of anti-TNF is visible in patient non-responders to azathioprine or methotrexate, with a significant decrease in activity (fig. 1) and surgery (fig. 2) throughout the years 2000–2006. In UC, there is at the present time no indication of a decreased colectomy rate in our patients. This may be due to the fact that anti-TNF has been used more recently in UC, with a delay of about 5 years when compared to CD. Finally, we have learnt that for maintaining clinical and endoscopic remission, both thiopurines and anti-TNF should be permanently used [32, 33].

In total, there are some signals of an effect of immunosuppressants and anti-TNF on the natural history of IBD; however, when regarding a cohort of patients, the improvement seems modest. A plausible explanation is that these therapies are introduced too late, while lesions have become irreversible. Thus there is a need to reconsider our current therapeutic strategies.

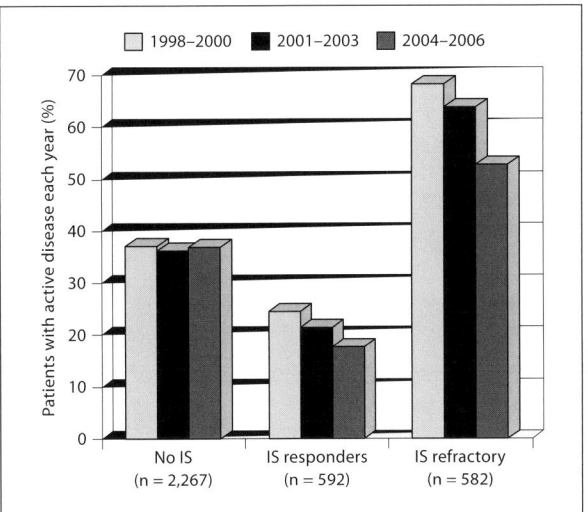

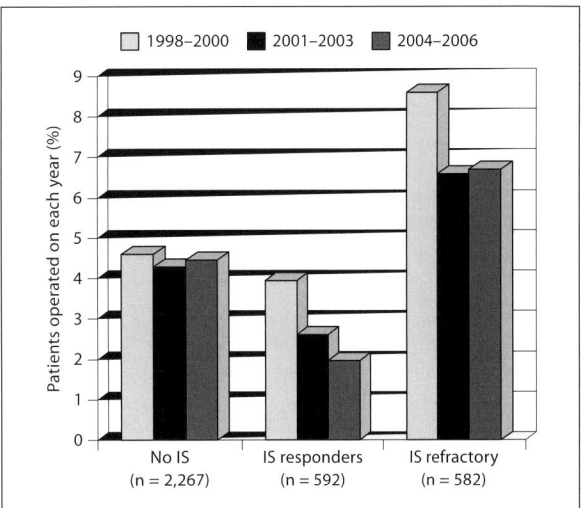

Fig. 1. Percentage of patients with active disease for every calendar year during 3 consecutive years over the period 1998–2006, in three groups of patients defined by their response to first-line immunosuppressive therapy (IS). Responders were defined as patients who were inactive the year following the introduction of IS, and refractory as those who were active the year following the introduction of IS. The year of diagnosis was excluded from analysis. The numbers indicate the number of patients in each group during the year 2006.

Fig. 2. Percentage of patients having intestinal surgery for every calendar year during 3 consecutive years over the period 1998–2006, in three groups of patients defined by their response to first-line immunosuppressive therapy (IS). For further details, see figure 1.

New Strategies

Defining Subgroups of Patients Needing Aggressive Therapies

Early introduction of immunosuppressants or anti-TNF in all patients would result in the overtreatment of a large proportion (30–50%) who will not develop a disabling disease. Besides, not every patient will respond to thiopurines, methotrexate, or anti-TNF. Thus there are two needs: (1) Recognizing at an early stage patients with the highest risk of developing a disabling disease or complications. This was addressed by our study searching predictors of disabling CD; the predictors were young age, perianal lesions, and steroid therapy during the first flare [34]. Prognosis is much more difficult to predict in UC patients, although the intensity of the first attack and pancolitic location are probably pejorative. (2) Selecting the best responders. In the SONIC trial, patients with ulcerative lesions on colonoscopy and with high CRP values benefited more from anti-TNF than other patients [35]. We believe that in these selected patients early aggressive therapies are warranted, and they should be maintained at least several years because the effect of these drugs ceases when they are stopped. The famous step-up versus top-down trial did not show major differences between the groups because anti-TNF were stopped in the top-down arm [32].

Treat Lesions Not Symptoms

The model of the postoperative recurrence following ileocecal resection in CD as described by Olaison et al. [36] and Rutgeerts et al. [37] clearly demonstrates that the development of preanastomotic inflammatory lesions in the neoterminal ileum progresses in a few years from aphthae to larger ulcers and stricture. Clinical symptoms occur 2–3 years after the development of first ulcerations. Infliximab has been shown to prevent those endoscopic lesions when started postoperatively and maintained during the year following surgery [38]. This model may be applied to unoperated CD. Treatment should be started with the goal to heal lesions for preventing symptoms. Mucosal healing is probably not a sufficient objective and healing of the whole width of the intestinal wall should be achieved, as it has been shown that thickening of the neoterminal ileum is associated with subsequent development of surgical recurrence [39]. Thus one can imagine to check regularly a patient for the presence of intestinal ulcerations and thickening, using non-invasive techniques (CRP, ferritin, fecal calprotectin, videocapsule and MRI) and to treat as early as possible an asymptomatic patient in order to prevent the development of symptoms and complications.

Conclusion

To conclude, although at present there is no evidence that our current therapeutic strategies are able to radically change the course of both CD and UC, particularly the need for surgery, times are changing. A more narrow surveillance and an aggressive therapeutic approach in selected patients are expected to have an impact on the evolution and complications of IBD. As experiences with immunosuppressants and anti-TNF are reassuring regarding their long-term safety, comparative strategies and trials are needed to prescribe the right drug at the right time to the right patient.

Disclosure Statement

The author declares that he is consultant for Abbott International.

References

1 Rutgeerts P, Vermeire S, Van Assche G: Biological therapies for inflammatory bowel diseases. Gastroenterology 2009;136:1182–1197.
2 Cosnes J, Cattan S, Blain A, et al: Long-term evolution of disease behavior of Crohn's disease. Inflamm Bowel Dis 2002;8:244–250.
3 Louis E, Collard A, Oger AF, Degroote E, Aboul Nasr El Yafi FA, Belaiche J: Behaviour of Crohn's disease according to the Vienna classification: changing pattern over the course of the disease. Gut 2001;49:777–782.
4 Vermeire S, Van Assche G, Rutgeerts P: Perianal Crohn's disease: classification and clinical evaluation. Dig Liver Dis 2007;39:959–962.
5 Schwartz DA, Loftus EV Jr, Tremaine WJ, et al: The natural history of fistulizing Crohn's disease in Olmsted County, Minnesota. Gastroenterology 2002;122:875–880.
6 Cosnes J: Crohn's disease phenotype, prognosis, and long-term complications: what to expect? Acta Gastroenterol Belg 2008;71:303–307.
7 Sachar DB, Bodian CA, Goldstein ES, et al: Is perianal Crohn's disease associated with intestinal fistulization? Am J Gastroenterol 2005;100:1547–1549.
8 Oberhuber G, Stangl PC, Vogelsang H, Schober E, Herbst F, Gasche C: Significant association of strictures and internal fistula formation in Crohn's disease. Virchows Arch 2000;437:293–297.
9 Munkholm P, Langholz E, Davidsen M, Binder V: Disease activity courses in a regional cohort of Crohn's disease patients. Scand J Gastroenterol 1995;30:699–706.
10 Mekhjian HS, Switz DM, Melnyk CS, Rankin GB, Brooks RK: Clinical features and natural history of Crohn's disease. Gastroenterology 1979;77:898–906.
11 Sands BE, Arsenault JE, Rosen MJ, et al: Risk of early surgery for Crohn's disease: implications for early treatment strategies. Am J Gastroenterol 2003;98:2712–2718.
12 Andersson P, Olaison G, Bodemar G, Nystrom PO, Sjodahl R: Surgery for Crohn colitis over a 28-year period: fewer stomas and the replacement of total colectomy by segmental resection. Scand J Gastroenterol 2002;37:68–73.
13 Galandiuk S, Kimberling J, Al-Mishlab TG, Stromberg AJ: Perianal Crohn disease: predictors of need for permanent diversion. Ann Surg 2005;241:796–802.
14 Canavan C, Abrams KR, Mayberry JF: Meta-analysis: mortality in Crohn's disease. Aliment Pharmacol Ther 2007;25:861–870.
15 Langholz E, Munkholm P, Davidsen M, Nielsen OH, Binder V: Changes in extent of ulcerative colitis: a study on the course and prognostic factors. Scand J Gastroenterol 1996;31:260–266.
16 Langholz E, Munkholm P, Davidsen M, Binder V: Course of ulcerative colitis: analysis of changes in disease activity over years. Gastroenterology 1994;107:3–11.
17 Hoie O, Wolters FL, Riis L, et al: Low colectomy rates in ulcerative colitis in an unselected European cohort followed for 10 years. Gastroenterology 2007;132:507–515.
18 Palli D, Trallori G, Saieva C, et al: General and cancer-specific mortality of a population-based cohort of patients with inflammatory bowel disease: the Florence Study. Gut 1998;42:175–179.
19 Dunckley P, Jewell D: Management of acute severe colitis. Best Pract Res Clin Gastroenterol 2003;17:89–103.
20 Wolters FL, Russel MG, Stockbrugger RW: Systematic review: has disease outcome in Crohn's disease changed during the last four decades? Aliment Pharmacol Ther 2004;20:483–496.
21 Jess T, Riis L, Vind I, et al: Changes in clinical characteristics, course, and prognosis of inflammatory bowel disease during the last five decades: a population-based study from Copenhagen, Denmark. Inflamm Bowel Dis 2007;13:481–489.
22 Cosnes J, Nion-Larmurier I, Beaugerie L, Afchain P, Tiret E, Gendre JP: Impact of the increasing use of immunosuppressants in Crohn's disease on the need for intestinal surgery. Gut 2005;54:237–241.
23 Travis SP, Farrant JM, Ricketts C, et al: Predicting outcome in severe ulcerative colitis. Gut 1996;38:905–910.
24 Truelove SC, Willoughby CP, Lee EG, Kettlewell MG: Further experience in the treatment of severe attacks of ulcerative colitis. Lancet 1978;2:1086–1088.
25 Lichtiger S, Present DH, Kornbluth A, et al: Cyclosporine in severe ulcerative colitis refractory to steroid therapy. N Engl J Med 1994;330:1841–1845.
26 D'Haens G, Geboes K, Ponette E, Penninckx F, Rutgeerts P: Healing of severe recurrent ileitis with azathioprine therapy in patients with Crohn's disease. Gastroenterology 1997;112:1475–1481.

27 Markowitz J, Grancher K, Kohn N, Lesser M, Daum F: A multicenter trial of 6-mercaptopurine and prednisone in children with newly diagnosed Crohn's disease. Gastroenterology 2000;119:895–902.
28 Vernier-Massouille G, Balde M, Salleron J, et al: Natural history of pediatric Crohn's disease: a population-based cohort study. Gastroenterology 2008;135:1106–1113.
29 Hanauer SB, Feagan BG, Lichtenstein GR, et al: Maintenance infliximab for Crohn's disease: the ACCENT I randomised trial. Lancet 2002;359:1541–1549.
30 Lichtenstein GR, Yan S, Bala M, Blank M, Sands BE: Infliximab maintenance treatment reduces hospitalizations, surgeries, and procedures in fistulizing Crohn's disease. Gastroenterology 2005;128:862–869.
31 Feagan BG, Panaccione R, Sandborn WJ, et al: Effects of adalimumab therapy on incidence of hospitalization and surgery in Crohn's disease: results from the CHARM study. Gastroenterology 2008;135:1493–1499.
32 D'Haens G, Baert F, van Assche G, et al: Early combined immunosuppression or conventional management in patients with newly diagnosed Crohn's disease: an open randomised trial. Lancet 2008;371:660–667.
33 Lemann M, Mary JY, Colombel JF, et al: A randomized, double-blind, controlled withdrawal trial in Crohn's disease patients in long-term remission on azathioprine. Gastroenterology 2005;128:1812–1818.
34 Beaugerie L, Seksik P, Nion-Larmurier I, Gendre JP, Cosnes J: Predictors of Crohn's disease. Gastroenterology 2006;130:650–656.
35 Colombel JF, Rutgeerts P, Reinisch W, et al: SONIC: a randomized double-blind controlled trial comparing Infliximab and infliximab plus azathioprine to azathioprine in patients with Crohn's disease naive to immunomodulators and biologic therapy. Gut 2008;57:A1.
36 Olaison G, Smedh K, Sjodahl R: Natural course of Crohn's disease after ileocolic resection: endoscopically visualised ileal ulcers preceding symptoms. Gut 1992;33:331–335.
37 Rutgeerts P, Geboes K, Vantrappen G, Beyls J, Kerremans R, Hiele M: Predictability of the postoperative course of Crohn's disease. Gastroenterology 1990;99:956–963.
38 Regueiro M, Schraut W, Baidoo L, et al: Infliximab prevents Crohn's disease recurrence after ileal resection. Gastroenterology 2009;136:441–450.
39 Sampietro GM, Corsi F, Maconi G, et al: Prospective study of long-term results and prognostic factors after conservative surgery for small bowel Crohn's disease. Clin Gastroenterol Hepatol 2009;7:183–191.

Primary Sclerosing Cholangitis: A Clinical Case

Natalya B. Gubergrits

M. Gorky National Medical University, Donetsk, Ukraine

Key Words
Primary sclerosing cholangitis · Monozygotic twins · Non-specific ulcerative colitis · PSC, first-degree relatives

Abstract
The basic hypotheses of pathogenesis of primary sclerosing cholangitis (PSC) are discussed, i.e. genetically conditioned pathology, autoimmune pathology, the result of inflammatory reaction in bile ducts, and cholangiopathy. A clinical case of monozygotic twins with association of PSC and non-specific ulcerative colitis (NUC) is presented. The first twin had a severe course of PSC and a mild course of NUC; he died due to bacterial complications of cholangitis. The second twin, patient B, had an opposite situation, a severe course of NUC, while PSC was suspected only after determination of cholestasis biochemical markers. As soon as cholestasis was revealed, patient B was administered Ursofalk and Budenofalk (in 2001). He received Salofalk as a basic therapy for NUC. Repeated liver biopsy in 2005 showed no progression of PSC, but minimal biochemical signs of cholestasis were present in 2009. It is therefore necessary to study the first-degree relatives of patients with PSC.

Copyright © 2009 S. Karger AG, Basel

Primary sclerosing cholangitis (PSC) is a severe progressing chronic disease of the liver accompanied by significant cholestasis as a result of inflammation and fibrosis of predominantly large bile ducts. In PSC, there is a significantly increased risk of colorectal cancer, cholangiocarcinoma and several other malignant tumors [1]. PSC etiology is still unclear despite the severe course of the disease and frequent complications. There are a number of hypotheses of PSC pathogenesis, the main ones include the following [2–4]: PSC genetically conditioned pathology [2, 3, 5] and PSC autoimmune pathology [4, 6]. PSC is the result of an inflammatory reaction in bile ducts due to infectious agents entering the liver from the large intestine through portal veins [7–10], while PSC cholangiopathy predominantly involves large bile ducts, i.e., it is related to bile duct pathologies which primarily affect cholangiocytes with further development of cholestasis [11, 12].

In our clinic we examined and treated 2 monozygotic twins and paid special attention to the hypothesis of genetic predisposition to PSC development. This hypothesis has been proven with a high occurrence of the disease among first-degree relatives (0.7%) and siblings (1.5%), which is 100 times higher than among the general population [5]. Furthermore, an association of PSC with a certain major histocompatibility complex (MHC) and non-MHC alleles [13–20] was found. Such haplotypes as DR B1*1301, DR B1*0301, DR B1*1501, MICA*008 and some others are closely associated with PSC [13–15]. However, some published data discredit the genetic basis of PSC. The association with some human leukocyte antigen (HLA) haplotypes is weak and not obligatory; studies on non-HLA polymorphisms are either reproducible or contradictory [13].

Although PSC is frequently associated with inflammatory bowel diseases (IBD), especially with non-specific ulcerative colitis (NUC), there is no genetic basis for such an association and of a connection between the HLA system and IBD [1]. IBD is diagnosed in PSC in 55–80% of cases, and vice versa, PSC is revealed in IBD only in 3–6% of cases [1, 13].

In 2001 we observed male patient K, 25 years old, who suffered from PSC complicated with bacterial cholangitis and secondary biliary cirrhosis of the liver. Seven years earlier a diagnosis of NUC with predominant affection of sigmoid colon and rectum with minimal activity of the disease was made. During the patient's stay in the clinic, NUC happened to be in a remission phase. Treatment with cephalosporins of third-generation metronidazole and ursodeoxycholic acid was ineffective. Anemia of mixed etiology (hemolytic and iron-deficient) grew progressively worse; additional symptoms appeared: significant arthralgia and myalgia, severe malabsorption. Endoscopic retrograde cholangiopancreatography (ERCP) was not conducted due to the patient's severe state. Liver punch biopsy showed the following: significant intra- and extracellular cholestasis especially on the lobules' periphery; bile accumulation in bile tract ducts; evident sclerosis with significant dilation of portal tracts; albuminous and vacuolar degeneration of hepatocytes; multiple piecemeal and bridge-like necroses; forming of false lobules; significant lymphohistiocytic infiltration with considerable quantity of segmentonuclear leukocytes including those with glycogen; leukocytes in lumen and in the walls of bile ducts. Conclusion: bacterial cholangitis, chronic hepatitis resulting in cirrhosis, with significant activity. The patient died due to sepsis that developed on the background of multiple abscesses of the liver.

Patient K had a twin brother (patient B) – they were monozygotic twins. In patient B, NUC developed at the age of 16 and its clinical course was more severe than in brother K: exacerbations were more frequent, with significant bleeding; colonoscopy showed involvement of the entire left half of the large intestine. Patient B did not have clinical signs of PSC in 2001. In view of the significant immunogenetic predisposition to PSC, both brothers underwent immunogenotypic analysis, which revealed allele DR B1*1301. Biochemistry of patient B showed elevation of alkaline phosphatase (normal: 7), γ-glutamyltransferase (normal: 6), an alanine aminotransferase (normal: 1.7) on the background of a normal bilirubin level. At the time of the first examination, patient B had NUC in the remission phase. Both brothers had perinuclear antineutrophil cytoplasmic antibodies in their blood. Patient B underwent liver biopsy twice – in 2001 and 2005. *Results of the first biopsy:* sclerosis and proliferation of bile duct epithelium, large cellular infiltrates around ducts, symptom of 'onion skin'. ERCP: sclerosing cholangiopancreatitis. A diagnosis of PSC in combination with NUC was made.

We would like to make a point of the presence of sclerosing cholangiopancreatitis and steatorrhea in patient K. The main pancreatic duct could be affected in case of PSC. On the other hand, large bile ducts could be involved in the case of autoimmune pancreatitis (AIP) [1, 21, 22]. In differential diagnosis between PSC and AIP, the different localization of strictures of common bile duct and main pancreatic duct plays an important role. Furthermore, PSC is frequently associated with NUC, while AIP only rarely; pancreas is not enlarged in PSC, but the course of AIP could be developed on the basis of pseudotumorous pancreatitis type, which means enlargement of the pancreas head; corticosteroids have a minor effect in PSC, but in AIP they are of high efficacy [21, 22]. Taking into account that our patient has a combination of sclerosing cholangitis with NUC and the pancreas was of normal size, we decided that strictures of the main pancreatic duct are extrahepatic manifestations of PSC. Steatorrhea is therefore a result of pancreatic duct involvement and a decrease of the amount of bile in duodenal lumen.

In patient B, the diagnosis was PSC, i.e. NUC involving the left side of the large intestine, moderate activity, and exacerbation stage. Chronic pancreatitis with mild excretory insufficiency of the pancreas was observed.

Since early 2001, patient B has been administered the following treatment: Ursofalk 20 mg/kg constantly, Salofalk 1 g/day in courses of 6–7 months with interruptions for 2–3 months, and Budenofalk 6 mg/day permanently. Taking into account steatorrhea, patient B constantly takes Creon 120,000 U FIP per day.

We chose the ursodeoxycholic acid (UDCA) preparation Ursofalk on the basis of evidence-based studies. Four placebo-controlled studies were conducted. They showed that UDCA application leads to a significant decrease of activity of alkaline phosphatase, γ-glutamyltransferase and transaminases; in three studies there was a decrease of bilirubin blood level, and in three studies a reduction of inflammatory infiltrates in periportal tracts on the background of the same degree of biliary duct changes. A positive influence of UDCA on the intensity of clinical manifestations (itching and general weakness) remains doubtful. Treatment should be permanent, i.e. lifelong. Treatment interruption leads to relapses [1].

Ordinary high doses of UDCA are prescribed in PSC. Rost et al. [23] studied 86 bile samples obtained from 56 patients with PSC; the UDCA dosage was 10–32 mg/kg. Saturation of bile with UDCA increased depending on dose elevation, but at a dose of 22–25 mg/kg a concentration plateau formed, so a further dose increase was inadvisable. Cullen et al. [24] showed that only with a high dosage of UDCA (30 mg/kg) could an increased lifespan of 1–4 years be reached in PSC patients. The authors assessed the histological changes in liver according to the Ludwig scale, which includes inflammation activity and fibrosis grade. According to this scale, on the background of UDCA therapy with a dose of 30 mg/kg over 2 years, the histological state of the liver remained stable and an improvement was even noticed (19%). In a study reported by Stiehl et al. [25], the Mayo Risk Score remained stable throughout the long period of therapy with UDCA. Components of the Mayo Risk Score include age, serum bilirubin level, prothrombin time, serum albumin concentration, and presence of edema and ascites.

PSC – precancerous pathology: the risk of cholangiocarcinoma in PSC is increased by 161 times, the risk of colorectal cancer by 10 times, and the risk of pancreatic cancer by 14 times. *Incidence of cholangiocarcinoma:* in PSC it is 6–20% and in colorectal cancer 9% after 10 years and 50% after 25 years. The colorectal cancer risk is also considerably higher in NUC in combination with PSC than in NUC without PSC [1, 13]. It was shown that UDCA is an effective remedy for colorectal cancer and cholangiocarcinoma prophylaxis in PSC patients [1, 13]. Stiehl et al. [26] showed that a combination of UDCA and endoscopic dilatation of bile ducts led to a decreased incidence of cholangiocarcinoma of 2.8%. *Absence of UDCA therapy:* this is an independent predictor of cholangiocarcinoma development, while application of UDCA significantly decreases its risk [27]. Long therapy with UDCA (>6 years) decreases the risk of cholangiocarcinoma depending on the duration of treatment [28]. Application of 8–10 mg/kg UDCA over 3 years reduces the frequency of relapses of large intestine adenomas by 12% and the frequency of determination of high-grade dysplasia by 39% [29]. Evaluation of results of studies conducted in Germany where patients were observed over 8 years showed that a combination of endoscopic dilatation of bile ducts and therapy with UDCA significantly increased patients' life span, even without liver transplantation [30].

Taking into account insufficient efficacy of systemic corticosteroids in PSC and the high probability of osteoporosis due to steatorrhea in our patient, we decided to prescribe budesonide (Budenofalk). Several pilot studies were conducted regarding the effectiveness of budesonide in PSC treatment. For example, Angulo et al. [31] examined 21 patients with PSC who received budesonide 9 mg/day during a year. The results obtained were a significant decrease of alkaline phosphatase and AST activity; also, the budesonide effect remained for over 3 months after drug withdrawal.

Results of the second liver biopsy of patient B (in 2005): there was no PSC progression, but infiltration around the ducts even decreased. There were no exacerbations of NUC during the past 3 years. Currently, patient B does not have any itching or jaundice, but mild reduction of fecal elastase-1 remains. Biochemistry at the beginning of 2008 was: alkaline phosphatase 1.5–3, γ-glutamyltransferase 2.5–3, alanine aminotransferase up to 1.5, and normal bilirubin. The patient is on a transplant waiting list.

To conclude, it is necessary to study first-degree relatives and siblings of patients with PSC, especially in case a patient has a monozygotic twin. In our clinic, timely diagnosed PSC in one of the co-twins allowed us to improve the course of the disease and avoid complications for 7 years.

Disclosure Statement

The author declares that no financial or other conflict of interest exists in relation to the content of this article.

References

1 Leuschner U: Autoimmunkrankheiten der Leber und Overlapsyndrome. Bremen, Uni-Med Verlag, 2001.
2 O'Mahony CA, Vierling JM: Etiopathogenesis of primary sclerosing cholangitis. Semin Liver Dis 2006;26:3–21.
3 Worthington J, Cullen S, Chapman R: Immunopathogenesis of primary sclerosing cholangitis. Clin Rev Allergy Immunol 2005; 28:93–103.
4 Saarinen S, Olerup O, Broome U: Increased frequency of autoimmune diseases in patients with primary sclerosing cholangitis. Am J Gastroenterol 2000;95:3195–3199.
5 Bergquist A, Lindberg G, Saarinen S, Broome U: Increased prevalence of primary sclerosing cholangitis among first-degree relatives. J Hepatol 2005;42:252–256.
6 Angulo P, Peter JB, Gershwin ME, DeSotel CK, Shoenfeld Y, Ahmed AE, et al: Serum autoantibodies in patients with primary sclerosing cholangitis. J Hepatol 2000;32: 182–187.

7 Bjornsson E, Cederborg A, Akvist A, Simren M, Stotzer PO, Bjarnason I: Intestinal permeability and bacterial growth of the small bowel in patients with primary sclerosing cholangitis. Scand J Gastroenterol 2005;40: 1090–1094.

8 Pohl J, Ring A, Stremmel W, Stiehl A: The role of dominant stenoses in bacterial infections of bile ducts in primary sclerosing cholangitis. Eur J Gastroenterol Hepatol 2006;18: 69–74.

9 Bjornsson ES, Kilander AF, Olsson RG: Bile duct bacterial isolates in primary sclerosing cholangitis and certain other forms of cholestasis – a study of bile cultures from ERCP. Hepatogastroenterology 2000;47: 1504–1508.

10 Kulaksiz H, Rudolph G, Kloeters-Plachky P, Sauer P, Geiss H, Stiehl A: Biliary *Candida* infections in primary sclerosing cholangitis. J Hepatol 2006;45:711–716.

11 Tietz PS, Larusso NF: Cholangiocyte biology. Curr Opin Gastroenterol 2006;22:279–287.

12 Lazandis KN, Strazzabosco M, Larusso NF: The cholangiopathies disorders of biliary epithelia. Gastroenterology 2004;127:1565–1577.

13 Weismüller TS, Wedemeyer J, Kubicka S, Strassburg CP, Manns MP: The challenges in primary sclerosing cholangitis – aetiopathogenesis, autoimmunity, management and malignancy. Hepatology 2008;48(suppl 1):38–57.

14 Norris S, Kondeatis E, Collins R, Satsangi J, Clare M, Chapman R, et al: Mapping MHC-encoded susceptibility and resistance in primary sclerosing cholangitis the role of MICA polymorphism. Gastroenterology 2001;120: 1475–1482.

15 Donaldson PT, Norris S: Evaluation of the role of MHC class II alleles, haplotypes and selected amino acid sequences in primary sclerosing cholangitis. Autoimmunity 2002; 35:555–564.

16 Henckaerts L, Fevery J, Van Stecnbergen W, Verslype C, Yap P, Nevens F, et al: CC-type chemokine receptor 5-Δ32 mutation protects against primary sclerosing cholangitis. Inflamm Bowel Dis 2006;12:272–277.

17 Eri R, Jonsson JR, Pandeya N, Purdie DM, Clouston AD Martin N, et al: CCR5-Δ32 mutation is strongly associated with primary sclerosing cholangitis. Genes Immun 2004; 5:444–450.

18 Yang X, Cullen SN, Li JH, Chapman RW, Jewell DP: Susceptibility to primary sclerosing cholangitis is associated with polymorphisms of intercellular adhesion molecule-1. J Hepatol 2004;40:375–379.

19 Bowlus CL, Karlsen TH, Broome U, Thorsby E, Vatn M Schrumpf E, et al: Analysis of MAdCAM-1 and ICAM-1 polymorphisms in 365 Scandinavian patients with primary sclerosing cholangitis. J Hepatol 2006;45: 704–710.

20 Gallegos-Orozco JF, Yurk CE, Wang N, Rakela J, Charlton MR, Cutting GR, et al: Lack of association of common cystic fibrosis transmembrane conductance regulator gene mutations with primary sclerosing cholangitis. Am J Gastroenterol 2005;100: 874–878.

21 Nakazawa T, Ohara H, Sano H, Ando T, Imai H, Takada H, et al: Difficulty in diagnosing autoimmune pancreatitis by imaging findings. Gastrointest Endosc 2007;65:99–108.

22 Pickartz T, Mayerle J, Lerch MM: Autoimmune pancreatitis. Nat Clin Pract Gastroenterol Hepatol 2007;4:314–323.

23 Rost C, Rudolph G, Klœters-Plachky P, Stiehl A: Effect of high-dose ursodeoxycholic acid on its biliary enrichment in primary sclerosing cholangitis. Hepatology 2004;40: 693–698.

24 Cullen SN, Rust C, Fleming K, Beuers U, Chapman RW: High-dose ursodeoxycholic acid for the treatment of primary sclerosing cholangitis is safe and effective. J Hepatol 2006;44(suppl):A635.

25 Stiehl A, Walker S, Stiehl L, Rudolph G, Hofmann WJ, Theilmann L: Effect of ursodeoxycholic acid on liver and bile duct disease in primary sclerosing cholangitis. A 3-year pilot study with a placebo-controlled study period. J Hepatol 1994;20:57–64.

26 Stiehl A, Rudolph G, Klœters-Plachky P, Sauer P, Walker S: Development of dominant bile duct stenoses in patients with primary sclerosing cholangitis treated with ursodeoxycholic acid: outcome after endoscopic treatment. J Hepatol 2002;36:151–156.

27 Brandsaeter B, Isoniemi H, Broome U, Olausson M, Backman L, Hansen B, et al: Liver transplantation for primary sclerosing cholangitis; predictors and consequences of hepatobiliary malignancy. J Hepatol 2004; 40:815–822.

28 Rudolph G, Klœters-Plachky P, Rost D, Stiehl A: The incidence of cholangiocarcinoma in primary sclerosing cholangitis after long-time treatment with ursodeoxycholic acid. Eur J Gastroenterol 2007;19: 487–491.

29 Alberts DS, Martinez ME, Hess LM, Einspahr JG, Green SB, Bhattacharyya AK, et al: Phase III trial of ursodeoxycholic acid to prevent colorectal adenoma recurrence. J Natl Cancer Inst 2005;97:846–853.

30 Stiehl A, Rudolph G, Sauer P, Benz C, Stremmel W, Walker S, Theilmann L: Efficacy of ursodeoxycholic acid treatment and endoscopic dilation of major duct stenoses in primary sclerosing cholangitis. An 8-year prospective study. J Hepatol 1997;26:560–566.

31 Angulo P, Batts KP, Jorgensen RA, LaRusso NA, Lindor KD: Oral budesonide in the treatment of primary sclerosing cholangitis. Am J Gastroenterol 2000;95:2333–2337.

Surveillance and Screening of Primary Sclerosing Cholangitis

Amr El Fouly   Alexander Dêchene   Guido Gerken

Gastroenterology and Hepatology Department, Essen University Hospital, Essen, Germany

Key Words
Primary sclerosing cholangitis, surveillance · Cholangiocarcinoma, imaging techniques · Cholangioscopy, ERC brush cytology · EUS fine-needle biopsy

Abstract
Primary sclerosing cholangitis (PSC) represents an idiopathic chronic cholestatic liver disease due to inflammatory destruction of the biliary tree. Clinically, the progressive disease leads to biliary cirrhosis in association with cholangiocarcinoma in 6–20% of the patients. Currently, liver transplantation remains the only life-extending treatment option in end-stage disease. However, due to the high risk of carcinoma development, PSC patients should be tightly screened and evaluated including newer technologies like endoscopic ultrasound-guided fine-needle aspiration biopsy and cholangioscopy including cytology and direct biopsy of the biliary mucosal lesions.

Copyright © 2009 S. Karger AG, Basel

Introduction

Primary sclerosing cholangitis (PSC) is defined as an idiopathic, chronic, cholestatic, liver disease characterized by inflammatory destruction of the biliary tree. Males have a higher incidence (60–80%), and it is common among the middle-aged population (30–60 years). The clinical course is very variable; progressive obliteration of the biliary tree leads to biliary cirrhosis and its complications in a significant proportion of patients [1–3]. The most dismal sequel of PSC is the occurrence of hepatobiliary carcinomas, especially cholangiocarcinoma (CCA) in 6–20% of patients [4–9]. Additionally, PSC is closely linked to inflammatory bowel disease (IBD), particularly ulcerative colitis, which is found in approximately two-thirds of patients with PSC [10]. The etiology of PSC is still unknown. Although it is associated with multiple autoantibodies, PSC is not a typical autoimmune disease and responds poorly to immunosuppressive therapies. In children, however, the clinical course and treatment of PSC might be different, in particular the overlap of PSC with autoimmune hepatitis is more often found in children than in adults [11–13]. Currently, liver transplantation remains the only life-extending treatment option in cases of end-stage PSC, and recently in combination with neoadjuvant radiochemotherapy in CCA [14].

Geographical Distribution of PSC

In a recent study, the incidence and prevalence of PSC have been found to be more common than previously believed. Scandinavian countries have the highest number

Table 1. Epidemiology of PSC [16]

Region	Time	Incidence (per 100,000/year)	Prevalence (per 100,000/year)
Norway	1986–1995	1.3	8.5
Wales, UK	1984–2003	0.9	12.7
Minnesota, USA	1976–2000	0.9	13.6
Spain[1]	1984–1988	0.07	0.22
Singapore[2]	1989–1998	NA	1.3
Alaska, USA	1983–2000	0	0

NA = Not available.
[1] Based on a questionnaire sent to gastroenterologists in parts of the country.
[2] Ten cases diagnosed over a 10-year period, giving a maximum prevalence of 1.3.

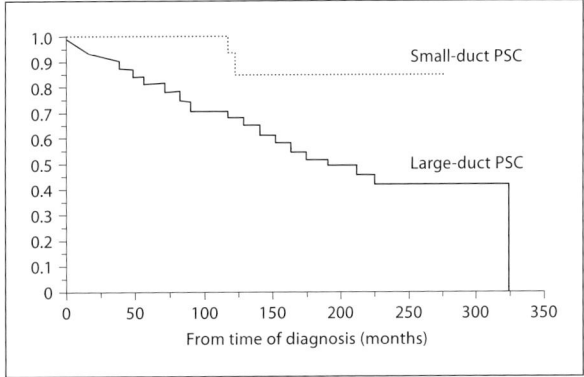

Fig. 1. Kaplan-Meier estimated survival curves for patients with small-duct and large-duct PSC (p < 0.01) [35].

of PSC patients, and it is considered as the single leading cause for liver transplantation [15]. The incidence is 0.9–1.3 per 100,000 in Northern Europe [16–18] and the USA [19], but <0.1 per 100,000 in Southern Europe [20] and Asia [21]. The survival rate of PSC ranges from 12 to 17 years, so that the prevalence of this disease in these same surveys ranges from 8 to 14 per 100,000 persons in Northern Europe and the USA, but is 1.3 or less in Southern Europe and Asia. The situation in Africa is unknown [16–22] (table 1).

Pathogenesis of PSC

The main cause of PSC is still unknown. Genetic abnormalities of the immune regulation, viral infection, toxins from intestinal bacteria, bacteria in the portal venous system and toxic bile acids from intestinal bacteria could have a role in the pathogenesis of PSC. However, immunopathogenetic mechanisms are likely involved because an association with human leukocyte antigen (HLA) complex haplotypes, multiple autoantibodies, and the presence of IBD is found in more than 80% of PSC patients [23, 24]. Correspondingly, an increased prevalence of HLA class I A1 as well as HLA class II B8 and DR3 is observed in PSC patients [25, 26]. Rapid disease progression in the presence of DR4 has been described but was subsequently discussed rather controversially [27–30].

PSC is associated with multiple autoantibodies, but most closely with atypical perinuclear antineutrophil cytoplasmic antibody (33–87%), antinuclear antibody (7–77%) and anti-smooth muscle antibody (13–20%), and there is no proof that these autoantibodies play a pathological role in the development of PSC.

PSC – Clinical Consequences and Prognosis

PSC is a disease with a variable clinical course, with progressive obliteration of the biliary tree leading to biliary cirrhosis and its complications such as portal hypertension and liver failure [3, 31]. Therefore, the clinical presentation of those patients could range between asymptomatic patients, symptomatic, advanced liver disease and/or malignancy (CCA) which may occur at any time, and they will require liver transplantation within a short time to those who remain asymptomatic for decades. Median survival from time of diagnosis to death or liver transplantation is estimated to be between 9 and 18 years and increases to 26 years if only death is used as a single endpoint [3, 8, 10, 31–33]. Asymptomatic patients have a significantly better prognosis than those with symptoms, but up to 17% of asymptomatic patients present with cirrhosis on liver biopsy at the time of diagnosis [10, 34].

The Kaplan-Meier estimated survival curve in figure 1 [35] shows longer survival rates have been demonstrated in patients with small-duct PSC compared to large-duct disease, with p < 0.01 statistical significance, and no development of CCA was found. Some patients, however, progress to classic PSC and/or end-stage liver disease with consequent necessity of OLT [36–38].

Table 2. Role of tumor markers in PSC [40]

	Sensitivity, %	Specificity, %	PPV, %	NPV, %
CA19-9	63 (38)	50 (81)	16 (38)	90 (91)
CEA	33	85	29	88

Sensitivity, specificity, positive predictive value (PPV) and negative predictive value (NPV) for CCA, using 37 ng/ml as the cut-off level for CA19-9 and 5 ng/ml for CEA. The values in parentheses show the same data but with a cut-off level of 200 ng/ml for CA19-9.

On the basis of clinical variables proven to correlate independently with prognosis, predicting survival is of great importance for defining a strategy of therapy and for timing OLT. Thus, many prognostic models and risk scores have been constructed. Most of the models include age and serum bilirubin. Kim et al. [39] developed the revised Mayo score on the basis of the course of disease in multicenter large number of PSC patients [40].

In this score, the need for liver biopsy has been eliminated, and thus the most important drawback of previous models is avoided. However, the mainstay of diagnosis has been cholangiography, and therefore it seems obvious to develop predictors based on cholangiographic abnormalities. A recent study from the Netherlands demonstrated that a cholangiographic classification system reflects disease stage and has the potential to serve as a predictor in determining prognosis [8]. In a more recent study with 273 PSC patients, consecutively, cholangiographic changes including the distribution of PSC manifestation as well as the presence of dominant bile duct stenosis were included together with other clinical parameters in a novel prognostic model ('PSC score') [3]. Compared with the Model for End-Stage Liver Disease score, revised Mayo score, and Child-Pugh score, the PSC score has the highest concordance index [3]. Nevertheless, the major limitation of all prognostic models is the inability to predict CCA development.

Role of Tumor Markers in PSC

Tumor markers play a limited role in early detection of CCA in PSC patients. Björnsson et al. [40] have screened a group of CCA patients with concomitant PSC for serum tumor markers (CA19-9 and CEA). They found only 56% had CA19-9 values above the upper reference value (37 ng/ml) and only 33% had values >300 ng/ml – the cut-off value suggested by the King's College Hospital group [40]. The PSC patients with IBD but without CCA had higher levels of CA19-9 (171 ng/ml) compared with patients without a concomitant IBD (56 ng/ml), although the difference did not reach statistical significance.

As shown in table 2, the sensitivity of CA19-9 in detecting CCA in the PSC patients (cut-off value 37 ng/ml) is only 63%, and the sensitivity of CEA was lower, although the specificity was relatively high. When the cut-off value of 200 ng/ml for CA19-9 was used, the sensitivity was lower (38%), but, as might be expected, a higher specificity (81%) was detected. However, the positive predictive value was only 38% when using 200 ng/ml as the upper normal range in those PSC patients [40, 41]. Nichols et al. [42] demonstrated 89% sensitivity and 86% specificity for CA19-9 in the same situation, using a cut-off value of 100 ng/ml. Benign extrahepatic cholestatic disease has been shown to increase the serum levels of CA19-9, with decreasing levels after the resolution of the cholestatic picture [43]. In benign cholestasis, a correlation has been demonstrated between CA19-9 and serum alkaline phosphate levels [43, 44].

Imaging in PSC

The diagnosis of PSC is based on characteristic cholangiographic changes in ERCP or PTC with supportive clinical, laboratory and pathologic findings. The imaging hallmarks are multiple segmental intra- and extrahepatic strictures, diverticular outpouchings, beaded ducts and a pruned appearance of the biliary tree as shown in figure 2. The strictures can be as short as 1–2 mm or may be several centimeters [45, 46].

In a recent case-control study by Fulcher et al. [47] showing the ability of MRC to distinguish PSC specifically in comparison to those with other hepatobiliary diseases, sensitivities of 85–88% and specificities of 92–97% were achieved. However, it is recognized that MRC has limitations in evaluating non-dilated ducts. Normal third- and fourth-order intrahepatic ductal branches are not well demonstrated in a large proportion of patients with current techniques. MRC is likely insensitive to early changes of PSC, particularly in non-dilated ducts. On the other hand, MRC is relatively superior to ERCP in demonstrating dilated ducts above an obstruction. The investigators have noted that in some cases MRC may be deficient in determination of length of strictures below an obstructed duct [48].

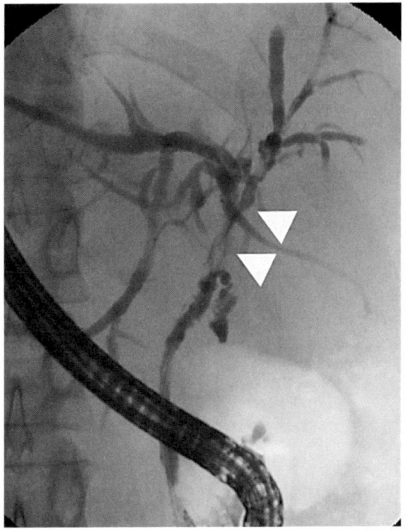 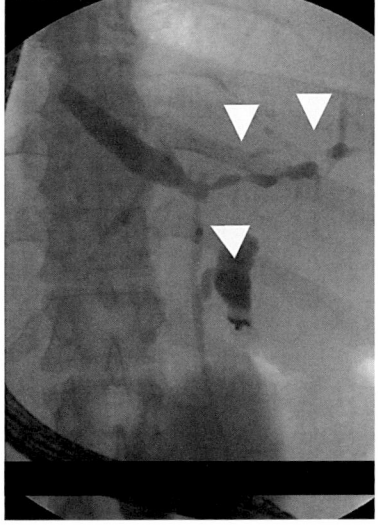 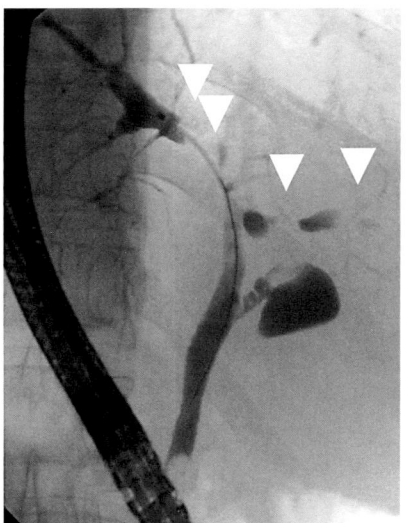

Common bile duct stenosis Common bile duct and right hepatic duct Right and left hepatic ducts

Fig. 2. Different types of PSC in ERC.

A full hepatic MRI has not only a role in initial diagnosis of PSC, but it also provides additional information about the status of the liver, spleen, varices, ascites, etc. CCA is a challenging outcome with PSC patients, and its diagnosis is difficult by ERCP. In respect to the role of MRC versus ERC in differentiation between CCA and benign stricture, Ashok [49] had retrospectively reviewed 89 patients (75 with CCA and 14 with benign cause of stricture) to assess the appearance of bile duct stricture. Final diagnosis was based on biopsy findings/surgical exploration. The sensitivity, specificity and accuracy of the two methods for the differentiation between malignant and benign strictures were 96, 85 and 91% respectively for MRCP and 80, 75 and 78% respectively for ERCP. Accuracy of MRCP is not only comparable but is also better than that of ERCP, especially in CCA. Hepatic MRI in combination with MRC and MR angiography can also provide a complete pretransplant evaluation in these patients.

Preoperative high-resolution CT scan (HRCT) accurately predicts resectability in patients with hilar CCA. Identification of specific radiographic features, in particular major vascular involvement and peritoneal abnormalities, is now used to avoid unnecessary laparotomy. Aloia et al. [50] performed a prospective study with 32 consecutive patients who underwent laparotomy for the diagnosis of hilar CCA. After preoperative assessment by helical HRCT (two contrast phases, rapid intravenous contrast bolus, 2.5 mm section thickness), 44% of the patients were unresectable (due to metastases) and 56% had resectable CCA. HRCT correctly predicted resectability in 17 of 18 patients who underwent therapeutic laparotomy (sensitivity 94%, specificity 79%). The negative predictive value (NPV) and positive predictive value (PPV) were 92 and 85%, respectively.

Positron emission tomography (PET) and positron emission and computed tomography (PET-CT) play no role in distinguishing between PSC and CCA. However, they could have role in evaluation and staging of CCA patients preoperatively. Kim [51] is leading a comparative study of 123 patients with suspected CCA between dynamic computed tomography (CT) and magnetic resonance imaging/magnetic resonance cholangiopancreatography (MRI/MRCP) with magnetic resonance (MR) angiography versus PET/PET-CT. The overall values for sensitivity, specificity, PPV, NPV, and accuracy of PET-CT in primary tumor detection were 84.0, 79.3, 92.9, 60.5, and 82.9%, respectively. PET-CT demonstrated no statistically significant advantage over CT and MRI/MRCP in the diagnosis of primary tumor, but it revealed significantly higher accuracy over CT in the diagnosis of regional lymph node metastases (75.9 vs. 60.9%, p = 0.004) and distant metastases (88.3 vs. 78.7%, p = 0.004).

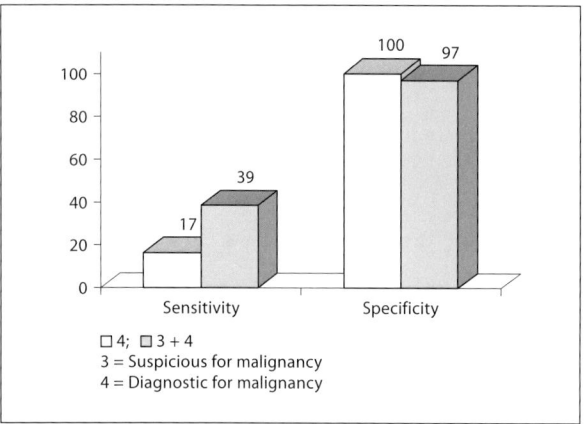

Fig. 3. Sensitivity and specificity of brush cytology in detection of CCA in PSC according to the traditional histological classification [52].

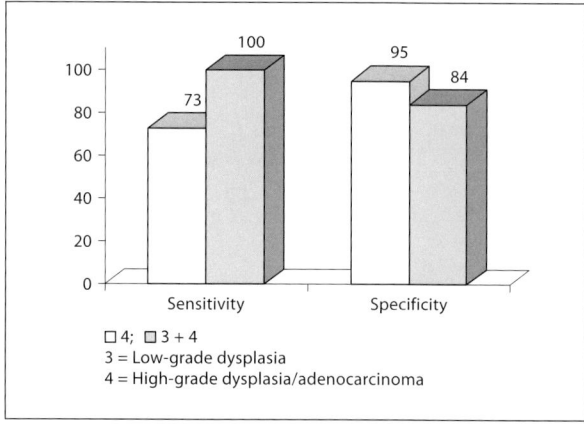

Fig. 4. Sensitivity and specificity of Brush cytology in detection of CCA in PSC patients according to the WHO histological classification [53].

Role of Cytology in PSC

In a prospective cytological analysis of 86 PSC patients, cytological diagnosis was classified according to traditional histological classification into four categories: (1) negative for malignancy, (2) atypical favoring reactive changes due to inflammation, (3) suspicious for malignancy, and (4) diagnostic for malignancy. When only specimens interpreted as diagnostic of malignancy were considered positive, the overall sensitivity was only 17%, but the specificity was perfect at 100%. If the specimens also interpreted as suspicious for malignancy were considered positive for cancer, the sensitivity increased to 39% and the specificity dropped minimally to 97% as shown in figure 3 [52]. Boberg et al. [53] have established accepted criterion for dysplasia in PSC at their institution. They examined the utility of biliary brush cytology in the diagnosis of CCA in patients with PSC. Cytology specimens were collected during ERC by stricture brushing and retrieved from a biliary stent after removal.

The WHO histological classification of tumors of the gallbladder and extrahepatic ducts [54] are classified into the following categories: (1) insufficient material for diagnosis, (2) normal and/or irregular non-dysplastic changes, indefinite for dysplasia, (3) low-grade dysplasia, and (4) high-grade dysplasia/adenocarcinoma. Accordingly, the sensitivity and specificity of brush cytology for the diagnosis of CCA were 100 and 84%, respectively, when low- and high-grade dysplasias were detected. They also observed a decrease in sensitivity and increase of specificity to 73 and 95%, respectively, for high-grade dysplasia/adenocarcinoma only (fig. 4) [53].

Nowadays, digital imaging analysis (DIA) and fluorescence in situ hybridization (FISH) are two cytological techniques that have been shown to have a promising and significant increase in diagnostic sensitivity of biliary tract malignancy over cytology while maintaining a high specificity of cytology [55, 56]. Both techniques are based on identifying aneuploidy, a hallmark of cancer [57]. DIA is a technique that uses a microscopic camera to quantify the amount of cellular DNA by measuring the intensity of nuclei stained with Feulgen dye, a cytochemical stain that stoichiometrically binds to nuclear DNA [58]. This technique is therefore able to quantitate aneuploidy in small cell populations. FISH is a technique that utilizes fluorescently labeled DNA probes to detect the chromosome number in cells and has been shown to detect malignancy in cytologic specimens from different body sites [59–61].

Therefore, in a prospective analysis of 86 PSC patients [52], the sensitivity and specificity were analyzed for DIA and FISH in samples where brush cytology was neither positive nor suspicious for malignancy. In this analysis, DIA had a sensitivity of 14% in tumors and a specificity of 88%. Thus, an additional 14% of tumors would be identified by employing DIA routinely while preserving the specificity of routine cytology (fig. 5). On the other hand, FISH had more than 60% sensitivity and 87% specificity

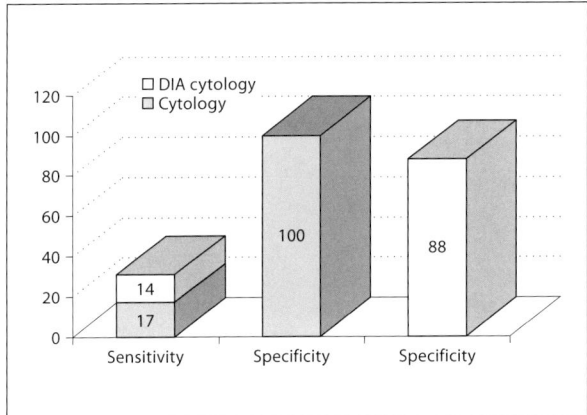

Fig. 5. Sensitivity and specificity of brush cytology versus DIA cytology in detection of CCA in PSC patients according to the traditional histological classification [52].

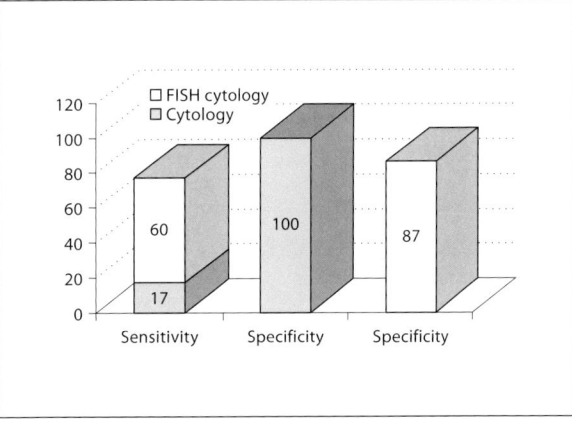

Fig. 6. Sensitivity and specificity of brush cytology versus FISH cytology in detection of CCA in PSC patients according to the traditional histological classification [52].

when brush cytology was neither positive nor suspicious of malignancy (fig. 6); therefore, FISH appears to be a more valuable adjunct to cytology in PSC with suspecting CCA.

Role of Molecular Markers in PSC

The addition of immunohistochemical examination for molecular markers such as p53 and K-ras mutation analysis did not improve the results in a previous study of brush cytology in PSC [62].

Role of Cholangioscopy in PSC

Reliable differentiation between benign and malignant dominant stenoses in PSC is challenging and very difficult, but it is very important to select the appropriate therapeutic modality, especially once an individual patient is considered to be a candidate for liver transplantation. Specific histological or cytological characteristics are required for a diagnosis of CCA; therefore, different techniques have recently been used together or in parallel with endoscopic brush cytology in order to improve results [63].

Recently, cholangioscopy has played an important role in early diagnosis of CCA and for definitive screening of small mucosal biliary lesions detected in non-icteric patients and has been helpful in diagnosing early malignant changes in patients with persistent PSC. Mapping biopsy for superficially spreading CCA is helpful in defining the proximal and distal extension of the tumor for further staging [64].

Tischendorf et al. [65] are leading a prospective screening of biliary stenotic lesions in patients with PSC in order to determine the diagnosis of CCA in PSC patients with dominant bile duct stenotic lesions, using cholangiography versus cholangioscopy comparing the cholangioscopic diagnosis with that of ERC. In this study, cholangiographic classification of the dominant bile duct stenoses resulted in a sensitivity of 66% and a specificity of 51% for malignancy that certainly is not sufficient for accurately determining the nature of a dominant bile duct stenosis. However, transpapillary cholangioscopy correctly identified 92% of the malignant stenoses and 93% of the benign stenoses, resulting in a sensitivity of 92%, a specificity of 93%, an accuracy of 93%, a PPV of 79%, and a NPV of 97% (as shown in table 3). The cholangioscopic appearances of mucosal changes were described and compared with the histological findings for the lesions.

In most of the CCA patients (75%), cholangioscopy revealed a polypoid or villous intraductal mass, while the minority has irregular and ulcerated mucosa. In the single patient with a false-negative diagnosis of malignant stenosis, erosive mucosal changes were noted in the stenotic area. On the other hand, benign stenoses were caused either by scarred strictures or by inflammatory

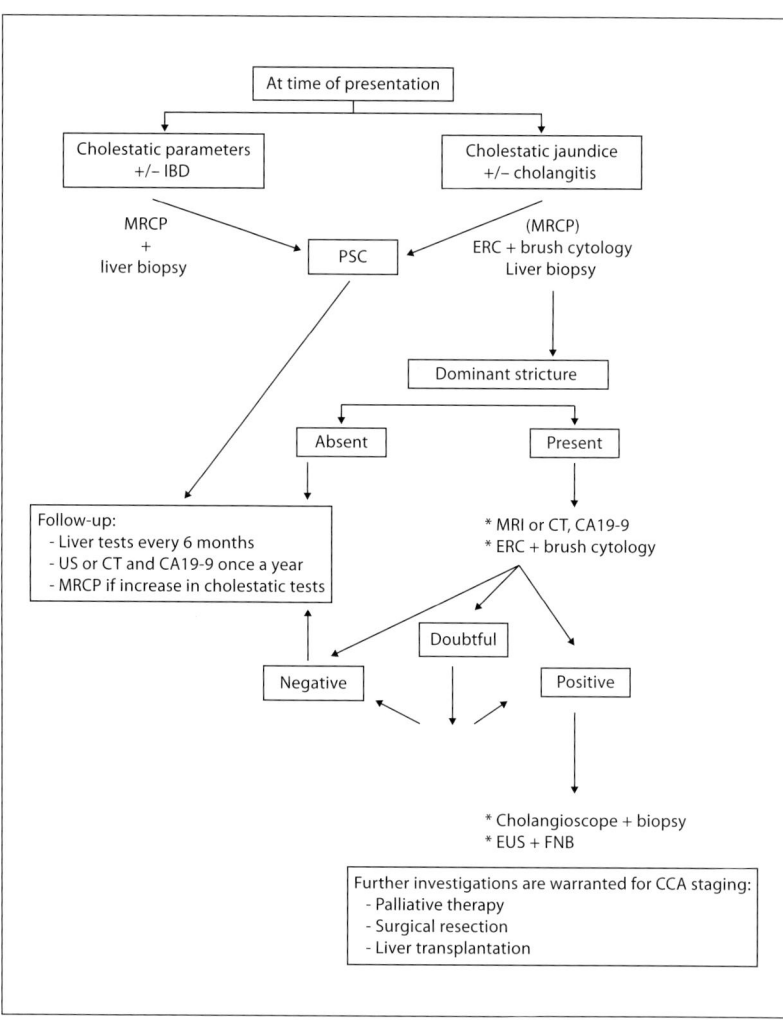

Fig. 7. Screening algorithm of PSC patients [68, 69].

Table 3. Role of endoscopic retrograde cholangiography (ERC) and cholangioscopy in differentiation between malignant and benign bile duct stenoses in patients with PSC (n = 53) [65]

	ERC, %	Cholangioscopy, %	p
Sensitivity	66	92	0.25
Specificity	51	93	<0.001
Accuracy	55	93	<0.001
PPV	29	79	<0.001
NPV	84	97	0.025

PPV = Positive predictive value; NPV = negative predictive value.

lesions, and the mucosa in the stricture segment was smooth and no surface irregularities were noted during cholangioscopy. The cholangioscopic findings in inflammatory stenoses ranged from vulnerable mucosa with redness to erosive and ulcerous mucosal changes with fibrinous coats. However, a combination of scarred and inflammatory characteristics was found in several cases. No complications directly attributable to cholangioscopy, such as biliary bleeding or bacterial cholangitis, were documented. The most important value of cholangioscopy is the direct macroscopic evaluation of the biliary tree in addition to directed targeted biopsies for further histopathological evaluation.

Role of EUS in PSC

After unsuccessful ERC brush cytology in PSC patients, experts considered the role of EUS-guided FNA (EUS-FNA) as a final option to exclude malignant biliary stenosis. Therefore, DeWitt et al. [66] screened 24 patients with PSC who underwent irrelevant ERCP brush cytology. The final diagnosis was determined by surgical pathology or the results of EUS-FNA at follow-up. EUS visualized a mass in 23 (96%) patients, including 13 in whom previous imaging detected no lesion. EUS-FNA demonstrated malignancy in 17 of 24 (71%) patients. No complications were noted. Pathology results from 8 of 24 (33%) patients who underwent surgery showed hilar CCA (n = 6), gallbladder cancer (n = 1), and a benign, inflammatory stricture (n = 1). Sensitivity, specificity, PPV, NPV, and accuracy of EUS-FNA were 77, 100, 100, 29, and 79%, respectively. And also in another study including 28 patients, sensitivity, specificity, PPV, NPV, and accuracy were 86, 100, 100, 57, and 88%, respectively. EUS-FNA had a positive impact on patient management in 84% of patients: preventing surgery for tissue diagnosis in patients with inoperable disease (n = 10), facilitating surgery in patients with unidentifiable cancer by other modalities (n = 8), and avoiding surgery in benign disease (n = 4) [67].

EUS-FNA is a sensitive method for the diagnosis of PBS following negative results or unsuccessful ERC brush cytology. The low NPV does not permit reliable exclusion of malignancy following a negative biopsy.

Screening Algorithm for PSC

As shown in figure 7 [68, 69], PSC patients should be closely screened and evaluated from the time of diagnosis in order to improve survival and final outcome. Evaluation of the liver state is mandatory and tight screening for early detection of CCA is warranted. This screening algorithm shows how to use the previously mentioned diagnostic and screening tools to tackle a case of PSC.

Disclosure Statement

The authors declare that no financial or other conflict of interest exists in relation to the content of this article.

References

1 Chapman RW, Marborgh BA, Rhodes JM, et al: Primary sclerosing cholangitis: a review of clinical features, cholangiography and hepatic histology. Gut 1980;21:870–877.
2 LaRusso NF, Wiesner RH, Ludwig J, et al: Primary sclerosing cholangitis. N Engl J Med 1984;310:899–903.
3 Tischendorf JJW, Hecker H, Krüger M, et al: Characterization, outcome, and prognosis in 273 patients with primary sclerosing cholangitis: a single-center study. Am J Gastroenterol 2007;102:107–114.
4 Wee A, Ludwig J, Coddey R, et al: Hepatobiliary carcinoma associated with primary sclerosing cholangitis and chronic ulcerative colitis. Hum Pathol 1985;16:719–726.
5 Rosen CB, Nagorney DM, Wiesner RH, et al: Cholangiocarcinoma complicating primary sclerosing cholangitis. Ann Surg 1991;213:21–25.
6 Farrant JM, Hayllar KM, Wilkinson ML, et al: Natural history and prognostic variables in primary sclerosing cholangitis. Gastroenterology 1991;100:1710–1717.
7 Broomé U, Olsson R, Lööf L, et al: Natural history and prognostic factor in 305 Swedish patients with primary sclerosing cholangitis. Gut 1996;38:610–615.
8 Ponsioen CY, Vrouenraets SME, Prawirodirdjo W, et al: Natural history of primary sclerosing cholangitis and prognostic value of cholangiography in a Dutch population. Gut 2002;51:562–566.
9 Tischendorf JJW, Meier PN, Strassburg C, et al: Characterization and clinical course of hepatobiliary carcinoma in patients with primary sclerosing cholangitis. Scand J Gastroenterol 2006;41:1227–1234.
10 Wiesner RH, Grambsch PB, Dickson ER, et al: Primary sclerosing cholangitis: natural history, prognostic factors and survival analysis. Hepatology 1989;10:430–436.
11 Wilschanski M, Chait P, Wade JA, et al: Primary sclerosing cholangitis in 32 children: clinical, laboratory, and radiographic features, with survival analysis. Hepatology 1995;22:1415–1422.
12 Gregorio GV, Portmann B, Karani J, et al: Autoimmune hepatitis/sclerosing cholangitis overlap syndrome in childhood: a 16-year prospective study. Hepatology 2001;33:544–553.

13 Feldstein AE, Perrault J, El-Youssif M, et al: Primary sclerosing cholangitis in children: a long-term follow-up study. Hepatology 2003; 38:210–217.
14 Graziadei IW, Wiesner RH, Marotta PJ, et al: Long-term results of patients undergoing liver transplantation for primary sclerosing cholangitis. Hepatology 1999;30:1121–1127.
15 Schrumpf E, Boberg KM: Epidemiology of primary sclerosing cholangitis. Best Pract Res Clin Gastroenterol 2001;15:553–562.
16 LaRusso NF, Shneider BL, Black D, et al: Primary sclerosing cholangitis: summary of a workshop. Hepatology 2006;44:746–764.
17 Boberg KM, Aadland E, Jahnsen J, et al: Incidence and prevalence of primary biliary cirrhosis, primary sclerosing cholangitis, and autoimmune hepatitis in a Norwegian population. Scand J Gastroenterol 1998;33:99–103.
18 Kingham JGC, Kochar N, Gravenor MB: Incidence, clinical pattern, and outcomes of primary sclerosing cholangitis in South Wales, United Kingdom. Gastroenterology 2004;126:1929–1930.
19 Bambha K, Kim WR, Talwalker J, et al: Incidence, clinical spectrum, and outcomes of primary sclerosing cholangitis in a United States community. Gastroenterology 2003; 125:1364–1369.
20 Escorsell A, Pares A, Rodes J, et al: Epidemiology of primary sclerosing cholangitis in Spain. Spanish Association for the Study of the Liver. J Hepatol 1994;21:787–791.
21 Ang TL, Fock KM, Ng TM, et al: Clinical profile of primary sclerosing cholangitis in Singapore. J Gastroenterol Hepatol 2002;17:908–913.
22 Hurlburt KJ, McMahon BJ, Deubner H, et al: Prevalence of autoimmune liver disease in Alaska Natives. Am J Gastroenterol 2002;97:2402–2407.
23 Angulo P, Peter JB, Gershwin ME, et al: Serum autoantibodies in patients with primary sclerosing cholangitis. J Hepatol 2000;32:182–187.
24 Worthington J, Cullen S, Chapman R: Immunopathogenesis of primary sclerosing cholangitis. Clin Rev Allergy Immunol 2005; 28:93–103.
25 Norris S, Kondeatis E, Collins R, et al: Mapping MHC-encoded susceptibility and resistance in primary sclerosing cholangitis: the role of MICA polymorphism. Gastroenterology 2001;120:1475–1482.
26 Donaldson PT, Norris S: Evaluation of the role of MHC class II alleles, haplotypes and selected amino acid sequences in primary sclerosing cholangitis. Autoimmunity 2002; 35:555–564.
27 Mehal WZ, Lo YM, Wordsworth BP, et al: HLA DR4 is a marker for rapid disease progression in primary sclerosing cholangitis. Gastroenterology 1994;106:160–167.

28 Olerup O, Olsson R, Hultcrantz R, Broomé U: HLA-DR and HLA-DQ are not markers for rapid disease progression in primary sclerosing cholangitis. Gastroenterology 1995;108:870–878.
29 Donaldson PT: Genetics of liver disease: immunogenetics and disease pathogenesis. Gut 2004;53:599–608.
30 Zein CO, Lindor KD, Angulo P: Prevalence and predictors of esophageal varices in patients with primary sclerosing cholangitis. Hepatology 2004;39:204–210.
31 Farrant JM, Hayllar KM, Wilkinson ML, et al: Natural history and prognostic variables in primary sclerosing cholangitis. Gastroenterology 1991;100:1710–1717.
32 Broomé U, Olsson R, Lööf L, et al: Natural history and prognostic factor in 305 Swedish patients with primary sclerosing cholangitis. Gut 1996;38:610–615.
33 Helzberg JH, Petersen JM, Boyer JL: Improved survival with primary sclerosing cholangitis. A review of clinicopathologic features and comparison of symptomatic and asymptomatic patients. Gastroenterology 1987;92:1869–1875.
34 Okolicsanyi L, Fabris L, Viaggi S, et al: Primary sclerosing cholangitis: clinical presentation, natural history and prognostic variables: an Italian multicentre study. Eur J Gastroenterol Hepatol 1996;8:685–691.
35 Björnsson E, Boberg KM, Cullen S, et al: Patients with small duct primary sclerosing cholangitis have a favourable long-term prognosis. Gut 2002;51:731–735.
36 Angulo P, Maor-Kendler Y, Lindor KD: Small-duct primary sclerosing cholangitis: a long-term follow-up study. Hepatology 2002; 35:1494–1500.
37 Björnsson E, Boberg KM, Cullen S, et al: Patients with small duct primary sclerosing cholangitis have a favourable long-term prognosis. Gut 2002;51:731–735.
38 Broomé U, Glaumann H, Lindström E, et al: Natural history and outcome in 32 Swedish patients with small duct primary sclerosing cholangitis (PSC). J Hepatol 2002;36:586–589.
39 Kim WR, Therneau TM, Wiesner RH, et al: Revised natural history model for primary sclerosing cholangitis. Mayo Clin Proc 2000; 75:688–694.
40 Björnsson E, Kilander A, Olsson R: CA19-9 and CEA are unreliable markers for cholangiocarcinoma in patients with primary sclerosing cholangitis. Liver 1999;19:501–508.
41 Ramagje K, Donaghay, Farranj MT, et al: Serum tumor markers for the diagnosis of cholangiocarcinoma in primary sclerosing cholangitis. Gastroenterology 1995;108:865–869.
42 Nichols JC, Goresg J, Larusson F, et al: Diagnostic role of serum CA19-9 for cholangiocarcinoma in patients with primary sclerosing cholangitis. Mayo Clin Proc 1993;68:874–879.

43 Basso D, Meggiatto T, Fabris C, et al: Extrahepatic cholestasis determines a reversible increase of glycoproteic tumour markers in benign and malignant diseases. Eur J Clin Invest 1992;22:800–804.
44 Maestranzi S, Przemioslo R, Mitchell H, et al: The effect of benign and malignant liver disease on the tumour markers CA19-9 and CEA. Ann Clin Biochem 1998;35:99–103.
45 Haider AM, Bret PM: The role of magnetic resonance cholangiography in primary sclerosing cholangitis. J Hepatol 2000;33:659–660.
46 Angulo P, Pearce DH, Johnson CD, et al: Magnetic resonance imaging in patients with biliary disease, its role in primary sclerosing cholangitis. J Hepatol 2000;33:520–527.
47 Fulcher AS, Turner MA, Franklin KJ, et al: Primary sclerosing cholangitis: evaluation with MR cholangiography: a case-control study. Radiology 2000;215:71–80.
48 Ernst O, Asselah T, Sergent G, et al: MR cholangiography in primary sclerosing cholangitis. Am J Roentgenol 1998;171:1027–1030.
49 Ashok KS: Role of MRCP versus ERCP in bile duct cholangiocarcinoma and benign stricture. Biomed Imaging Interv J 2007;3:e12–e545.
50 Aloia TA, Charnsangavej C, Faria S, et al: High-resolution computed tomography accurately predicts resectability in hilar cholangiocarcinoma. Am J Surg 2007;193:702–706.
51 Kim JY, Kim MH, Lee TY, et al: Clinical role of ^{18}F-FDG PET-CT in suspected and potentially operable cholangiocarcinoma: a prospective study compared with conventional imaging. Am J Gastroenterol 2008;103:1145–1151.
52 Moreno Luna LE, Kipp B, Halling K, et al: Advanced cytologic techniques for the detection of malignant pancreatobiliary strictures. Gastroenterology 2006;131:1064–1072.
53 Boberg KM, Jebsen P, Clausen OP, et al: Diagnostic benefit of biliary brush cytology in cholangiocarcinoma in primary sclerosing cholangitis. J Hepatol 2006;45:568–574.
54 Albores-Saavedra J, Henson DE, Sobin LH: The WHO histological classification of tumors of gallbladder and extrahepatic bile ducts. A commentary on the second edition. Cancer 1992;70:410–414.
55 Baron TH, Harewood GC, Rumalla A, et al: A prospective comparison of digital image analysis and routine cytology for the identification of malignancy in biliary tract stricture. Clin Gastroenterol Hepatol 2004;2:214–219.
56 Kipp BR, Stadheim LM, Halling SA, et al: A comparison of routine cytology and fluorescence in situ hybridization for the detection of malignant bile duct strictures. Am J Gastroenterol 2004;99:1675–1681.

57 Duesberg PH: Are cancers dependent on oncogenes or on aneuploidy? Cancer Genet Cytogenet 2003;143:89–91.
58 Sebo TJ: Digital image analysis. Mayo Clin Proc 1995;70:81–82.
59 Kipp BR, Karnes RJ, Brankley SM, et al: Monitoring intravesical therapy of superficial bladder cancer using fluorescence in situ hybridization. J Urol 2005;173:401–404.
60 Gu M, Ghafari S, Zhao M: Fluorescence in situ hybridization for HER-2/neu amplification of breast carcinoma in archival fine-needle aspiration biopsy specimens. Acta Cytol 2005;49:471–476.
61 Shibata T, Uryu S, Kokubu A, et al: Genetic classification of lung adenocarcinoma based on array-based comparative genomic hybridization analysis: its association with clinicopathologic features. Clin Cancer Res 2005;11:6177–6185.
62 Ponsioen CY, Vrouenraets SME, van Milligen de Witt AWM, et al: Value of brush cytology for dominant strictures in primary sclerosing cholangitis. Endoscopy 1999;31:305–309.
63 Lindberg B, Arnelo U, Bergquist A, et al: Diagnosis of biliary strictures in conjugation with endoscopic retrograde cholangiopancreatography, with special reference to patients with primary sclerosing cholangitis. Endoscopy 2002;34:909–916.
64 Nimura Y: Staging cholangiocarcinoma by cholangioscopy. HPB (Oxford) 2008;10:113–115.
65 Tischendorf JJ, Krüger M, Trautwein C, et al: Cholangioscopic characterization of bile duct stenoses in PSC. Endoscopy 2006;38:665–669.
66 DeWitt J, Misra VL, Leblanc JK, et al: EUS-guided FNA of proximal biliary strictures after negative ERCP brush cytology results. Gastrointest Endosc 2006;64:325–333.
67 Eloubeidi MA, Chen VK, Jhala NC, et al: Endoscopic ultrasound-guided fine-needle aspiration biopsy of suspected cholangiocarcinoma. Clin Gastroenterol Hepatol 2004;2:209–213.
68 Fevery J, Verslype C, Lai G, et al: Incidence, diagnosis, and therapy of cholangiocarcinoma in patients with primary sclerosing cholangitis. Dig Dis Sci 2007;52:3123–3135.
69 Weber A, Schmid RM, Prinz C: Diagnostic approaches for cholangiocarcinoma. World J Gastroenterol 2008;14:4131–4136.

Medical Management of Crohn's Disease: Treatment Algorithms 2009

Stephen B. Hanauer

Medicine and Clinical Pharmacology, Section of Gastroenterology, Hepatology, and Nutrition, University of Chicago Medical Center, Chicago, Ill., USA

Key Words
Crohn's disease, goals · Crohn's disease, medical management · Treatment algorithms

Abstract
There has been a continual evolution of therapy for Crohn's disease (CD) over the past decade since the introduction of biological therapies targeting tumor necrosis factor-α. Conventional agents continue to be safe and effective for patients with mild to moderately active CD and, in population series, less than half of the patients with CD require corticosteroid therapy. In contrast, patients presenting at young ages, those with extensive disease, deep ulcerations, transmural complications or extraintestinal complications that require corticosteroid therapy have a poor prognosis. Introduction of immunosuppressives late in the course or for patients with steroid-dependent or steroid-refractory disease have not changed the 'natural history' of CD or the need for eventual surgical resections. There is increasing evidence that early intervention with immunosuppressives or biologic agents at the same time as corticosteroids, or biologic agents targeting tumor necrosis factor or adhesion molecules, can have rapid and prolonged benefits, including steroid sparing, reductions in hospitalizations and, perhaps, reductions in the need for surgery. Treatment should be optimized according to the patient status and response with whichever level of therapy is introduced and maintained.

Copyright © 2009 S. Karger AG, Basel

Medical management of Crohn's disease (CD) is undergoing an evolution both related to evolving medical therapies, but also to treatment goals [1]. The current goals of treatment for CD are, primarily, clinical and include: induction and maintenance of response/remission according to clinical indices; prevention of complications related to the disease or therapy; improvement and maintenance of quality of life, and limiting the indications for surgery. Current 'guidelines' for the treatment of CD are based on evidence for 'induction of remission' and 'maintenance of remission' from clinical trials with single agents and advocate a 'step-up' approach to induction according to clinical 'severity' at entry into the trial [2, 3]. Patients with mild disease are treated with aminosalicylates (although their ultimate efficacy is controversial) or delayed-release budesonide; those with moderate-severe disease are treated with conventional corticosteroids; patients refractory to steroids receive a biologic anti-tumor necrosis factor (TNF) agent, and surgery is indicated for patients failing biologics. Patients can also be 'stepped up' in therapeutic class if they fail to respond to a less effective class figure 1.

The advantages of the 'step-up' approach are that many patients can be treated with less toxic agents reserving corticosteroids and biologics for patients with a demonstrable 'need' for more intensive therapy [4]. The approach also appears to minimize risk and may be cost-effective in the short term. However, potential disadvantages of the 'step-up' approach include the risk that

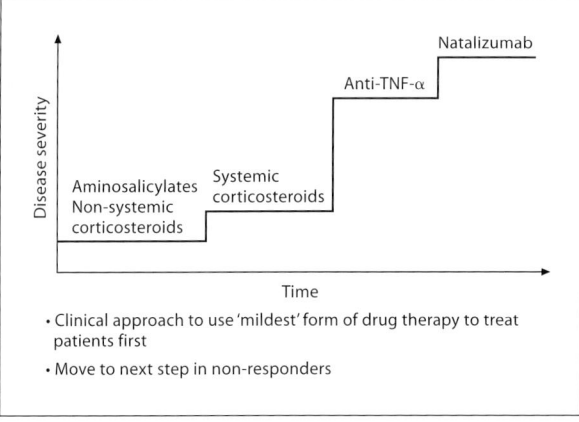

Fig. 1. Conventional approach to CD induction therapy.

patients must 'earn' a more effective therapy which decreases the quality of life before patients obtain an optimal response and the observations that conventional therapies have not altered the disease course towards transmural complications (strictures and fistulae) or the requisite for surgical resections. Hence, evaluation of the long-term economics of these conventional approaches needs to consider both direct and indirect costs of care over the lifetime of patients rather than simply accounting for the costs of a course of therapy.

While the field is moving towards a 'top-down', or 'early aggressive' management approach, it is important to consider that the majority of patients in population series never require corticosteroid management [5, 6]. Unfortunately, to date, we have not yet defined appropriate patient criteria to initiate a uniform early aggressive approach for every patient diagnosed with CD.

In addition, the concept of a therapeutic 'pyramid' for induction of response/remission based upon the severity of disease fails to take into account the concept that CD is a chronic, lifelong condition that requires both inductive and maintenance strategies. Furthermore, the therapy needed to induce remission will dictate what therapy will be effective (or ineffective) to maintain remission.

As an example, aminosalicylates, while efficacious for patients with mild to moderately active CD, may be effective at maintaining aminosalicylate-induced remissions (not yet studied in controlled clinical trials) [7]. In contrast, aminosalicylates are not effective at maintaining steroid-induced remissions. After corticosteroid induction, either immunosuppressants or biologics targeting TNF-α are required to maintain remissions. If anti-TNF agents are initiated to induce remissions, effective maintenance strategies will depend upon whether the patient is corticosteroid-naive or immunosuppressive-naive [8].

Another important consideration regarding the attainment of treatment goals in CD pertains to the duration of disease. CD is a transmural process that progresses towards the complications of stenoses and fistulae over the course [9, 10] (fig. 2).

At presentation, the majority of patients will have, primarily, an inflammatory phenotype that evolves over years towards the development of stricturing and fistulae. Therefore, since all current therapies target inflammatory mediators and none have had impact on fibrosis, it would be anticipated that intervention early in the course is more likely to have a significant impact than the introduction of therapies once a patient already has evidence of transmural complications. The impact of earlier intervention has been demonstrated both with conventional immunosuppressives and with biologic therapies.

A study of azathioprine in adult patients with chronic, active CD demonstrated that the addition of azathioprine to steroid-induction therapy maintained remissions in approximately 42% of patients after 1 year [11]. In contrast, a similar trial design in children with newly diagnosed CD who had never received corticosteroids reported that over 90% of children were in a clinical remission [12]. The difference between drug and placebo resulted was similar (~35%) for each trial, and hence the number needed to treat (~3); however, the absolute response rates between study populations were remarkably different (91 vs. 42%) (fig. 3, 4).

Studies with biologics in patients with chronic active CD also demonstrate consistency in demonstrating that patients with longer-duration disease are still more likely to respond than patients treated with placebo, but both the active treatment and placebo response rates decline with longer-duration disease [1, 4, 8, 13].

Enter biologic therapies with monoclonal antibodies or antibody fragments targeting TNF-α. There are currently three different biologic agents that are available in different countries [14]. Infliximab and adalimumab are IgG1 antibodies that have the potential to bind TNF in the circulation and on cell membranes, and induce apoptosis. Certolizumab pegol is a Fab' fragment bound to polyethylene glycol to maintain pharmacokinetics. All three have been evaluated in the induction and maintenance of patients with chronic active CD refractory to aminosalicylates, corticosteroids or immunosuppressives. The clinical trial designs leading to regulatory approval for these agents have demonstrated that open-la

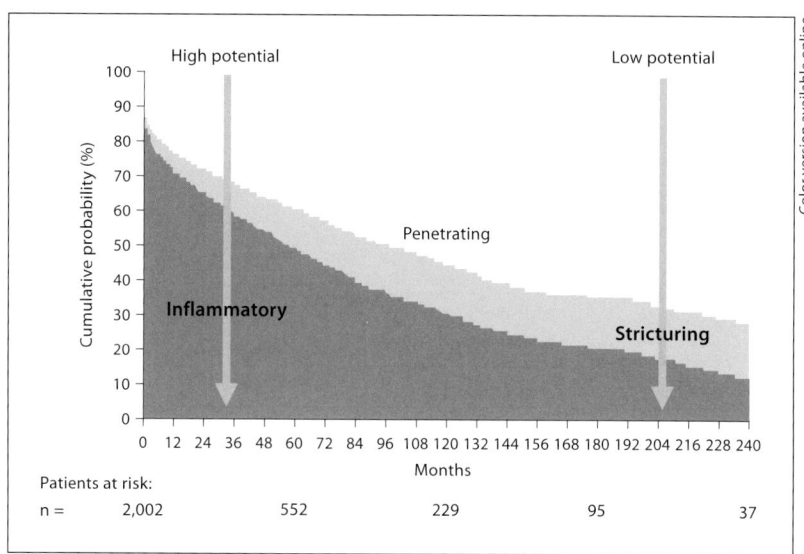

Fig. 2. Impact of therapy will depend on degree of structural damage and velocity of progression [from 9].

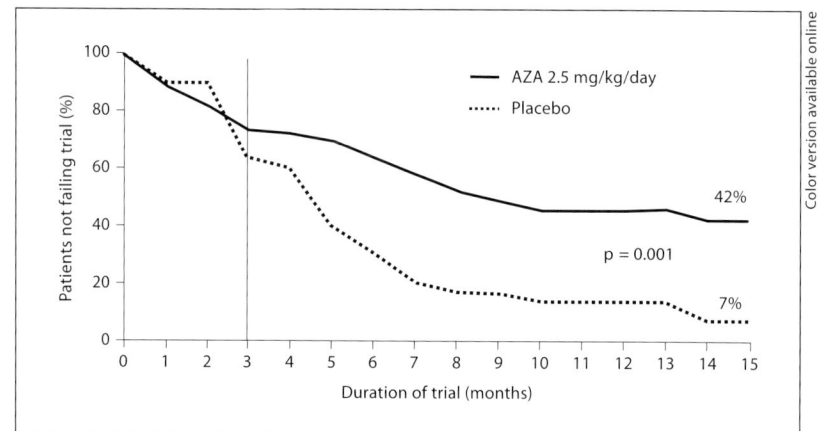

Fig. 3. Efficacy of AZA as CD maintenance therapy after steroids in adults. Remission induced by prednisolone tapered over 12 weeks. Inclusion: patients were not steroid-dependent [from 11].

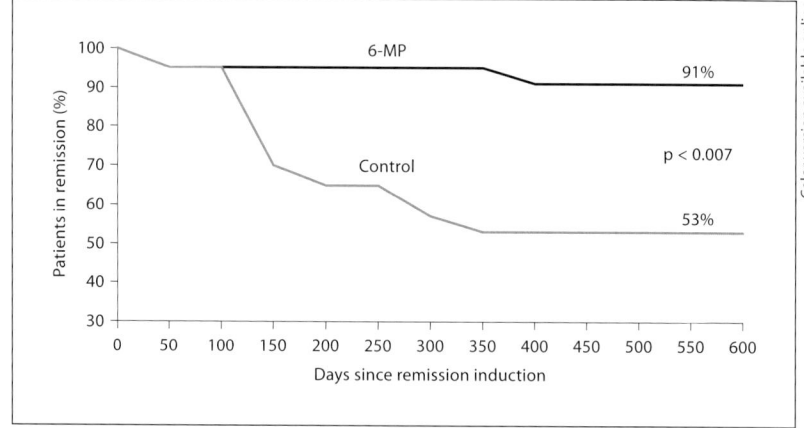

Fig. 4. Efficacy of 6-MP as CD maintenance therapy after steroids in steroid-naive children (n = 55). At baseline, patients received prednisone plus either 6-MP or placebo. Steroids tapered after induction of remission [from 12].

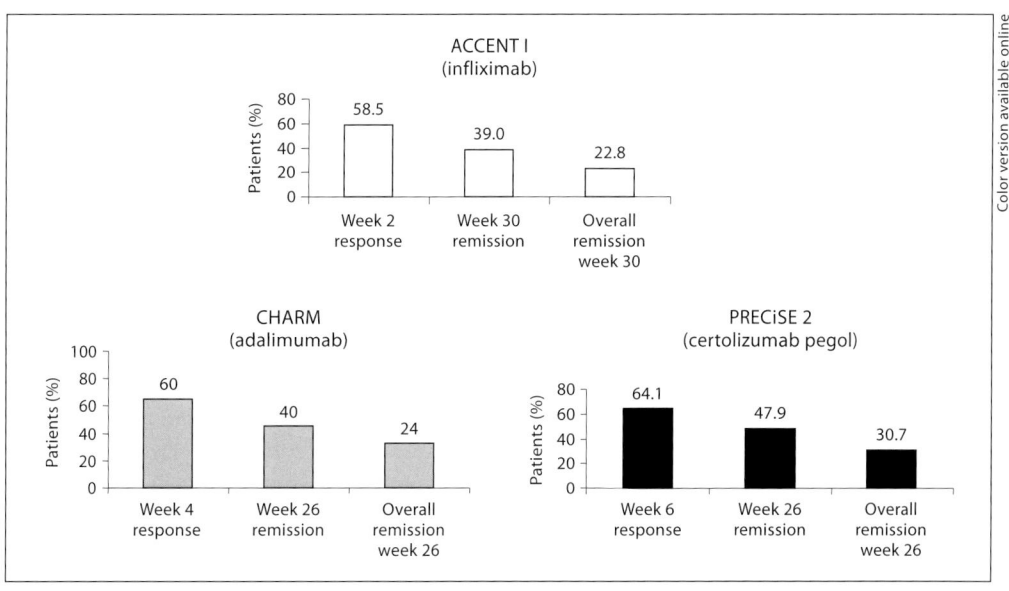

Fig. 5. Comparing ACCENT I, CHARM and PRECiSE 2 results.

bel induction with randomization of responders to maintenance therapy with active drug versus placebo have been the most efficient trial design [4]. Indeed, maintaining responders on long-term therapy mimics clinical practice in that non-responders are not 'exposed' to the risks (or costs) of ineffective treatment.

While studies directly comparing one agent with another have not been performed, comparing across trials demonstrates more similarity than differences. Acutely, approximately 60% of patients with active symptoms of CD despite a stable dose of aminosalicylates, corticosteroids, or immunosuppressants will have a significant reduction in the symptoms and signs that is maintained by regular dosing over 6–12 months [4, 8] (fig. 5).

Unfortunately, in the pivotal phase III studies, only 25–30% of patients will be in a steroid-free remission, although, in clinical experience [8], the long-term response rate is closer to 60% improving patient selection (confirmation of active mucosal disease) and dose modification (according to dose or dosing interval).

Most recently, three novel clinical trials using biologic agents have attempted to assess the impact of early aggressive intervention with biologic therapy as well as the role of concomitant therapy with biologics and immunosuppressants. In the 'top-down, step up' trial reported by D'Haens et al. [15], steroid-naive patients with relatively newly diagnosed CD were randomized to receive (a) an inductive course of corticosteroids followed by weaning or (b) and inductive course of infliximab. Patients who relapsed with corticosteroid tapering were given a second course of steroids and, if they relapsed, were then administered either azathioprine or placebo. If azathioprine failed to maintain remissions, patients could be treated, episodically, with infliximab. Patients induced with infliximab were also treated with azathioprine maintenance. If patients relapsed, they were allowed to receive episodic infliximab. The endpoints of the studies were clinical remission, steroid exposure and mucosal healing. While there were no statistical differences in remission rates at 1 year, patients treated with infliximab induction had significantly less steroid exposure and a remarkable rate of mucosal healing (70 vs. 30%) after 2 years. The trial suggests that corticosteroids, while efficacious at inducing clinical remission, may impair long-term mucosal healing rates.

The other two trials explored the role of concomitant immunosuppressants with infliximab to induce or maintain clinical remissions. The SONIC trial [16] randomized immunosuppressant-naive patients with *active* CD to receive: infliximab induction and maintenance monotherapy; azathioprine monotherapy, or infliximab induction and maintenance combined with azathioprine. In contrast to the pivotal phase III trials with infliximab, adalimumab or certolizumab pegol that revealed no statistical differences in outcome (or adverse effects) when the biologic was added to patients with active disease *despite* immunosuppressive therapy, the combination of infliximab plus azathioprine in immunosuppressive-naive patients with active disease was superior to monother-apy.

In contrast, the COMMITT trial [17] enrolled CD patients with chronic active CD who were induced into clinical remission with corticosteroids and were then randomized to infliximab induction and maintenance monotherapy, or combination therapy with infliximab induction/maintenance in combination with methotrexate. In patients with steroid-induced remissions, the combination of infliximab and methotrexate was no more beneficial than infliximab monotherapy in allowing a regimented steroid taper over 14 weeks and in maintaining remission over 1 year.

The reconciliation of these different clinical trial results suggests that combination therapy with steroids + infliximab, steroids + immunosuppressives, or infliximab + immunosuppressive are more efficacious than monotherapy for induction and maintenance of CD. Whether or not the combination of a biologic and immunosuppressive for immunosuppressive-naive patients is required for long-term maintenance or whether one agent can be withdrawn after a stable remission has been achieved remains to be established since evolving data suggest that long-term combination therapy may increase the risk of opportunistic infections and neoplasia [18–20].

Clinical trials need to be translated into clinical practice and the heterogeneity of patients and concomitant medications will require prospective assessment of patient subgroups and predictive factors to define optimal treatment strategies. Thus far, the consistency of an early aggressive approach with combination therapy appears to apply to patients with sufficiently severe disease to require corticosteroids. Patients who require steroid induction can be maintained with concomitant thiopurines or methotrexate [11, 12, 21]. Alternatively, results from the trial of D'Haens et al. [15] suggest that steroid-naive patients may also be induced with infliximab and maintained on a thiopurine. The comparative efficacy of these two approaches has not been evaluated.

Immunosuppressive-naive patients with moderate-severe activity require combined immunosuppression to induce and maintain remissions: either steroids + anti-TNF biologic [17] or anti-TNF + immunosuppressive [16]. Whether or not combination therapy will be required long term or the immunosuppressant or biologic can be withdrawn, and in what time frame, remains to be established.

In contrast, patients who are steroid-refractory/dependent despite immunosuppressive therapy require induction and maintenance with a biologic therapy targeting TNF [22–24]. In this situation, withdrawal of the immunosuppressant after 1 year of remission can be considered [25]. Patients who lose response to a biologic agent targeting TNF should be re-evaluated to assess whether or not symptoms are due to inflammation. If there is persistent inflammation and there is no evidence of immunogenicity (patients respond to each treatment but lose response prior to the next infusion or injection) can be treated with dose increases or reduced intervals between anti-TNF administrations. Patients with evidence of immunogenicity to an anti-TNF agent can be treated with an alternative anti-TNF [26]. Patients who lose response and have no response to a second anti-TNF have the opportunity for natalizumab therapy in countries where the anti-adhesion molecule is available [27, 28].

As more therapies become available for the treatment of CD, our goals of therapy will continue to evolve. While at present our goals are primarily clinical, in the future therapies will be directed more at inducing and maintaining inflammatory remissions with additional goals of mucosal healing, disease modification (prevention of structural damage) and will include pharmacoeconomic endpoints until the eventual cause is identified, and we will be able to prevent the disease from developing in susceptible individuals.

Disclosure Statement

The author is a consultant for: Abbott Laboratories, Centocor, Schering Plough, UCB Pharma, Prometheus Laboratories, Elan/Biogen, Procter & Gamble, Ferring, Shire and Salix.

References

1 Vermeire S, van Assche G, Rutgeerts P: Review article: altering the natural history of Crohn's disease – evidence for and against current therapies. Aliment Pharmacol Ther 2007;25:3–12.
2 Lichtenstein GR, Hanauer SB, Sandborn WJ: Management of Crohn's disease in adults. Am J Gastroenterol 2009;104:465–484.
3 Travis SP, Stange EF, Lemann M, Oresland T, Chowers Y, Forbes A, et al: European evidence-based consensus on the diagnosis and management of Crohn's disease: current management. Gut. 2006;55(suppl 1):i16–i35.

4 Hanauer SB: Positioning biologic agents in the treatment of Crohn's disease. Inflamm Bowel Dis 2009 (in press).
5 Faubion WA Jr, Loftus EV Jr, Harmsen WS, Zinsmeister AR, Sandborn WJ: The natural history of corticosteroid therapy for inflammatory bowel disease: a population-based study. Gastroenterology 2001;121:255–260.
6 Munkholm P, Langholz E, Davidsen M, Binder V: Frequency of glucocorticoid resistance and dependency in Crohn's disease. Gut 1994;35:360–362.
7 Hanauer SB: The case for using 5-aminosalicylates in Crohn's disease: pro. Inflamm Bowel Dis 2005;11:609–612.
8 Rutgeerts P, Vermeire S, Van Assche G: Biological therapies for inflammatory bowel diseases. Gastroenterology 2009;136:1182–1197.
9 Beaugerie L, Seksik P, Nion-Larmurier I, Gendre JP, Cosnes J: Predictors of Crohn's disease. Gastroenterology 2006;130:650–656.
10 Cosnes J, Cattan S, Blain A, Beaugerie L, Carbonnel F, Parc R, et al: Long-term evolution of disease behavior of Crohn's disease. Inflamm Bowel Dis 2002;8:244–250.
11 Candy S, Wright J, Gerber M, Adams G, Gerig M, Goodman R: A controlled double-blind study of azathioprine in the management of Crohn's disease. Gut 1995;37:674–678.
12 Markowitz J, Grancher K, Kohn N, Lesser M, Daum F: A multicenter trial of 6-mercaptopurine and prednisone in children with newly diagnosed Crohn's disease. Gastroenterology 2000;119:895–902.
13 Van Assche G, Vermeire S, Rutgeerts P: Optimizing treatment of inflammatory bowel diseases with biologic agents. Curr Gastroenterol Rep 2008;10:591–596.
14 Clark M, Colombel JF, Feagan BC, Fedorak RN, Hanauer SB, Kamm MA, et al: American Gastroenterological Association Consensus Development Conference on the Use of Biologics in the Treatment of Inflammatory Bowel Disease, June 21–23, 2006. Gastroenterology 2007;133:312–339.
15 D'Haens G, Baert F, van Assche G, Caenepeel P, Vergauwe P, Tuynman H, et al: Early combined immunosuppression or conventional management in patients with newly diagnosed Crohn's disease: an open randomised trial. Lancet 2008;371:660–667.
16 Sandborn W, Rutgeerts P, Reinisch W, Kornbluth A, Lichtiger S, D'Haens G, et al: Sonic: a randomized, double-blind, controlled trial comparing infliximab and infliximab plus azathioprine to azathioprine in patients with Crohn's disease naïve to immunomodulators and biologic therapy. Am J Gastroenterol 2008;103:S436(A1117).
17 Feagan B, McDonald J, Panaccione R, Enns R, Bernstein CN, Ponich T, et al: A randomized trial of methotrexate in combination with infliximab for the treatment of Crohn's disease. Late breaking abstract DDW 2008. Gastroenterology 2008;135:294–296.
18 Toruner M, Loftus EV Jr, Harmsen WS, Zinsmeister AR, Orenstein R, Sandborn WJ, et al: Risk factors for opportunistic infections in patients with inflammatory bowel disease. Gastroenterology 2008;134:929–936.
19 Peyrin-Biroulet L, Colombel JF, Andborn WJ: Insufficient evidence to conclude whether anti-TNF therapy increases the risk of lymphoma in Crohn's disease. Clin Gastroenterol Hepatol 2009 (in press).
20 Shale M, Kanfer E, Panaccione R, Ghosh S: Hepatosplenic T-cell lymphoma in inflammatory bowel disease. Gut 2008;57:1639–1641.
21 Feagan BG, Fedorak RN, Irvine EJ, Wild G, Sutherland L, Steinhart AH, et al: A comparison of methotrexate with placebo for the maintenance of remission in Crohn's disease. North American Crohn's Study Group Investigators. N Engl J Med 2000;342:1627–1632.
22 Colombel JF, Sandborn WJ, Rutgeerts P, Enns R, Hanauer SB, Panaccione R, et al: Adalimumab for maintenance of clinical response and remission in patients with Crohn's Disease: the CHARM Trial. Gastroenterology 2007;132:52–65.
23 Hanauer SB, Feagan BG, Lichtenstein GR, Mayer LF, Schreiber S, Colombel JF, et al: Maintenance infliximab for Crohn's disease: the ACCENT I randomised trial. Lancet 2002;359:1541–1549.
24 Sandborn WJ, Feagan BG, Stoinov S, Honiball PJ, Rutgeerts P, Mason D, et al: Certolizumab pegol for the treatment of Crohn's disease. N Engl J Med 2007;357:228–238.
25 Van Assche G, Magdelaine-Beuzelin C, D'Haens G, Baert F, Noman M, Vermeire S, et al: Withdrawal of immunosuppression in Crohn's disease treated with scheduled infliximab maintenance: a randomized trial. Gastroenterology 2008;134:1861–1868.
26 Rutgeerts P, Vermeire S, Van Assche G: Biological therapies for inflammatory bowel diseases. Gastroenterology 2009;136:1182–1197.
27 Targan SR, Feagan BG, Fedorak RN, Lashner BA, Panaccione R, Present DH, et al: Natalizumab for the treatment of active Crohn's disease: results of the ENCORE Trial. Gastroenterology 2007;132:1672–1683.
28 Sandborn WJ, Colombel JF, Enns R, Feagan BG, Hanauer SB, Lawrance IC, et al: Natalizumab induction and maintenance therapy for Crohn's disease. N Engl J Med 2005;353:1912–1925.

Medical Management of Ulcerative Colitis

Gerhard Rogler

Division of Gastroenterology and Hepatology, Department of Visceral Medicine, University Hospital Zürich, Zürich, Switzerland

Key Words

Ulcerative colitis · Topical therapy · Medical management · Aminosalicylates · Inflammatory bowel disease · Systemic therapy

Abstract

Ulcerative colitis (UC) is a chronic and relapsing inflammation limited to the colonic mucosa and always involving the rectum with variable extension towards the cecum. The aim of medical treatment is to induce and maintain clinical remission. In contrast to Crohn's disease for which a 'top-down' or 'early aggressive' therapy is discussed, in UC the concept of a step-up treatment is still valid. This step-up approach includes local or systemic administration of 5-aminosalicylic acid as first-line therapy followed by topical or systemic steroid administration as well as azathioprine, 6-mercaptopurine, cyclosporine, and more recently anti-tumor necrosis factor monoclonal antibodies as options in refractory or chronic active disease. Colectomy may be necessary if medical treatments are unsuccessful or if complications develop. The decision about the individual therapy of UC is dependent on both disease activity and on disease location. Different therapy strategies are applied in ulcerative proctitis, left-sided colitis, pancolitis and fulminant colitis as well as in chronic active disease and maintenance of remission. This overview presents important concepts in the treatment of UC based on the published guidelines.

Copyright © 2009 S. Karger AG, Basel

Introduction

Ulcerative colitis (UC) besides Crohn's disease is the most important chronic inflammatory bowel disease. Its incidence in Europe is estimated to be 5–25 new patients per 100,000 inhabitants per year [1–5]. As its course and extent vary considerably, an individualized diagnostic approach and therapy are mandatory.

Clearly the therapeutic management of UC is focused on the induction and maintenance of remission. However, presently we face a discussion of whether clinical or endoscopical remission should be the final treatment goal. During relapses or flares of UC, pharmacological or surgical interventions are needed to re-establish remission. For the re-establishment of remission and achievement of long-term remission, strategies have to be employed that minimize steroid use and therapy-related side effects.

Treatment decisions are based on disease severity, i.e. mild, moderate or severe. The degree of inflammation is a crucial factor for the choice of the therapeutic procedures. In addition, the duration of the symptoms, preceding therapy/therapies, disease history as well as individual symptoms influence the therapy decision. The extent of the disease (pancolitis, left-sided colitis, rectosigmoiditis or proctitis) will clearly be of impact on the decision for a specific therapy. Symptoms indicating the severity of the disease flare – such as vomiting, signs of bowel obstruction, number of bowel movements, presence of blood, weight loss, high fever and abdominal tenderness and pain during defecation – are useful practical criteria of severity in everyday medical practice. Frequently, the efficacy of a topical local therapy is underestimated, or is not addressed, because of the rectal application.

The valid guidelines represent the basis on which the optimal therapy must be determined for the individual patient.

Medical Management of Acute Flares of Ulcerative Colitis

An acute flare of UC is usually characterized by typical clinical complaints, such as frequent bowel movements, bloody diarrhea and abdominal pain. It is frequently recommended to exclude an infectious colitis before starting any treatment. The impact and efficacy of such 'routine diagnostics', however, has never been really evaluated. A recent development is an increase in the incidence of *Clostridium difficile* colitis and CMV colitis among UC patients, especially under immunosuppressive conditions. This has to be kept in mind in patients that seem to have steroid-refractory UC.

The choice of therapy for acute flares or relapses of UC is based on the clinical presentation. The value of laboratory markers for the therapy decision is limited. As a minimum requirement, hemoglobin levels, leukocyte counts as well as general inflammation parameters such as thrombocyte counts, ESR or CRP should be determined [6]. 'Control colonoscopies' without therapeutic or prognostic consequences are not indicated and should not be performed during an acute flare of UC. Changes in the extension of the disease can also be proven by ultrasound in the hands of an experienced doctor.

In general, a step-up approach is recommended in all guidelines for the treatment of UC (fig. 1). An abundance of evidence exists that supports the use of aminosalicylates (5-ASA) in mild to moderate UC for the induction of remission. Corticosteroids are used in patients not responding to 5-ASA or in patients with more severe disease. Azathioprine (AZA) and 6-mercaptopurine (6-MP) have been shown to be useful in steroid-refractory patients.

Left-Sided Colitis, Rectosigmoiditis, Proctitis

Distal or left-sided UC with mild to moderate activity should be initially treated topically [7]. The rectal application of steroids (as enema or foam) is superior to placebo; however, 5-aminosalicylic acid (5 ASA) is superior to steroids in topical application [8, 9]. Consecutively,

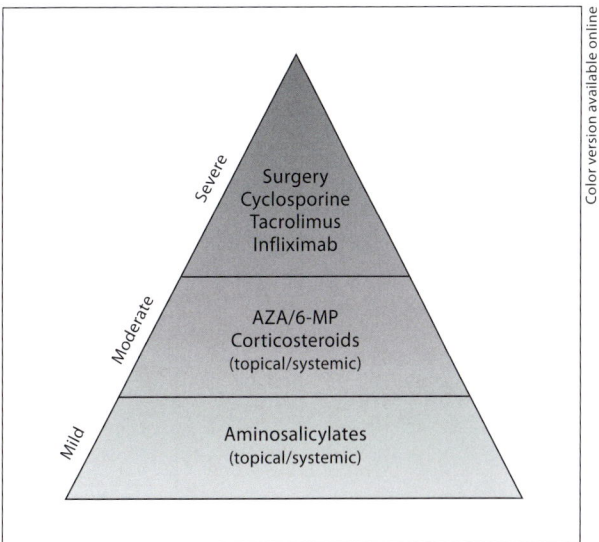

Fig. 1. Step-up therapy approach in UC.

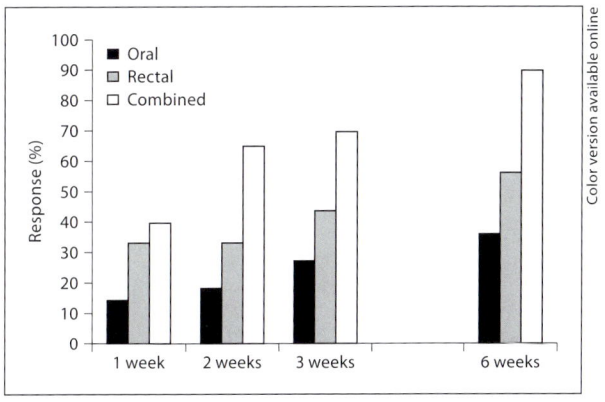

Fig. 2. Advantage of combination therapy of oral and rectal 5-ASA therapy over monotherapy (according to Safdi et al. [12]).

treatment of first choice in mild to moderate left-sided colitis or rectosigmoiditis are foams or enemas with 5-ASA (mesalamine) [7, 10]. During an acute flare of colitis, application of enemas is frequently uncomfortable due to the at times large volume (up to 100 ml), making them less well tolerated by the patients [11]. In patients with UC, the rectum is usually the side of the most severe inflammation. It contains the highest number of sensory nerves in the bowel. Therefore, it is easily conceivable that

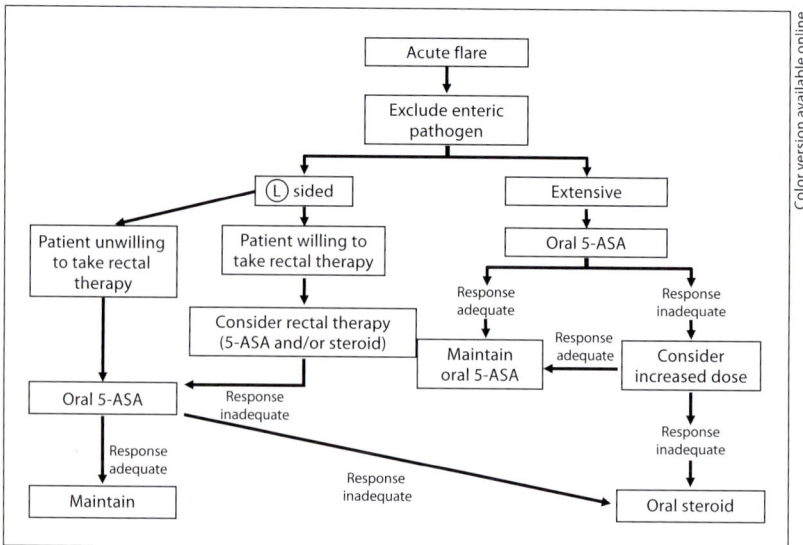

Fig. 3. Treatment algorithm for mild to moderate UC.

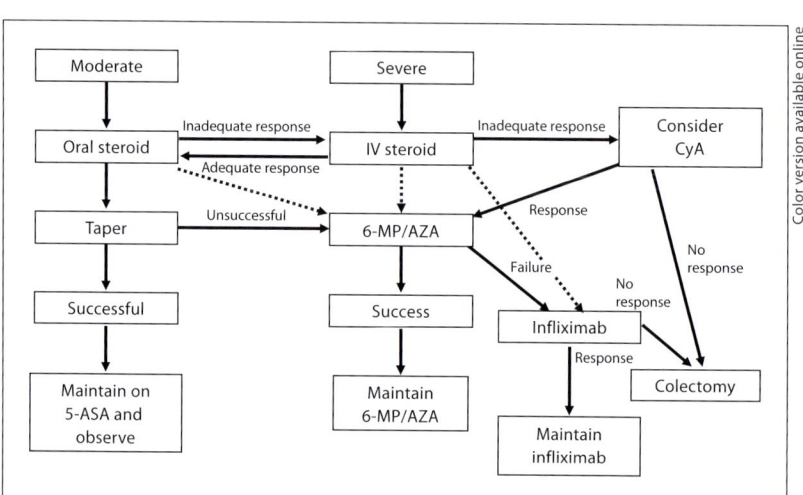

Fig. 4. Treatment algorithm for moderate to severe UC.

such a large volume of fluid will cause complaints. Foams are better accepted by the patients in general (potentially also due to the smaller volume). In ulcerative proctitis, 5-ASA suppositories should be used [11].

If the disease extends to the left colonic flexure, it appears to be recommendable to combine topical therapy with an oral 5-ASA preparation [12–14]. The recommended duration of treatment is at least 4 weeks [10, 15]. The minimal, but sufficient topical dose for the achievement of a remission is 1 g 5-ASA per day [14]. Higher doses up to 4 g/day have not been proven to be more effective [10, 15, 16]. If a topical therapy with 5-ASA over several weeks is ineffective, topical steroids should be added for at least 4 weeks [17, 18]. If the topical therapy finally fails, systemic steroids should be used [13, 19]. A severe flare of a distal colitis should primarily be treated orally with systemic steroids, if possible in combination with topical use of 5-ASA [13, 20] (fig. 2).

In different studies, initial steroid doses between 40 and 60 mg/day did not seem to exhibit remarkable differences in therapeutic efficacy [21].

Pancolitis

A mild to moderate flare of a pancolitis should initially be treated with oral 5-ASA [16, 22, 23] (fig. 3). 4 g 5-ASA per day are superior to 2 g. Usually it has been recommended that 5-ASA should be taken in three doses over the day. Newer studies from the last years indicate that the total daily dose can be taken at one time (e.g. in the morning) – or even should be taken at one time, as in some studies there was even increased efficacy under these conditions [24–26]. The possibility to take the whole dose at one time is also likely to increase patient compliance and adherence to therapy. From several studies we know that the main drawback of 5-ASA therapy (and probably the most important reason for therapy failure) is a reduced adherence due to the mode of intake and the number of tablets or capsules (up to 8 per day). With respect to this, new formulations as 'granules' or 'sachets' may also be of clear advantage.

During severe pancolitis or lack of response to a therapy with 5-ASA, systemic glucocorticoids should be used orally or intravenously (initially a 60-mg prednisone equivalent per day) [27, 28] (fig. 4). In patients requiring steroid therapy, the immediate outcomes are favorable, but the long-term outcome at 1 year is somewhat disappointing. About half of the patients with UC initially treated with steroids will require additional therapy after 1 year. A population-based study has shown that a year after the initial course of corticosteroid treatment, a prolonged steroid response is seen in only 49% of patients with UC. However, sometimes a second course of steroid therapy will induce remission again. In addition, numbers may change with sufficient and well-adhered maintenance therapy. Steroid dependence has been reported to develop in 22% of UC patients, with surgery being required in 29% of those patients. In general, a state of steroid dependence should clearly be avoided. Therefore, it is questionable whether this really can be a measure in clinical studies. Whether the steroids for pancolitis are given orally or intravenously should be decided with respect to the clinical presentation of the patient.

Usually steroids are combined with oral aminosalicylates, although the efficacy or advantage of such a combination has never been documented by appropriate clinical studies. The tapering of steroids has long been performed very schematically. Tapering regimes differing from country to country have been established. In the meantime it is accepted that tapering of steroids should be planned individually according to the patient's clinical symptoms. If no response can be achieved by the oral administration of steroids, a change to one course of intravenous administration is usually recommended. This could be justified with the assumption that during severe colitis there is increased peristalsis also of the small bowel and resorption of oral steroids could be reduced. Studies on the change of an oral steroid administration to an intravenous one do not exist; however, in the experience of most clinicians this approach has clinically worked for a number of patients. An intravenous therapy duration of 10 days is generally sufficient. If no improvement is observed within a period of 10 days, therapy has to be reconsidered and changed. Before the infliximab era, cyclosporine at a dose of 4 mg/kg·day i.v. was primarily recommended [28]. The Leuven group has shown that cyclosporine 2 mg/kg·day i.v. is equivalently effective [29]. Serum levels can be measured at any time during therapy, since by the continuous infusion steady-state levels are reached early. The ACT-1 and ACT-2 studies among others showed that the anti-tumor necrosis factor antibody infliximab (5 mg/kg in weeks 0, 2 and 8 and then every 8 weeks) is effective in severe UC [30–32]. The discussion at which time point in the step-up approach of severe UC treatment infliximab should be used is still ongoing [33]. New data also exist for a successful therapy with tacrolimus in this situation [34, 35]. Tacrolimus can be used in individual cases as an alternative to cyclosporine.

Medical Management of Severe Acute Colitis/Toxic Megacolon

A severe flare is characterized by the respective clinical symptoms which include systemic signs such as fever, tachycardia and anemia as well as increased inflammation parameters. Crucial symptoms are frequent bloody diarrhea, fever >38.5°C and weight loss. An abdominal X-ray should be performed to search for a dilation of the colon (toxic megacolon) [36].

A megacolon is present if the diameter of the colon transversum is >5.5 cm. Ultrasound can be a useful diagnostic supplement in this situation [36]. A sigmoidoscopy may be useful to exclude *C. difficile* colitis and CMV colitis. Since a fulminant colitis or a toxic megacolon can also occur on the basis of an intestinal infection, investigations on *C. difficile* toxin as well as an adequate CMV diagnostic (e.g. immunohistochemistry for pp65) should be performed [37–39]. For the treatment of a fulminant flare of UC, the patient should be hospitalized. An interdisciplinary approach between gastroenterologists and visceral surgeons is mandatory. A conservative therapy should only be performed if no contraindications exist [40].

Treatment can be started with a course of intravenous steroids, e.g. 4 × 100 mg hydrocortisone per day [41]. In addition to fluid and electrolyte substitution, parenteral nutrition may be indicated. If steroid therapy fails (no sufficient treatment response within 3–5 days) and a clear indication for surgery is not given, a therapy with intravenous cyclosporine (2 or 4 mg/kg·day as continuous infusion) may be applied [28, 42, 43]. As mentioned, infliximab has been proven to be an alternative in this situation in several studies [31, 44–46].

If intravenous cyclosporine is successful after 7–10 days, it is usually switched to oral therapy for maintenance of remission and combined with other immunosuppressants such as AZA (2.5 mg/kg·day) [43]. Oral cyclosporine cannot be expected to maintain remission for longer periods. Approximately 60–80% of the patients benefit on a long-term basis and for 40% of the patients colectomy can be avoided [43]. As an alternative to cyclosporine, tacrolimus has also been successfully used [34, 47]. This therapy should be reserved to centers with appropriate experience.

If the need for a rapid surgical intervention is possible, further corticosteroids should be avoided as steroids increase the risk of post-surgical (infectious) complications [48]. Parenteral nutrition should applied for fluid and electrolyte substitution. In controlled studies, however, this was not superior to enteral nutrition. Clearly, enteral nutrition cannot be used under subileus/ileus conditions. Controlled studies do not show an advantage of an additional administration of antibiotics; therefore, this should only be done if signs of infection/superinfection or peritonitis are present.

After achieving remission, AZA (2–2.5 mg/kg) can be used for maintenance therapy [49, 50]. A *Pneumocystis carinei/jiroveci* prophylaxis is recommended during the triple immunosuppression (cyclosporine, AZA and systemic steroids). The efficacy of such prophylaxis has not been proven so far [51]. If therapy fails, early colectomy should be performed. The clinical value of leukocyte apheresis is still a matter of discussion.

Medical Management of Chronic Active Ulcerative Colitis

A chronic active disease is characterized by the persistence of clinical symptoms (diarrhea, blood loss, pain) despite an adequate medical therapy. Also, a disease course that has shown some improvement upon therapy which is however not complete and permanent (<2 relapses/year) is termed a *chronic active disease*. A colonoscopy with biopsies and subsequent histology may be helpful in individual cases, e.g. for the exclusion of CMV colitis. In cases of severe, chronically active UC, the option of a colectomy should always be discussed with the patient.

If no colectomy is performed for the moment, an immunosuppression with AZA/6-MP may be useful [52, 53]. Newer studies indicate that infliximab can also be given if a fast therapy response is desired or necessary [32]. In individual cases the discrimination of a chronically active colitis and irritable bowel syndrome can be difficult. Particularly in therapy-refractory disease under immunosuppression, an appropriate diagnostic procedure must be undertaken to exclude CMV colitis. Oral systemic steroids should not be used as continuous therapy due to their side effects. In chronically active distal colitis, however, the long-term rectal administration of steroid enemas or foams may be acceptable due to their low systemic bioavailability.

A therapy failure on AZA therapy can at the earliest be diagnosed after 6 months of continuous administration. Maintenance therapy with AZA or 6-MP should be applied for 3–5 years [54, 55]. According to all available data, the administration of AZA during pregnancy is regarded as being safe. Upon administration of AZA/6-MP the leukocyte count and the transaminases must be controlled regularly if abdominal pain occurs. Additionally, serum lipase levels should be determined. After start of the immunosuppressive therapy, leukocyte counts and GPT values should be controlled after 1, 2, 4, 8 and 12 weeks, thereafter at least every 12 weeks. Upon AZA therapy, bone marrow suppression may occur, which must be discovered in time. With leukocyte numbers <2,500, AZA therapy should be terminated. After normalization of the values a therapy may be restarted with lower doses (e.g. 50 mg/day) under close supervision. Pancreatitis may occur usually in the first weeks of treatment and require immediate termination therapy. Minor increases in serum lipase or amylase without clinical symptoms are frequently observed in inflammatory bowel disease patients; their relevance remains obscure, an observing attitude is acceptable. A subsequent rise of serum liver enzymes under therapy is also a reason for termination of AZA/6-MP therapy.

The use of infliximab represents an important therapy alternative [32]. It is regarded to be safe and well tolerated, however, a tuberculosis skin test or lymphocyte stimulation test (such as QuantiFERON®) as well as a lung X-ray need to be performed prior to starting the therapy. It needs to be kept in mind that tuberculosis screening can be false-negative due to immunosuppression. Only 22% of patients will be in remission without the need of additional steroids according to the ACT-1 and ACT-2 data. On the other hand, treatment success is usually rapid and an improvement of the patients can be observed sometimes already on the day after the administration.

The administration of methotrexate can be considered in individual cases in adult patients but also in children [56]. The initial dose is 20–25 mg parenterally (oral, i.m., s.c.) every week (children: 15 mg/m² body surface). After achieving remission, a dose reduction to 10–15 mg/week is usually recommended. Regular blood cell counts must also take place under a therapy with methotrexate. For the monitoring of the potential hepatotoxicity, regular measurements of liver enzymes should be performed. Preexisting chronic liver disease or chronic lung disease represent contraindications for the therapy. The oral administration of tacrolimus (0.1–0.2 mg/kg b.w.) and the use of a leukocyte apheresis can be considered in individual cases.

Maintenance of Remission in Ulcerative Colitis

The definition of remission is based on clinical features. Criteria for remission are absence of diarrhea (>3 bowel movements/day), no visible blood in stools as well as no UC-associated intestinal or extraintestinal complaints. For maintenance of remission in patients with UC, first-line therapy is 5-ASA administered orally or rectally [57–59]. The combination of oral and rectal/topical therapy is superior to oral monotherapy (fig. 2). In the case of distal UC, evidence for the superiority of the rectal application exists [59].

The compliance or adherence on maintenance therapy is crucial for its success [60]. If more than two-thirds of the recommended dose is taken, the risk of a flare or relapse in the first year is only approximately 10–20% [61]. With respect to this, it is certainly favorable that newer studies point to the fact that the entire 5-ASA dosage can be taken at one time (e.g. either the morning or evening), i.e., the distribution into three doses is no longer necessary.

The effectiveness of the following minimal dosages has been demonstrated in clinical studies: (1) *oral administration*: SASP 2 g/day; 5-ASA 1.5 g/day; olsalazine 1.0 g/day, (2) *rectal administration*: left-sided colitis: 5-ASA enemas either 1 g/day or 4 g each third day or 4 g/day on the first 7 days of the month; proctitis: 5-ASA suppositories 2 × 500 mg/day or 1 g/day three times weekly.

Since individual patients prefer mesalazine foams as compared to enemas, this form of application can probably be given at a similar dosage, even if studies are not available for maintenance of remission with foam preparations. Maintenance therapy should be administrated for at least 2 years.

Upon incompatibility of 5-ASA, a probiotic pathogen preparation, e.g. *Escherichia coli* Nissle, can be used successfully for the maintenance of remission with a similar clinical efficacy [62, 63]. As alternatives for complicated UC, AZA/6-MP [53] and infliximab can be used for the maintenance of remission [32]. Systemic steroids should not be used for maintenance therapy. The increased efficacy of a combination of oral and rectal therapy with 5-ASA is well documented by clinical studies; however, most patients prefer monotherapy.

Disclosure Statement

The author has received research funding from Abbott, Essex, Falk, UCB, Ardeypharm and Lifor. The author is member of advisory boards for Abbott, Essex, Novartis and UCB.

References

1 Rao SS, Holdsworth CD, Read NW: Symptoms and stool patterns in patients with ulcerative colitis. Gut 1988;29:342–345.

2 Jones HW, Grogono J, Hoare AM: Surveillance in ulcerative colitis: burdens and benefit. Gut 1988;29:325–331.

3 Armitage EL, Aldhous MC, Anderson N, Drummond HE, Riemersma RA, Ghosh S, Satsangi J: Incidence of juvenile-onset Crohn's disease in Scotland: association with northern latitude and affluence. Gastroenterology 2004;127:1051–1057.

4 Turunen P, Kolho KL, Auvinen A, Iltanen S, Huhtala H, Ashorn M: Incidence of inflammatory bowel disease in Finnish children, 1987–2003. Inflamm Bowel Dis 2006;12:677–683.

5 Vind I, Riis L, Jess T, Knudsen E, Pedersen N, Elkjaer M, Bak Andersen I, Wewer V, Nørregaard P, Moesgaard F, Bendtsen F, Munkholm P: Increasing incidences of inflammatory bowel disease and decreasing surgery rates in Copenhagen City and County, 2003–2005: a population-based study from the Danish Crohn colitis database. Am J Gastroenterol 2006;101:1274–1282.

6 Descos L, Andre F, Andre C, Gillon J, Landais P, Fermanian J: Assessment of appropriate laboratory measurements to reflect the degree of activity of ulcerative colitis. Digestion 1983;28:148–152.
7 Gionchetti P, Amadini C, Rizzello F, Venturi A, Campieri M: Treatment of mild to moderate ulcerative colitis and pouchitis. Aliment Pharmacol Ther 2002;16(suppl 4):13–19.
8 Marshall JK, Irvine EJ: Rectal corticosteroids versus alternative treatments in ulcerative colitis: a meta-analysis. Gut 1997;40:775–781.
9 Campieri M, Gionchetti P, Belluzzi A, Brignola C, Migaldi M, Tabanelli GM, Bazzocchi G, Miglioli M, Barbara L: Efficacy of 5-aminosalicylic acid enemas versus hydrocortisone enemas in ulcerative colitis. Dig Dis Sci 1987;32:67S–70S.
10 Marshall JK, Irvine EJ: Rectal aminosalicylate therapy for distal ulcerative colitis: a meta-analysis. Aliment Pharmacol Ther 1995;9:293–300.
11 Campieri M, Gionchetti P, Belluzzi A, Brignola C, Tabanelli GM, Miglioli M, Barbara L: 5-Aminosalicylic acid as enemas or suppositories in distal ulcerative colitis? J Clin Gastroenterol 1988;10:406–409.
12 Safdi M, DeMicco M, Sninsky C, Banks P, Wruble L, Deren J, Koval G, Nichols T, Targan S, Fleishman C, Wiita B: A double-blind comparison of oral versus rectal mesalamine versus combination therapy in the treatment of distal ulcerative colitis. Am J Gastroenterol 1997;92:1867–1871.
13 Regueiro M, Loftus EV Jr, Steinhart AH, Cohen RD: Medical management of left-sided ulcerative colitis and ulcerative proctitis: critical evaluation of therapeutic trials. Inflamm Bowel Dis 2006;12:979–994.
14 Marshall JK, Irvine EJ: Putting rectal 5-aminosalicylic acid in its place: the role in distal ulcerative colitis. Am J Gastroenterol 2000;95:1628–1636.
15 Sutherland L, MacDonald JK: Oral 5-aminosalicylic acid for induction of remission in ulcerative colitis. Cochrane Database Syst Rev 2003:CD000543.
16 Sutherland L, Macdonald JK: Oral 5-aminosalicylic acid for induction of remission in ulcerative colitis. Cochrane Database Syst Rev 2006:CD000543.
17 Mulder CJ, Tytgat GN, Wiltink EH, Houthoff HJ: Comparison of 5-aminosalicylic acid (3 g) and prednisolone phosphate sodium enemas (30 mg) in the treatment of distal ulcerative colitis. A prospective, randomized, double-blind trial. Scand J Gastroenterol 1988;23:1005–1008.
18 Mulder CJ, Fockens P, Meijer JW, van der Heide H, Wiltink EH, Tytgat GN: Beclomethasone dipropionate (3 mg) versus 5-aminosalicylic acid (2 g) versus the combination of both (3 mg/2 g) as retention enemas in active ulcerative proctitis. Eur J Gastroenterol Hepatol 1996;8:549–553.
19 Lofberg R, Danielsson A, Suhr O, Nilsson A, Schioler R, Nyberg A, Hultcrantz R, Kollberg B, Gillberg R, Willen R, Persson T, Salde L: Oral budesonide versus prednisolone in patients with active extensive and left-sided ulcerative colitis. Gastroenterology 1996;110:1713–1718.
20 Katz JA: Medical and surgical management of severe colitis. Semin Gastrointest Dis 2000;11:18–32.
21 Baron JH, Connell AM, Kanaghinis TG, Lennard-Jones JE, Jones AF: Outpatient treatment of ulcerative colitis. Comparison between three doses of oral prednisone. Br Med J 1962;2:441–443.
22 Tremaine WJ, Schroeder KW, Harrison JM, Zinsmeister AR: A randomized, double-blind, placebo-controlled trial of the oral mesalamine (5-ASA) preparation, Asacol, in the treatment of symptomatic Crohn's colitis and ileocolitis. J Clin Gastroenterol 1994;19:278–282.
23 Schroeder KW, Tremaine WJ, Ilstrup DM: Coated oral 5-aminosalicylic acid therapy for mildly to moderately active ulcerative colitis. A randomized study. N Engl J Med 1987;317:1625–1629.
24 Kruis W, Kiudelis G, Racz I, Gorelov IA, Pokrotnieks J, Horynski M, Batovsky M, Kykal J, Bohm SK, Greinwald R, Muller R: Once-daily versus three-times-daily mesalazine granules in active ulcerative colitis: a double-blind, double-dummy, randomised non-inferiority trial. Gut 2009;58:233–240.
25 Kamm MA, Sandborn WJ, Gassull M, Schreiber S, Jackowski L, Butler T, Lyne A, Stephenson D, Palmen M, Joseph RE: Once-daily, high-concentration MMX mesalamine in active ulcerative colitis. Gastroenterology 2007;132:66–75.
26 Dignass AU, Bokemeyer B, Adamek HE, Mross MR, Vinter-Jensen L, Boerner N, Silvennoinen J, Tan TG, Oudkerk-Pool M, Stijnen T, Dietel P, Klugmann T, Veerman H: Maintenance therapy with once-daily 2 g mesalazine (Pentasa) treatment improves remission rates in subjects with ulcerative colitis compared to twice daily 1 g mesalazine: data from a randomised controlled trial. Gastroenterology 2008;134:A494.
27 Truelove SC, Witts LJ: Cortisone in ulcerative colitis; final report on a therapeutic trial. Br Med J 1955;2:1041–1048.
28 D'Haens G, Lemmens L, Geboes K, Vandeputte L, Van Acker F, Mortelmans L, Peeters M, Vermeire S, Penninckx F, Nevens F, Hiele M, Rutgeerts P: Intravenous cyclosporine versus intravenous corticosteroids as single therapy for severe attacks of ulcerative colitis. Gastroenterology 2001;120:1323–1329.
29 Van Assche G, D'Haens G, Noman M, Vermeire S, Hiele M, Asnong K, Arts J, D'Hoore A, Penninckx F, Rutgeerts P: Randomized, double-blind comparison of 4 versus 2 mg/kg intravenous cyclosporine in severe ulcerative colitis. Gastroenterology 2003;125:1025–1031.
30 Feagan BG, Reinisch W, Rutgeerts P, Sandborn WJ, Yan S, Eisenberg D, Bala M, Johanns J, Olson A, Hanauer SB: The effects of infliximab therapy on health-related quality of life in ulcerative colitis patients. Am J Gastroenterol 2007;102:794–802.
31 Regueiro M, Curtis J, Plevy S: Infliximab for hospitalized patients with severe ulcerative colitis. J Clin Gastroenterol 2006;40:476–481.
32 Rutgeerts P, Sandborn WJ, Feagan BG, Reinisch W, Olson A, Johanns J, Travers S, Rachmilewitz D, Hanauer SB, Lichtenstein GR, de Villiers WJ, Present D, Sands BE, Colombel JF: Infliximab for induction and maintenance therapy for ulcerative colitis. N Engl J Med 2005;353:2462–2476.
33 Tsai HH, Punekar YS, Morris J, Fortun P: A model of the long-term cost effectiveness of scheduled maintenance treatment with infliximab for moderate-to-severe ulcerative colitis. Aliment Pharmacol Ther 2008;28:1230–1239.
34 Ogata H, Matsui T, Nakamura M, Iida M, Takazoe M, Suzuki Y, Hibi T: A randomised dose finding study of oral tacrolimus (FK-506) therapy in refractory ulcerative colitis. Gut 2006;55:1255–1262.
35 Yamamoto S, Nakase H, Mikami S, Inoue S, Yoshino T, Takeda Y, Kasahara K, Ueno S, Uza N, Kitamura H, Tamaki H, Matsuura M, Inui K, Chiba T: Long-term effect of tacrolimus therapy in patients with refractory ulcerative colitis. Aliment Pharmacol Ther 2008;28:589–597.
36 Hoffmann JC, Schwandner O, Bruch HP: Ulcerative colitis. Fulminant disease (in German). Z Gastroenterol 2004;42:1002–1006.
37 Minami M, Ohta M, Ohkura T, Ando T, Ohmiya N, Niwa Y, Goto H: Cytomegalovirus infection in severe ulcerative colitis patients undergoing continuous intravenous cyclosporine treatment in Japan. World J Gastroenterol 2007;13:754–760.
38 Kojima T, Watanabe T, Hata K, Shinozaki M, Yokoyama T, Nagawa H: Cytomegalovirus infection in ulcerative colitis. Scand J Gastroenterol 2006;41:706–711.
39 Kambham N, Vij R, Cartwright CA, Longacre T: Cytomegalovirus infection in steroid-refractory ulcerative colitis: a case-control study. Am J Surg Pathol 2004;28:365–373.
40 Cima RR, Pemberton JH: Surgical indications and procedures in ulcerative colitis. Curr Treat Options Gastroenterol 2004;7:181–190.

41 Meyers S, Lerer PK, Feuer EJ, Johnson JW, Janowitz HD: Predicting the outcome of corticoid therapy for acute ulcerative colitis. Results of a prospective, randomized, double-blind clinical trial. J Clin Gastroenterol 1987; 9:50–54.
42 Lichtiger S, Present DH, Kornbluth A, Gelernt I, Bauer J, Galler G, Michelassi F, Hanauer S: Cyclosporine in severe ulcerative colitis refractory to steroid therapy. N Engl J Med 1994;330:1841–1845.
43 Cohen RD, Stein R, Hanauer SB: Intravenous cyclosporin in ulcerative colitis: a five-year experience. Am J Gastroenterol 1999;94: 1587–1592.
44 Jarnerot G: Infliximab or cyclosporine for severe ulcerative colitis. Gastroenterology 2006;130:287.
45 Hanauer SB: Infliximab or cyclosporine for severe ulcerative colitis. Gastroenterology 2005;129:1358–1359.
46 Jarnerot G, Hertervig E, Friis-Liby I, Blomquist L, Karlen P, Granno C, Vilien M, Strom M, Danielsson A, Verbaan H, Hellstrom PM, Magnuson A, Curman B: Infliximab as rescue therapy in severe to moderately severe ulcerative colitis: a randomized, placebo-controlled study. Gastroenterology 2005;128:1805–1811.
47 Baumgart DC, Pintoffl JP, Sturm A, Wiedenmann B, Dignass AU: Tacrolimus is safe and effective in patients with severe steroid-refractory or steroid-dependent inflammatory bowel disease – a long-term follow-up. Am J Gastroenterol 2006;101:1048–1056.
48 Aberra FN, Lewis JD, Hass D, Rombeau JL, Osborne B, Lichtenstein GR: Corticosteroids and immunomodulators: postoperative infectious complication risk in inflammatory bowel disease patients. Gastroenterology 2003;125:320–327.

49 Fernandez-Banares F, Bertran X, Esteve-Comas M, Cabre E, Menacho M, Humbert P, Planas R, Gassull MA: Azathioprine is useful in maintaining long-term remission induced by intravenous cyclosporine in steroid-refractory severe ulcerative colitis. Am J Gastroenterol 1996;91:2498–2499.
50 Sood A, Kaushal V, Midha V, Bhatia KL, Sood N, Malhotra V: The beneficial effect of azathioprine on maintenance of remission in severe ulcerative colitis. J Gastroenterol 2002;37:270–274.
51 Higgins RM, Bloom SL, Hopkin JM, Morris PJ: The risks and benefits of low-dose cotrimoxazole prophylaxis for *Pneumocystis pneumonia* in renal transplantation. Transplantation 1989;47:558–560.
52 Sands BE: Immunosuppressive drugs in ulcerative colitis: twisting facts to suit theories? Gut 2006;55:437–441.
53 Timmer A, McDonald J, Macdonald J: Azathioprine and 6-mercaptopurine for maintenance of remission in ulcerative colitis. Cochrane Database Syst Rev 2007:CD000478.
54 Mantzaris GJ, Sfakianakis M, Archavlis E, Petraki K, Christidou A, Karagiannidis A, Triadaphyllou G: A prospective randomized observer-blind 2-year trial of azathioprine monotherapy versus azathioprine and olsalazine for the maintenance of remission of steroid-dependent ulcerative colitis. Am J Gastroenterol 2004;99:1122–1128.
55 Lopez-Sanroman A, Bermejo F, Carrera E, Garcia-Plaza A: Efficacy and safety of thiopurinic immunomodulators (azathioprine and mercaptopurine) in steroid-dependent ulcerative colitis. Aliment Pharmacol Ther 2004;20:161–166.

56 Egan LJ, Sandborn WJ, Tremaine WJ, Leighton JA, Mays DC, Pike MG, Zinsmeister AR, Lipsky JJ: A randomized dose-response and pharmacokinetic study of methotrexate for refractory inflammatory Crohn's disease and ulcerative colitis. Aliment Pharmacol Ther 1999;13:1597–1604.
57 Sutherland L, Macdonald JK: Oral 5-aminosalicylic acid for maintenance of remission in ulcerative colitis. Cochrane Database Syst Rev 2006:CD000544.
58 Orchard T, Probert CS, Keshav S: Review article: maintenance therapy in patients with ulcerative colitis. Aliment Pharmacol Ther 2006;24(suppl 1):17–22.
59 Gionchetti P, Rizzello F, Morselli C, Tambasco R, Campieri M: Aminosalicylates for distal colitis. Aliment Pharmacol Ther 2006; 24(suppl 3):41–44.
60 Bergman R, Parkes M: Systematic review: the use of mesalazine in inflammatory bowel disease. Aliment Pharmacol Ther 2006;23: 841–855.
61 Kane SV, Cohen RD, Aikens JE, Hanauer SB: Prevalence of nonadherence with maintenance mesalamine in quiescent ulcerative colitis. Am J Gastroenterol 2001;96:2929–2933.
62 Bohm SK, Kruis W: Probiotics: do they help to control intestinal inflammation? Ann NY Acad Sci 2006;1072:339–350.
63 Kruis W, Fric P, Pokrotnieks J, Lukas M, Fixa B, Kascak M, Kamm MA, Weismueller J, Beglinger C, Stolte M, Wolff C, Schulze J: Maintaining remission of ulcerative colitis with the probiotic *Escherichia coli* Nissle 1917 is as effective as with standard mesalazine. Gut 2004;53:1617–1623.

Diagnostic and Treatment Algorithms of Ulcerative Colitis in Ukraine

I.N. Skrypnyk

Ukrainian Medical Stomatological Academy, Poltava, Ukraine

Key Words

Diagnostic algorithms · Treatment algorithms · Ulcerative colitis, diagnostics · Ulcerative colitis, pathogenesis · Ulcerative colitis, Ukraine

Abstract

Questions concerning the diagnosis and treatment of ulcerative colitis (UC) in Ukraine are described. In recent years, there has been considerable progress in conservative therapy and new drugs have been developed that provide persistent remission of the inflammatory process after long-term application in many cases. The results of our own investigation on the efficiency of rebamipide in the complex treatment of UC patients are presented. Optimization of treatment with substitution of mesalazine in tablet or granule form, especially with an additional rebamipide prescription and a once-daily administration of budesonide, leads to an increased effectiveness of treatment and improvement of quality of life in UC patients. In the future, development of new approaches in the pharmacotherapy of UC will use medications as a basic therapy with the purpose of achieving high-quality and effective 'convalescence of mucous membrane', including cytoprotectors, bilious acids, endogenous substances, stabilization of membranes, antihypoxants and correction of microbiocenosis disorders.

Copyright © 2009 S. Karger AG, Basel

Introduction

Ulcerative colitis (UC) is one of the most difficult and unsolved problems of modern medicine, and because of its severity, frequency of complications and lethality, it occupies one of the first places on the list of gastrointestinal tract diseases. There is an increasing tendency of UC frequency and an 'epidemic' is forecasted for Eastern Europe, including Ukraine. In Europe, UC morbidity has increased practically twofold in the last 10 years and comprises 8–12 cases per 100,000 inhabitants annually. The prevalence of UC has also had a tendency to grow and comprises 40–117 patients per 100,000 inhabitants [1].

The epidemiological indexes of this disease in Ukraine differ because of the predominance of its serious and complicated forms. The variety of clinical forms complicates diagnosis and estimation of activity of the process in the aggravation phase. Thus, the risk of complications rises due to inadequate treatment, the disability of patients being able to work, and the increase of lethality.

Pathogenesis

As the questions of etiology and pathogenesis of UC have not been studied too well, the development of early diagnosis principles of the disease is difficult. Recent decades are characterized by considerable expansion and deepening of concepts about the pathogenesis of intestine inflammatory diseases on the basis of the genetic and epidemiological research that has been conducted.

UC is a polyetiological disease in which the genetic predisposition plays a leading role, due to immunological mechanisms under the influence of stress factors, eating disorders and allergy. In the Donetsk region of Ukraine, a genetic predisposition of UC was found in 19.8% of cases, different types of allergy in 21.5%, and protracted chemical influences, related to the features of profession, in 6% cases. Immunological and eating disorders were observed in all patients [2].

60% of UC patients have a mild form of the disease, and the typical intermittent course of disease takes place in 30% of the patients. The existence of different types of UC is conditioned by genetic features (polymorphism of NOD2/CARD15 gene), the influence on the organism of external environmental factors, and patients having harmful habits [3]. It was recently determined that appendectomy as well as smoking reduce the risk of UC development associated with the severe course of the disease [4, 5]. Glycoprotein P plays a very important role in protecting against coli bacteria and toxins, and breaking the barrier's function for genotype 3435TT possessors can stipulate their predisposition to UC [6]. The important role of breaking the resistance of the intestine's mucous membrane-protective barrier in UC pathogenesis has been confirmed by the discovery of ASCA antibodies in the blood serum of these patients (antibodies to *Saccharomyces cerevisiae*). However, they are not a pathognomonic diagnostic UC index, because they are often found in UC patients' relatives who have no signs of this disease manifestation [3].

Diagnostics

The clinical picture consists of intestinal symptoms which are characteristic for all patients and intestinal indications are practically found in 50% of the patients. With the standardization of the clinical picture, the indexes of the clinical activity of Rachmilewitz and Mayo disease are presently used. However, these indexes are used for scientific research but not in doctors' surgeries in Ukraine. It is important to evaluate not only the prevalence of the inflammatory process in the colon and disease activity, but also the degree of gravity. Except for immune changes of patients with UC, a dysbalance of the cytokine regulation was revealed with a predominance of proinflammatory cytokines such as tumor necrotic factor-α (TNF-α), interleukins (IL)-1, -6, -8, -12 and a decrease of anti-inflammatory IL-4, -10, and -11 [7].

It is necessary to provide endoscopic research with a biopsy in dynamics. Capsule videoendoscopy is the most informative and objective method of investigation in this respect. Histological research is the standard in diagnosis of UC. For the patients with UC in the stage of remission, endoscopy of the colon must be provided not less than once during 6–8 months. Irrigography is an additional diagnostic method and allows to evaluate the prevalence of inflammation in colon in case it is not possible to perform colonoscopy.

High-quality determination of stool protein in feces as the most exact and sensible indicator of this disease activity is reasonable for the diagnosis of inflammatory diseases of the intestine and irritated intestine syndrome. Stool protein is produced by neutrocytes, and if patients suffer from intestinal inflammatory diseases, an increased amount secretes through the bowel wall as a result of leukocyte migration [8]. In UC feces stool protein, sensitivity is 94.1% and specificity is 80%. A marker is a more exact indicator of the inflammatory process than red corpuscles ($p < 0.01$) and C-reactive protein ($p < 0.001$). The level of feces stool protein correlates well with UC activity ($p < 0.001$) [9].

Treatment

The traditional and generally recognized tasks of treatment are to reduce disease activity, reduce expressed clinical symptoms, improve patients' quality of life, and prevent relapses. Before beginning treatment it is important to estimate therapy possibilities taking the following into account: localization and gravity of the process, presence of complications, response to the previously applied therapy is important to create an individual chart of the patient's treatment, and estimate the prospect of applied therapy.

Basic medicinal therapy of UC is conducted depending on the gravity of colitis and includes derivates of mesalazine, topical steroids (first-line), cytostatics and biological preparations (second-line). Basic UC therapy must be provided independent of the gravity of colitis according to ECCO recommendations. Mesalazine is prescribed in case of minimal activity at a dose of 3–4 g/day orally and is rectally independent of the process [10]. Mesalazine (Eudragit L) granules provide the prolonged liberation of active matter and have maximal contact with the mucous membrane of distal parts of the intestine [11].

Rectal application of steroids, mainly topical steroids, is indicated with the purpose of minimizing side effects [12]. We prescribe mesalazine 4–8 g/day and budesonide 9 mg/day in cases of moderate activity. A daily dose of 9 mg budesonide possesses greater efficiency if taken once daily over an 8-week period than if taken 3 mg three times a day. The efficiency with single dose of budesonide is related to a considerably higher concentration of preparation in blood serum and also higher absolute bioavailability [13]. We prescribe high doses of mesalazine, >8 g/day, in patients with severe forms of UC. The dose of budesonide is increased up to 18 mg/day, and we then combine it with steroids. Because of the ineffectiveness of mesalazine and budesonide application, high second-line doses are prescribed, e.g. immunosuppressors or biological therapy preparations. Difficulties of therapy are that 25–30% of patients are resistant to basic therapy with standard doses, and that the side effects due to systemic glucocorticoids and immunosuppressants are forecasted.

Azathioprine is suitable for chronic slack steroid-resistant and steroid-dependent active forms of UC treatment, supporting disease remission and cannot be used in acute situations. To achieve a maximal effect, 4–6 months are required. Prescribing azathioprine in a complex with steroids allows to reduce the preparation dose. However, prolonged azathioprine use leads to the development of colon neoplasia in UC patients [14].

The observation in patients who had taken azathioprine for 7 years testifies the necessity of conducting colectomy in 88% of the cases. Patients who did not take azathioprine had better results [15]. Short-term cyclosporine treatment is effective in steroid-dependent UC and is an alternative treatment for glucocorticoid therapy in patients with a severe attack. In glucocorticoid and cytostatic refractory forms of UC, inhibitors of TNF-α are used such as adalimumab and certolizumab – the clinical effects of application of which are similar to that of in-fliximab. According to the results of two placebo-controlled reports [16, 17], infliximab application leads to a clinical improvement and remission in patients with severe intensity and middle gravity intensity of UC, which did not react to standard therapy. However, currently the US FDA has only approved natalizumab. The future perspective is application of recombinant human IL-10 [2].

The ultimate goal of treatment nowadays is removing or improving patients' complaints and symptoms, prophylaxis or reducing complications and in the future 'convalescence' of mucous membrane and development of etiotropic therapy. A promising trend in UC treatment is the use of cytoprotectors, which will lead to an increased resistance of the bowels' mucosal epithelial cells. Rebamipide is a novel agent that stimulates mucosal epithelial cell regeneration by increasing the expression of epithelial growth factor. We examined 25 patients with an average severe course of UC (the index of clinical activity 6–12; endoscopic index 4 according to Rachmilewitz, 1989) who were divided into three groups depending on curative complexes: group I (n = 9): mesalazine (tablets) 3 g/day and budesonide 9 mg/day taken 3 times; group II (n = 8): mesalazine (granules) 3 g/day and budesonide 9 mg/day taken once; group III (n = 8): mesalazine (granules) 3 g/day and budesonide 9 mg/day taken once + rebamipide 300 mg/day.

Clinical, endoscopic assessments were made at baseline and the end of the study and symptoms were recorded on a daily basis. The primary endpoint was introduction of clinical remission and clinical improvement was also measured using the UC disease activity index. The exchange of fuco- and sialoproteins was estimated according to their concentration in blood and the level of their excretion with urine, taking into account the state of the patients. Studying the state of the protective mucous barrier in intestinal inflammatory diseases is particularly important, as well as establishing any damage as a result of inflammation and ulceration.

The largest number of patients in the clinical remission phase after 8 weeks of therapy was recorded: in group III, 6 patients (75%), in group II, 5 patients (62.5%), and in group I, 5 patients (55.6%). The duration of clinical remission was: 24.7 ± 1.4 days in group I, 27.5 ± 1.7 days in group II, and 30.7 ± 1.8 days in group III ($p > 0.05$). Endoscopic remission was detected in 3 (33.3%) patients of group I, in 4 (50%) patients of group II, and in 5 (62.5%) patients of group III.

An increased concentration of N-acetylneuraminic acid was detected in the patients of all groups as well as a 1.8 times decrease of the blood fucose level in connection with albumin ($p < 0.05$). The prescription of curative complexes leads to a reduction of N-acetylneuraminic acid of 1.4 times and in fucose to an increase of 1.5 times in blood, which is significantly expressed in group III ($p < 0.05$). The same changes were detected in the examination of excretion of fucose in urine.

During a previously conducted multicenter research in patients with medially severe and severe UC, it was found that rebamipide's efficiency in enemas was similar to the effect of 5-aminosalicylic acid on the background of basic therapy in the disease activity index, endoscopic index score, endoscopic grading scale, and biopsy score [18]. Analogous results were obtained by the research of Ogata et al. [19] in which rebamipide's efficiency in enemas was observed in UC through strengthening the expressiveness of intercellular protein of claudin-1 in the intestine's epithelial cells. Rebamipide has a broad spectrum of pharmacological actions that include suppression of neutrophil functions and stimulation of mucosal epithelial cell regeneration. Thus, rebamipide renders a protective effect on the mucous membrane of intestine by strengthening the expressiveness of epithelial factor of growth, reducing peroxide oxidation in the mucous membrane of intestine, stimulating regeneration of the mucous membrane of intestine, and suppressing the function of neutrophils [20, 21].

When comprising treatment complexes for UC patients, it is necessary to take into account the presence of viral and bacterial superinfections that can imitate an intensification of the disease. Probiotic preparations of *Lactobacillus* GG are effective and safe for UC patients in a composition of antirecurrent complexes in combination with mesalazine. *Lactobacillus* GG treatment is more effective than standard therapy on the basis of mesalazine with regard to duration; it is free from intensification ($p < 0.05$) and can be used as a component of antirecurrent therapy [22].

Determining the important role of mucous barrier resistance of intestine in UC, pathogenesis serves as a basis for optimization of medical complexes with the use of antibacterial preparations, probiotics, phosphatidylcholine and preparations of bilious acids. In inflammatory diseases of the bowel, the protective ability of mucous membrane collapses with inflammation and ulceration that is related to the cooperation between the immune system, genetic predisposition and environment.

In experimental colitis using rat models, an increase of bacterial translocation is registered which diminishes when melatonin is administered. In the group of animals with experimental colitis that were given melatonin, there is a marked decrease of the TNF-α concentration, caspase-3 activity and endotoxin level in blood serum [23]. Essential phospholipids are prescribed with the purpose of strengthening the resistance of epithelial cell membranes in the intestine, improving their plasticity and also such effects as antioxidative, disaggregational effect, immunomodulation on a cellular level, restoring damaged membrane structures of the cell, and increasing prostaglandin synthesis [24–26]. Thus, simultaneously essential phospholipids render a hepatoprotective effect that is extremely important during the protracted therapy with aminosalicylates and glucocorticoids.

An important direction in the realization of the concept of 'convalescence of mucous membrane' is prescribing antihypoxants with the purpose of removing tissue hypoxia and improving blood circulation into the mucous membrane of the intestine. The preparation of choice is a deproteinized hemoderivate which provides an increase of the energetic potential of cells (an increase of 5 times the cell consumption of glucose), reduces inflammatory-cellular infiltration, anabolism action, improves blood supply and removes tissue hypoxia.

The influence of UC on quality of life, related to the health of patients, was estimated for 26 patients in an Italian university clinic study [27]. Three questionnaires given to the patients at the ambulatory visit were used, namely SF-36 (general well-confirmed method of measuring of quality of life, related to the health), SCL-90 (for the evaluation of the psychological state of patients) and the Holmes-Rahe scale (for evaluation of vital stress situations). The decrease of quality of life, related to health, and general severity of psychological symptoms is set in UC patients and irritable intestine syndrome. Thus, the gravity of the last vital stress situation is considered as being more difficult in irritable intestine syndrome patients in comparison with UC. The basic task of treatment is not only induction of remission and temporal removal of symptoms, but also maintenance of protracted remission, maintenance of the patient's quality of life and prophylaxis of new malignant formations of the colon [28].

Conclusion

Thus, optimization of the curative complexes with the substitution of mesalazine in tablet or granule form, especially with an additional rebamipide prescription, as a once-daily dose of budesonide will lead to an increase of treatment effectiveness and improvement of overall quality of life in UC patients. In the future, development of new approaches in the pharmacotherapy of UC will use medications on the background of basic therapy with the purpose of achieving high-quality and effective 'convalescence of mucous membrane', including cytoprotectors (rebamipide), bilious acids (ursodeoxycholic acid), endogenous substances (melatonin), stabilization of membranes (phosphatidylcholine), antihypoxants (deproteinized hemoderivate) and correction of microbiocenosis disorders.

Disclosure Statement

The author declares that no financial or other conflict of interest exists in relation to the content of this article.

References

1 Rogala L, Miller N, Graf LA, Rawsthorne P, Clara I, Walker JR, Lix L, Ediger JP, McPhail C, Bernstein CN: Population-based controlled study of social support, self-perceived stress, activity and work issues, and access to healthcare in inflammatory bowel disease. Inflamm Bowel Dis 2008;23:98–101.

2 Dorofeev AE: Diagnostic and Treatment of the Gastroenterological Diseases. Donetsk, Nord-Press, 2009.

3 Scholmerich J: Ulcerative Colitis and Crohn's Disease. Abstr Falk Workshop on Digestive Diseases: State of the Art and Daily Practice, Santiago de Chile, 2008, pp 15–16.

4 Beaugerie L, Massot N, Carbonnel F, Cattan S, Gendre JP, Cornes J: Impact of cessation of smoking on the course of ulcerative colitis. Am J Gastroenterol 2001;96:2113–2116.

5 Cornes J, Carbonnel F, Beaugerie L, Blain A, Reijasse D, Gendre JP: Effect of appendicectomy on the course of ulcerative colitis. Gut 2002;51:803–807.

6 Schwab M, Schaffeler E, Marx C, Fromm MF, Kaskas B, Metzler J, Stange E, Herfarth H, Scholmerich J, Gregor M, Walker S, Carcorbi I, Roots I, Brinkmann U, Zanger UM, Eichelbaum M: Association between the C3435T MDR1 gene polymorphism and susceptibility for ulcerative colitis. Gastroenterology 2003;124:26–33.

7 Baumgart DC, Carding SR: Inflammatory bowel disease: cause and immunobiology. Lancet 2007;369:1627–1640.

8 Tibble JA, Bjarnason I: Fecal calprotein as an index of intestinal inflammation. Drugs Today 2001;37:85–96.

9 Mikhaylova Y, Pimanov SI, Voropayev Y, Timashova VR: The fecal marker of ulcerative colitis. Rus J Gastroenterol Hepatol Coloproctol 2007;17:60–63.

10 Farup PG, Hilterleitner TA, Lukas M, Heburne X, Rachmilewitz D, Campieri M, Meier R, Keller R, Rathbone B, Oddsson E: Mesalazine 4 g daily given as prolonged-release granules twice daily and four times daily is at least as effective as prolonged-release tablets four times daily in patients with ulcerative colitis. IBD 2001;7:237–242.

11 Kruis W: The optimal dose of 5-aminosalicylic acid in active ulcerative colitis: a dose-finding study with newly developed mesalamine. Clin Gastroenterol Hepatol 2003;1:36–43.

12 Faubion WA, Loftus RV, Harmessen WS: The natural history of corticosteroid therapy for inflammatory bowel disease: a population-based study. Gastroenterology 2001;121:255–260.

13 Kolkman JJ, Molmann HW, Molmann AC: Evaluation of oral budesonide in the treatment of active distal ulcerative colitis. Drugs Today 2004;40:589–601.

14 Hawthorne AB, Logan R NA, Hawkey CJ: Randomized controlled trial of azathioprine withdrawal in ulcerative colitis. Br Med J 1992;305:20–22.

15 Moskovitz DN, Van Assche G, Maenhout B, Arts J, Ferrante M, Vermeire S, Rutgeerts P: Incidence of colectomy during long-term follow-up after cyclosporine-induced remission of severe ulcerative colitis. Clin Gastroenterol Hepatol 2006;4:760–765.

16 Probert C, Hearing S, Schreiber S: Infliximab in moderately severe glucocorticoid-resistant ulcerative colitis: a randomized controlled trial. Gut 2003;52:998–1002.

17 Rutgeerts P, Sandborn WJ, Feagan BG: Infliximab for induction and maintenance therapy for ulcerative colitis. N Engl J Med 2005;353:2462–2476.

18 Miyata M, Satoh M, Kasugai K, Kakumi S, Mori T, Onishi M: Rebamipide enema versus 5-aminosalicylic acid enema for distal ulcerative colitis: a randomized controlled trial. Gut 2006;55(suppl 5):A128.

19 Ogata H, Kamada N, Inoue N, Matsui T, Hibi T: A randomized, multicentre pilot study comparing mesalazine enemas and rebamipide enemas for active ulcerative colitis. Gut 2006;55(suppl 5):A129.

20 Kobayashi T, Zinchuk VS, Garcia del Saz E: Suppressive effect of rebamipide, an anti-ulcer agent, against activation of human neutrophils exposed to formyl-methionyl-leucyl-phenylalanine. Histol Histopathol 2000;15:1067–1076.

21 Masamure A, Yoshida M, Sakai Y, et al: Rebamipide inhibits ceramide-induced interleukin-8 production in Kato III human gastric cancer cells. J Pharmacol Exp Ther 2001;298:485–494.

22 Zocco MA, Zileri dal Verme L, Cremonini F, Piscaglia AC, Nista EC, Candelli M, Novi M, Cazzato IA, Ojetti V, Armuzzi A, Gasbarrini G, Gasbarrini A: Efficacy of lactobacillus GG in maintaining remission of ulcerative colitis. Aliment Pharmacol Ther 2006;23:1567–1574.

23 Akcan A, Kucuk C, Sozuer E, Esel D, Akyildiz H, Akgun H, Muhtaroglu S, Aritas Y: Melatonin reduces bacterial translocation and apoptosis in trinitrobenzene sulphonic acid-induced colitis of rats. World J Gastroenterol 2008;14:918–924.

24 Pankov R, Markovska T, Antonov P: Influence of membrane phospholipids composition and structural organization on spontaneous lipid transfer between membranes. Gen Physiol Biophys 2006;25:313–324.

25 Kingsley M: Effects of phophatidylserine supplementation on exercising humans. Sports Med 2006;36:557–669.

26 Skrypnyk I: Optimization of the treatment of the alcoholic liver disease patients in association with atherosclerosis. Gut 2007;56(suppl 3):A269.

27 Pace F, Molteni P, Bollani S, Sarzi-Puttini P, Stockbrugger R, Porro GB, Drossman DA: Inflammatory bowel disease versus irritable bowel syndrome: a hospital-based, case-control study of disease impact on quality of life. Scand J Gastroenterol 2003;38:1031–1038.

28 Van Assche G: Communication and beliefs of quality of life and mucosal healing treatment goal in everyday practice: results of a large pan-European survey of physicians treating inflammatory bowel disease. Gut 2007;56(suppl 3):A162.

Therapy- and Non-Therapy-Dependent Infectious Complications in Inflammatory Bowel Disease

Hans-Jörg Epple

Medical Clinic I, Gastroenterology, Rheumatology, Infectiology, Charité – Universitätsmedizin Berlin, Campus Benjamin Franklin, Berlin, Germany

Key Words
Inflammatory bowel disease, infectious complications · Non-therapy-dependent infections · Therapy-dependent infections · Immunosuppressive therapy, infection prevention

Abstract
Background: Patients with inflammatory bowel disease (IBD) are susceptible to infections. **Results:** Independently from immunomodulatory therapy, IBD predisposes to infectious complications. Thus, the incidence of *Clostridium difficile* infection is increased in IBD patients, and a significant proportion of these patients contracts *C. difficile* infection outside the hospital and without precedent antibiotic use. Cytomegalovirus infection has been reported in corticosteroid-naive patients with ulcerative colitis, and infectious gastroenteritis has been linked to initiation and exacerbation of IBD. Finally, in Crohn's disease there is a substantial risk for abscess formation, and urinary tract infections occur more frequently than in a non-IBD control population. Apart from the disease process itself, factors that predispose to infectious complications in IBD are malnutrition, advanced age, immunosuppressive medications, leukopenia from immunosuppressive medications, and surgery. However, the main risk for infections is clearly related to the use of immunosuppressive agents such as corticosteroids, azathioprine, methotrexate, cyclosporine, and TNF-blocking biologicals. A wide spectrum of infectious complications has been reported in patients treated with these medications, including viral (e.g. CMV, VZV, EBV), bacterial (e.g. *Mycobacteria*, *Listeria*, staphylococci), fungal (e.g. *Pneumocystis jiroveci*, *Aspergillus*, *Candida*, *Cryptococcus*) and protozoal *(Toxoplasma)* pathogens. The greatest risks obviously relate to the combined use of immunomodulating agents rather than to individual drugs. The risk of infections is also aggravated by an insufficient immunization status as frequently observed in patients with IBD. **Conclusion:** Physicians treating patients with IBD must be aware of the risk for infectious complications in these patients as well as of strategies to minimize them.

Copyright © 2009 S. Karger AG, Basel

Introduction

Infectious complications are a significant cause of morbidity and mortality in inflammatory bowel disease (IBD). Increased rates of infection-related and respiratory deaths have been reported in patients with IBD in Scandinavia [1–6]. The risk for infections may be related to the disease process itself, its complications and/or the use of immunosuppressive medications. In patients without IBD, certain risk factors have been found to predispose to opportunistic infections. These include acquired or inherited immune deficiency states, malnutrition, leukopenia, diabetes mellitus, and target organ diseases such as chronic structural airway disease. Some of these also apply for patients with IBD. As shown in table 1, factors

Table 1. Risk factors for infectious complications in IBD patients [7]

Non-therapy-dependent
   IBD (MC > CU)
   Malnutrition
   Advanced age
Therapy-dependent
   Operations
   Immunosuppressive therapy
   Leukopenia from immunosuppressive therapy

increasing the risk for infections in IBD patients are either associated with therapeutic modalities such as immunosuppressive therapy and operations or independent from these like IBD in its own right, malnutrition, and age [7]. Intercurrent infections in IBD patients pose a difficult problem for several reasons. They often present in an atypical way, are potentially hazardous to the patient's health status, are difficult to treat and may preclude from effective therapy in cases of active IBD. Therefore, knowledge of therapy- and non-therapy-dependent infectious complications in IBD including appropriate diagnostic, therapeutic and preventive strategies are important for each gastroenterologist treating patients with IBD.

Non-Therapy-Dependent Infections

IBD independently predisposes to infectious complications. For example, a major complication of fistulizing Crohn's disease is the formation of abscesses, which most frequently develop in the perianal location, but may also occur intraabdominally or intrahepatically [8–10]. Early abscess detection followed by immediate effective treatment is crucial for patient safety. Standard diagnostic procedures for perianal fistular disease are examination under anesthesia and magnetic resonance imaging or endoscopic ultrasound [11]. After a diagnosis of abscess has been confirmed by imaging techniques, treatment modalities are percutaneous drainage with concurrent antimicrobial therapy or surgery. Most patients treated initially with percutaneous drainage will later have to undergo resective surgery [11].

Although there are no controlled studies investigating the risk for urinary tract infection in IBD, urinary tract infections have been frequently reported in patients with Crohn's disease [12, 13]. In some Crohn patients, these infections occur secondary to enterovesicular fistulas [13]. Bowel resection seems to be another risk factor for the development of cystitis [12]. Therefore, Crohn patients should be frequently asked for urinary symptoms, and a urinalysis should be performed in each patient with suggestive symptoms or before initiation of immunosuppressive therapy. Symptoms such as pneumaturia or fecaluria are almost diagnostic for the presence of an enterovesicular fistula, which should also be searched for in cases of positive polymicrobial urine culture or frequently recurrent cystitis.

Numerous studies described an association of enteric infections with relapse of IBD. Pathogens involved include *Clostridium difficile*, *Salmonella* spp., *Shigella* spp., *Campylobacter* spp., *Escherichia coli*, cytomegalovirus and *Entamoeba histolytica* [14–18]. The problem of cytomegalovirus reactivation in IBD is covered in another contribution to this issue [see article by I. Zaytsev]. Enteric infections are not only regarded as potential triggers of IBD flares, but there also is evidence for a role of infectious diarrhea in the initiation of IBD [19, 20]. Still, comparative data on the prevalence of enteric pathogens associated with diarrheal relapse of IBD are sparse. In a retrospective cohort study from London, about 10% of relapses were associated with infections, 5.5% being due to *C. difficile* and the remainder to other organisms like *Campylobacter*, *Salmonella* and *E. histolytica* [14]. The high prevalence of *C. difficile* in this study came as a surprise because earlier reports published during the 1980s found a low prevalence of *C. difficile* infection in IBD patients. Therefore, the contribution of *C. difficile* infection to morbidity and mortality of patients with IBD was considered to be low and specific testing for this pathogen was not warranted in IBD patients experiencing colitis flare. Recent reports indicate that this recommendation no longer is correct. Thus, up to 20% of IBD flares were associated with a positive stool ELISA for *C. difficile* toxins [21]. This change coincides with the changed epidemiology for *C. difficile* infection showing increased incidence and mortality in numerous studies from the USA and Europe. In a recent study from a tertiary referral population of IBD patients, between 2000 and 2005 a significant increase in the number and rate of IBD patients with *C. difficile* infection was found [22]. Moreover, a diagnosis of IBD was associated with an increased risk for *C. difficile infection*, and *C. difficile* infection aggravated the clinical course of IBD in a significant number of patients, with increased risk for hospitalization as well as colectomy [23, 24]. In summary, in IBD patients with diarrhea, routine stool tests for enteric pathogens, parasites, and *C. difficile* toxins A and B should be performed. Only in the absence of risk factors for enteric infection (such as

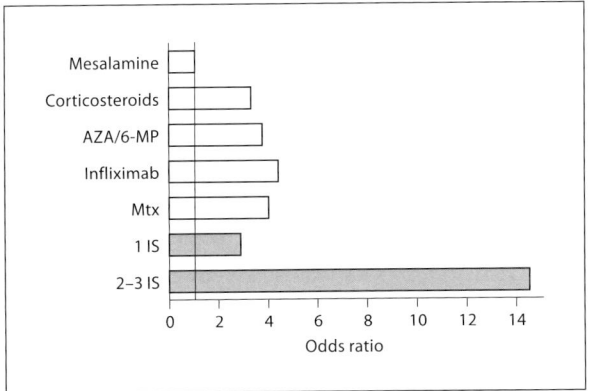

Fig. 1. Association between use of immunosuppressive medication and odds for opportunistic infection. 1 IS = Use of single immunosuppressive medication; 2–3 IS = combined use of two or three immunosuppressive medications (according to Toruner et al. [25]).

Table 2. Opportunistic infections reported with immunosuppressive therapy in patients with IB [26]

Viral	Herpes zoster Herpes simplex CMV EBV HPV	Protozoal	*Toxoplasma* *Coccidiodides* *Leishmania*
Bacterial	*C. difficile* *E. coli* *Salmonella* spp. *S. pneumoniae* *M. tuberculosis* Non-tuberculous MB *Legionella* spp. *L. monocytogenes* *Nocardia*	Fungal	*Candida* *P. jiroveci* *Aspergillus* spp. *Histoplasma* *Cryptococcus* spp. *Blastomyces* *Coccidiodides*

previous antibiotic therapy, history of infectious diarrhea, travel history, fever) and if the presenting symptoms fulfill the patient-individual pattern of a diarrheal flare may a thorough diagnostic workup for infectious diarrhea be omitted.

Therapy-Dependent Infections

Anti-inflammatory and immunomodulatory medications are indispensible in the management of IBD. Unfortunately, the medications used – corticosteroids, purine analogues, methotrexate, cyclophosphamide, cyclosporine, tacrolimus and anti-TNF drugs – are all associated with infections. In a recent case-control study performed in IBD patients, the use of corticosteroids, AZA/6-MP, and infliximab were all associated with an increased risk for development of opportunistic infections [25]. In multivariate analysis, the odds for development of an opportunistic infection were increased by these drugs by a factor of 3. Moreover, when used in combination, these drugs synergistically increased the likelihood of an opportunistic infection with a calculated odds ratio of 14, if two or three drugs were combined (fig. 1) [25]. These observations add further evidence – if needed – to the plausible notion that opportunistic infections are important iatrogenic complications of immunomodulatory therapy and that the risk for opportunistic infection correlates with the level of immunosuppression.

A broad spectrum of opportunistic and non-opportunistic pathogens has been attributed to the immunomodulatory therapies in IBD (table 2). Modulated by host immune status, co-medication and exposition to certain pathogens, all different kinds of infections may occur with every immunosuppressive regimen [26]. Still, due to their mechanism of action, drugs such as corticosteroids, AZA/6-MP, MTX, cyclosporine and TNF antagonists predispose to a certain degree for infection with certain pathogens. For example, as a result of T-lymphocyte apoptosis, purine antimetabolites predispose to infection by herpes viruses such as cytomegalovirus, varicella zoster virus, herpes simplex virus or Epstein-Barr virus [25]. Glucocorticosteroids exert less obvious effects on lymphocytes, but inhibit neutrophil macrophage function. Therefore, immunosuppression with corticosteroids is associated with a markedly increased risk for *Candida* infections at mucosal surfaces [25]. Due to their inhibiting action on granuloma formation, TNF antagonists are strongly associated with the risk for reactivation of granulomatous infections [27]. If such reactivation occurs, inhibited granuloma formation often leads to atypical manifestations like extrapulmonary tuberculosis.

In general, the diagnostic approach in patients with infectious complications should therefore be guided by localizing symptoms as well as by any identified disposition for infection with certain pathogens. Furthermore, the indication for anti-TNF-based therapies should carefully be weighed against the potential risk for reactivation of granulomatous infections. In particular, testing for latent tuberculosis by tuberculin skin test or interferon-γ release assay is mandatory for IBD patients planned for anti-TNF therapy. Patients identified with latent tuberculosis should receive prophylactic INH-treatment (start 1 month prior to anti-TNF, total duration 9 months, alternatively 4 months of rifampin), and patients with suspected or proven active tuberculosis should not receive anti-TNF treatment but rather be treated for tuberculosis with a standard four-drug regimen [28].

Prevention of Infections in IBD Patients on Immunosuppressive Therapy

In light of the increased risk for infection and its associated mortality in immunosuppressed patients with IBD [2], prevention rather than treatment of infection seems most desirable in these patients. As outlined in a recent review by Viget et al. [26], the preventive strategy is based on risk identification, vaccination, and prophylactic treatment of bacterial, fungal or viral infections.

Risk identification includes a systematic diagnostic workup prior to immunosuppression including a comprehensive history (e.g. travel history, contact with infectious patients, history of VZV, HSV, EBV, and CMV infection, vaccination status), clinical examination focused on detection of possible local or systemic infection, laboratory tests (e.g. complete blood count, CRP, urinalysis, serology for CMV, HSV, VZV, HBV, HCV, and HIV), tuberculin skin testing and chest X-ray.

Vaccination is warranted against pneumococcal disease, influenza (annually), and HBV. Varicella vaccine should also be considered for seronegative patients but only be administered before immunosuppression has been started, because the varicella vaccine is an attenuated life vaccine which – like other life vaccines – is contraindicated in patients on immunosuppression. In respect to the growing concern regarding HPV infection in young women with IBD, it seems likely that HPV vaccination will also be recommended in the future to this patient group. Presently however, no data are available regarding the immunogenicity and duration of HPV vaccination in IBD patients on immunosuppressive therapy.

Preemptive therapy for latent tuberculosis has been dealt with before (see above). Data on chemoprophylaxis for *Pneumocystis jiroveci* pneumonia in IBD patients are scarce. Extrapolating from other groups of immunocompromised patients, it is recommended by many experts for patients treated with multiple immunosuppressants and those with a CD4 T-cell count of <300 cells/μl. The agent of choice is trimethoprim-sulfamethoxazole, 480 mg daily. Alternative regimens are aerolized pentamidine, dapsone or atovaquone. Patients with chronic hepatitis B infection or HIV infection should be treated with antivirals before immunosuppressive therapy is started. Furthermore, continual aciclovir or valaciclovir treatment should be considered in patients who have more than four episodes of HSV disease per year [26].

Disclosure Statement

The author declares that no financial or other conflict of interest exists in relation to the content of this article.

References

1 Ekbom A, Helmick CG, Zack M, et al: Survival and causes of death in patients with inflammatory bowel disease: a population-based study. Gastroenterology 1992;103: 954–960.
2 Hutfless SM, Weng X, Liu L, et al: Mortality by medication use among patients with inflammatory bowel disease, 1996–2003. Gastroenterology 2007;133:1779–1786.
3 Jess T, Loftus EV Jr, Harmsen WS, et al: Survival and cause specific mortality in patients with inflammatory bowel disease: a long-term outcome study in Olmsted County, Minnesota, 1940–2004. Gut 2006;55:1248–1254.
4 Jess T, Gamborg M, Munkholm P, et al: Overall and cause-specific mortality in ulcerative colitis: meta-analysis of population-based inception cohort studies. Am J Gastroenterol 2007;102:609–617.
5 Persson PG, Bernell O, Leijonmarck CE, et al: Survival and cause-specific mortality in inflammatory bowel disease: a population-based cohort study. Gastroenterology 1996; 110:1339–1345.
6 Winther KV, Jess T, Langholz E, et al: Survival and cause-specific mortality in ulcerative colitis: follow-up of a population-based cohort in Copenhagen County. Gastroenterology 2003;125:1576–1582.
7 Aberra FN, Lichtenstein GR: Methods to avoid infections in patients with inflammatory bowel disease. Inflamm Bowel Dis 2005; 11:685–695.
8 Hurst RD, Molinari M, Chung TP, et al: Prospective study of the features, indications, and surgical treatment in 513 consecutive patients affected by Crohn's disease. Surgery 1997;122:661–668.
9 Keighley MR, Eastwood D, Ambrose NS, et al: Incidence and microbiology of abdominal and pelvic abscess in Crohn's disease. Gastroenterology 1982;83:1271–1275.

10 Mir-Madjlessi SH, McHenry MC, Farmer RG: Liver abscess in Crohn's disease. Report of four cases and review of the literature. Gastroenterology 1986;91:987–993.
11 Schwartz DA, Wiersema MJ, Dudiak KM, et al: A comparison of endoscopic ultrasound, magnetic resonance imaging, and exam under anesthesia for evaluation of Crohn's perianal fistulas. Gastroenterology 2001; 121:1064–1072.
12 Ben-Ami H, Ginesin Y, Behar DM, et al: Diagnosis and treatment of urinary tract complications in Crohn's disease: an experience over 15 years. Can J Gastroenterol 2002;16: 225–229.
13 Gruner JS, Sehon JK, Johnson LW: Diagnosis and management of enterovesical fistulas in patients with Crohn's disease. Am Surg 2002; 68:714–719.
14 Mylonaki M, Langmead L, Pantes A, et al: Enteric infection in relapse of inflammatory bowel disease: importance of microbiological examination of stool. Eur J Gastroenterol Hepatol 2004;16:775–778.
15 Hermens DJ, Miner PB Jr: Exacerbation of ulcerative colitis. Gastroenterology 1991; 101:254–262.
16 Kochhar R, Ayyagari A, Goenka MK, et al: Role of infectious agents in exacerbations of ulcerative colitis in India. A study of *Clostridium difficile*. J Clin Gastroenterol 1993; 16:26–30.
17 Weber P, Koch M, Heizmann WR, et al: Microbic superinfection in relapse of inflammatory bowel disease. J Clin Gastroenterol 1992;14:302–308.
18 Szilagyi A, Gerson M, Mendelson J, et al: *Salmonella* infections complicating inflammatory bowel disease. J Clin Gastroenterol 1985;7:251–255.
19 Ruigomez A, Garcia Rodriguez LA, Panes J: Risk of irritable bowel syndrome after an episode of bacterial gastroenteritis in general practice: influence of comorbidities. Clin Gastroenterol Hepatol 2007;5:465–469.
20 Porter CK, Tribble DR, Aliaga PA, et al: Infectious gastroenteritis and risk of developing inflammatory bowel disease. Gastroenterology 2008;135:781–786.
21 Meyer AM, Ramzan NN, Loftus EV Jr, et al: The diagnostic yield of stool pathogen studies during relapses of inflammatory bowel disease. J Clin Gastroenterol 2004;38:772–775.
22 Issa M, Ananthakrishnan AN, Binion DG: *Clostridium difficile* and inflammatory bowel disease. Inflamm Bowel Dis 2008;14:1432–1442.
23 Issa M, Vijayapal A, Graham MB, et al: Impact of *Clostridium difficile* on inflammatory bowel disease. Clin Gastroenterol Hepatol 2007;5:345–351.
24 Ananthakrishnan AN, McGinley EL, Binion DG: Excess hospitalisation burden associated with *Clostridium difficile* in patients with inflammatory bowel disease. Gut 2008;57: 205–210.
25 Toruner M, Loftus EV, Jr., Harmsen WS, et al: Risk factors for opportunistic infections in patients with inflammatory bowel disease. Gastroenterology 2008;134:929–936.
26 Viget N, Vernier-Massouille G, Salmon-Ceron D, et al: Opportunistic infections in patients with inflammatory bowel disease: prevention and diagnosis. Gut 2008;57:549–558.
27 Wallis RS, Broder MS, Wong JY, et al: Granulomatous infectious diseases associated with tumor necrosis factor antagonists. Clin Infect Dis 2004;38:1261–1265.
28 Wallis RS. Anti-tuberculosis treatment and infliximab. Respir Med 2005;99:1620–1622.

Laparoscopic Management of Inflammatory Bowel Disease

Raul J. Rosenthal   Badma Bashankaev   Steven D. Wexner

Cleveland Clinic Florida, Weston, Fla., USA

Key Words
Laparoscopy · Inflammatory bowel disease · Terminal ileum

Abstract
The goal of the surgical management of Crohn's disease is to improve quality of life. Surgical management is generally reserved for patients who developed complications of the disease or who are unresponsive to or develop complications from aggressive medical therapy. Friable mesentery, inflammatory phlegmons, fistulas, abscesses, and adhesions from previous surgeries pose a surgical challenge to the laparoscopic approach. The laparoscopic approach to terminal ileal Crohn's disease is feasible and safe even in cases complicated by fistulas with previous abdominal surgery or recurrent disease. This approach is associated with an increased operative time compared to laparotomy, however, offers significant advantages over open ileocolic resection in terms of pulmonary function, length of hospital stay, duration of postoperative ileus, cosmesis, postoperative small bowel obstruction, and early postoperative complications. Laparoscopy is also associated with decreased overall hospitalization costs and improved patient satisfaction. Therefore, the laparoscopic approach for patients with Crohn's disease should be considered as the preferred operative approach.

Copyright © 2009 S. Karger AG, Basel

Laparoscopic Treatment of Crohn's Disease

The goal of the surgical treatment of Crohn's disease is to improve quality of life. Surgery is generally reserved for patients who develop complications of the disease such as strictures and fistulas or who are unresponsive to or develop complications from aggressive medical therapy. Markedly thickened bowel loops, thickened and friable mesentery, inflammatory phlegmons, fistulas, abscesses, and adhesions from previous surgeries pose a surgical challenge to the laparoscopic approach.

Studies of Crohn's Disease

In 1996, Reissman et al. [1] reported their early experience of laparoscopy in 29 patients with terminal ileitis. A mean length of the hospital stay was 5.2 days and an overall morbidity rate was 10%. A further study of Reissman et al. [2] assessed a series of 51 patients with Crohn's disease. The mean length of hospital stay was 5.1 days. The overall conversion and complication rates were 14% each, and there was no mortality. Alabaz et al. [3a] retrospectively compared the safety, outcome, and feasibility of laparoscopic-assisted and conventional laparotomy for ileocolic resection in Crohn's disease. The length of hospitalization was significantly longer in the laparotomy group (9.6 vs. 7 days) with no difference in the morbidity rate (16.7 vs. 15.3%) and conversion (11%). Patients in the laparoscopically-assisted group returned to work faster

(3.7 weeks) compared with 8.2 weeks in the laparotomy group, had better cosmetic results and improved social and sexual lives.

Hamel et al. [4] showed the feasibility and safety of laparoscopically-assisted subtotal colectomy in patients with Crohn's disease compared to ileocolic resection. Although there were more intraoperative complications in the subtotal colectomy group (29 vs. 7%), the hospital stay was similar (8.8 days) and the postoperative complication rate was not significantly different (29 and 18%, respectively).

Laparoscopic management of Crohn's disease is complicated by fistulas, abscess, or strictures and is therefore especially challenging. Watanabe et al. [5] reviewed 25 laparoscopic operations in 20 patients with a total of 31 intestinal fistulas. The complication and conversion rates were 16% each. The median hospital stay was 8 days.

Duepree et al. [6] compared 21 patients who had a laparoscopic ileocolic resection with 24 patients who had an open resection. The median length of hospital stay was significantly shorter in the laparoscopic group compared to the open group (3 and 5 days, respectively). Resumption of oral intake and intestinal function were faster in the laparoscopic group, and there was no difference in the complication rate between the groups (14.3 and 16.7%, respectively). Benoist et al. [7] compared the postoperative outcome of 24 laparoscopic ileocolic resections with 32 open cases. There were no significant differences between the two groups in the morbidity and mortality rates, operative time, resumption of bowel function, hospital stay, and postoperative morphine requirement.

Young-Fadok et al. [9] matched 33 cases of laparoscopic ileocolic resections with 33 open resections. They found significantly shorter length of hospital stay, a shorter period of narcotic use, and reduced time to regular diet in the laparoscopic group compared to the laparotomy group without any significant differences in the complication rates.

Long-term outcomes following laparoscopic ileocolic resections were assessed in several studies. Alabaz et al. [3a] reported significantly more symptomatic bowel obstructions in the laparotomy group compared to the laparoscopic group in a mean follow-up of 30 months (31 vs. 8%, respectively). Bergamaschi et al. [3b] compared 39 patients who underwent laparoscopic ileocolic resection with 53 patients who had previously undergone open resection by the same surgeons at the same institution in terms of small bowel obstruction and recurrence rates at a follow-up of 5 years. They reported a significantly lower rate of small bowel obstruction following laparoscopy (11.1 vs. 35.4% following laparotomy) with no differences in the recurrence rates (27.7 and 29.1%, respectively).

Milsom et al. [8a] compared the short-term outcome of 31 patients in the laparoscopic group versus 29 in the laparotomy group. They found a significantly faster recovery of pulmonary function and fewer minor complications in the laparoscopic group compared to the laparotomy group (13 and 28%, respectively). However, there were no significant differences in the amount of morphine used, return of bowel function parameters, or the median length of stay between the two groups.

Thaler et al. [8b] showed that long-term quality of life is significantly reduced in patients with CD at long-term follow-up after both laparoscopic and open surgery and lower than in the general healthy population. Irrespective of the surgical procedure, recurrence was the single significant predictor of quality of life in this study.

Several studies have conducted economic analysis of surgery for ileocolic Crohn's disease. Duepree et al. [6] demonstrated significantly lower direct cost per case for the laparoscopic group compared to the open group. Young-Fadok et al. [9] showed significantly lower direct and indirect costs in the laparoscopic group compared to the laparotomy group.

Laparoscopic experience has improved over recent years. However, Hamel et al. [10] showed no differences in either morbidity or conversion between the earlier and the latter time periods of the experience, suggesting maintenance of a plateau after the initial experience.

Summarizing the Approach

The laparoscopic approach to terminal ileal Crohn's disease is feasible and safe even in cases complicated by fistulas or in patients with previous abdominal surgery or recurrent disease. This approach is associated with an increased operative time compared to laparotomy; however, it offers significant advantages over open ileocolic resection in terms of pulmonary function, length of hospital stay, duration of postoperative ileus, cosmesis, postoperative small bowel obstruction, and early postoperative complications. Laparoscopy is also associated with decreased overall hospitalization costs and improved patient satisfaction. Therefore, the laparoscopic approach for patients with Crohn's disease should be considered as the preferred operative approach.

Laparoscopic Surgery for Ulcerative Colitis and Familial Adenomatous Polyposis

The surgical approach to the treatment of mucosal ulcerative colitis (MUC) and familial adenomatous polyposis (FAP) has dramatically evolved; restorative proctocolectomy with the construction of an ileal reservoir emerged as the treatment of choice to manage these conditions [11, 12]. In the case of MUC, procedures like appendicostomy and ileostomy, aimed to decompress the colon, were followed by safe treatment options like subtotal colectomy and completion proctectomy [11]. For decades, FAP, a condition with a 100% risk of colorectal cancer in untreated individuals, was managed with total proctocolectomy and permanent stoma, the only efficacious treatment to lower cancer mortality and morbidity [13]. However, living with a permanent stoma was not an attractive option for many of these patients and diverse attempts to avoid a permanent stoma were undertaken. Procedures like straight ileoanal anastomosis were performed in the mid 20th century but with poor functional outcomes [11, 14]. In 1976, Parks and Nicholls [15] described the technique of ileal reservoir-anal anastomosis after total proctocolectomy in 8 patients with MUC, obtaining satisfactory results in 4 out of 5 patients available to follow-up by the time of publication. During the last 30 years, restorative proctocolectomy with ileal pouch-anal anastomosis (IPAA) has become the standard surgical treatment for patients with MUC and FAP [11–13, 16–21] and several modifications to the original technique have been advocated including changes to the shape of the pouch itself [12, 13]. In the original technique, a transanal mucosectomy followed by a pouch-anal hand-sewn anastomosis was performed [12, 15]. Alternatively, closure of the rectum with a stapler and completion of the anastomosis with a circular stapler placed through the staple line – the so-called double-stapling technique – was described by Knight and Griffen [22] and was intended to preserve the anal transition zone, hence achieving better functional results [11–13]. Temporary diverting loop ileostomy has been routinely used as a protective measure. However, several studies have proposed the single stage pouch as a safe alternative [18, 23–25].

Laparoscopic surgery was originally introduced by gynecologists mainly with diagnostic purposes. General surgeons adopted this technique [26] and virtually all abdominal procedures have been successfully completed laparoscopically. Laparoscopic colectomy and IPAA (Lap-IPAA) for the treatment of MUC and FAP was intended to take advantage of the benefits of laparoscopy such as early bowel function recovery, decreased pain, less adhesions, shorter hospital stay and better cosmesis [13]. However, these benefits were not as obvious with such a complex and technically demanding undertaking. In 1992, Wexner et al. [26] published the results of a prospective trial in which they compared the results of 5 patients who underwent open versus 5 patients who underwent laparoscopic-assisted total abdominal colectomy. In this short, early series, parameters like length of surgery, length of ileus and hospital stay were longer for the laparoscopic group; no morbidity or mortality were seen. In another study by the same authors [27], in which 5 patients with MUC were treated using the laparoscopic approach, operative time was significantly longer and only a shorter length of incision but no recognizable advantages in terms of morbidity or hospital length of stay were observed. Schmitt et al. [28] compared duration of ileus and of hospitalization in 22 patients who underwent laparoscopic-assisted colectomy and 20 age, gender, and diagnosis-matched controls who underwent standard colectomy and they found that neither the length of time for ileus resolution nor the length of hospitalization were reduced in the laparoscopic group concluding that Lap-IPAA failed to provide any of the theoretical advantages described for other laparoscopic procedures. Other series of patients with MUC or FAP treated with laparoscopic TPC + IPAA are listed in table 1 [17, 18, 29–34].

Marcello et al. [35] compared laparoscopic versus open restorative proctocolectomy by using a case-matched design that included 40 patients, 20 consecutive laparoscopic cases (13 MUC, 7 FAP) and 20 open cases (13 MUC, 7 FAP) and found that operative time was significantly longer but bowel function returned more quickly and the length of stay was shorter in laparoscopic cases. Dunker et al. [16] matched 16 patients who underwent a Lap-

Table 1. Laparoscopic TPC + IPAA (case series)

Group	Year	Patients	Mean OR time	Morbidity
Tucker [34]	1995	4	5 h, 27 min	Not stated
Liu [31]	1995	5	8 h	20%
Hildebrandt [30]	1998	5	6 h	0
Santoro [33]	1999	5	6 h, 4 min	0
Pace [32]	2002	13	4 h, 25 min	46%
Hasegawa [29]	2002	18	6 h	33.3%
Ky [18]	2002	32	5 h, 15 min	34%
Kienle [17]	2003	59	5 h, 20 min	18%

IPAA with 19 patients who had a conventional IPAA. No differences were found in functional outcome and quality of life, and satisfaction with the cosmetic result of the scar was significantly higher in the laparoscopic-assisted group compared with the conventional group. They found that neither functional outcome nor quality of life of Lap-IPAA were different from conventional IPAA. In the long term, better cosmesis was the most important advantage after laparoscopic surgery. In a case-control study, Marcello et al. [36] published results in which 19 patients who underwent laparoscopic total colectomy were compared to 29 patients who underwent open total colectomy for acute colitis. This study aimed to determine the safety and efficacy of laparoscopic colectomy in patients in the acute setting when compared with those individuals undergoing conventional urgent colectomy. The authors found that operative times were significantly longer in the laparoscopic group but bowel function returned more quickly and the length of stay was shorter, and therefore concluded that the technique was feasible and safe in patients with acute nonfulminant colitis and could lead to a faster recovery than conventional resection. Ky et al. [18] addressed the issue of the feasibility of a one-stage laparoscopic-assisted restorative proctocolectomy in patients with MUC and FAP; 32 (29 MUC and 3 FAP) patients who underwent such a procedure over a 24-month period were followed up prospectively for short- and long-term complications and functional outcome. The 11 postoperative complications included were 1 pelvic abscess, and 1 pouch leak requiring reoperation (1 temporary ileostomy and 1 transpouch drainage). In this study, it was concluded that one-stage laparoscopic-assisted restorative proctocolectomy could be performed effectively and safely. In 2005, Larson et al. [20] published the results of a study designed to assess the operative, functional, and quality-of-life outcomes in patients with MUC or FAP with a minimum of 1 year follow-up after undergoing Lap-IPAA versus open IPAA. Patients were matched by age, gender, body mass index, and indication. Postoperative morbidity occurred in 6% of the laparoscopic cases and 12% of the open cases. Functional outcome after a minimum of 1 year revealed equivalent median day and median nocturnal number of stools and quality of life was equivalent as well. It was concluded that the function and quality-of-life outcomes for patients undergoing Lap-IPAA seemed to be equivalent to the open experience. Also, in 2006, Larson et al. [19] released their results on a study in which 100 Lap-IPAA patients were case-matched to 200 open IPAA patients by age, operation, gender, date of operation, and body mass index and operative and postoperative outcomes at 90 days were compared. The laparoscopic conversion rate was 6%. Median operative time was longer for the Lap-IPAA group. Lap-IPAA patients had shorter median time to regular diet, time to ileostomy output, length of stay, and decreased IV narcotic use. Postoperative morbidity was equivalent and readmission rates were equal. The authors concluded that Lap-IPAA is equivalent to open IPAA in terms of safety and feasibility. In addition, Lap-IPAA provided significant improvements in short-term recovery outcomes. Other series of patients with MUC or FAP treated with laparoscopic TPC + IPAA versus open TPC + IPAA are grouped in table 2 [28, 37, 38]. All of these studies have the common denominator of a highly skilled surgical team operating on very carefully selected patients.

Among the proved benefits of laparoscopic-assisted restorative proctocolectomy and IPAA for the treatment of MUC and FAP are shorter length of hospital stay with shorter ileus and faster recovery and milder postoperative pain. In addition, a better cosmesis is attributable to this approach. On the other hand, significantly longer operative times have to be expected. However, due to the complexity of this procedure, a steep and longer learning curve is expected before it can be routinely and safely undertaken. Prospective randomized studies are optimal before this complex procedure can be considered the best option for the surgical management of these diseases.

Table 2. TPC + IPAA, laparoscopic vs. open (other series)

Author	Year	Surgery	Patients	MUC/FAP	Op. time min	Morbidity, %	Hosp. stay days
Schmitt [28]	1994	Lap.	22	16/6	240	68	8.7
		Open	20	15/5	120	35	8.9
Araki [37]	2001	Lap.	21	21	215	33.3	3.6
		Open	11	11	198	45.5	3.9
Hashimoto [38]	2001	Lap.	11	6/5	443	64	24.1
		Open	13		422	38	31.3

Disclosure Statement

S.D. Wexner is a consultant for Covidien, received a consultant fee from Karl Storz, Ethicon, and honoraria and stock options from Power Medical Interventions. R.J. Rosenthal is a consultant and received educational grants from Ethicon, Covidien and Karl Storz.

References

1 Reissman P, et al: Laparoscopic surgery in the management of inflammatory bowel disease. Am J Surg 1996;171:47–51.
2 Reissman P, et al: Laparoscopic surgery in Crohn's disease. Indications and results. Surg Endosc 1996;10:1201–1204.
3a Alabaz O, et al: Comparison of laparoscopically assisted and conventional ileocolic resection for Crohn's disease. Eur J Surg 2000;166:213–217.
3b Bergamaschi R, Pessaux P, Arnaud JP: Comparison of conventional and laparoscopic ileocolic resection for Crohn's disease. Dis Colon Rectum 2003;46:1129–1133.
4 Hamel CT, et al: Laparoscopic surgery for inflammatory bowel disease. Surg Endosc 2001;15:642–645.
5 Watanabe M, et al: Successful application of laparoscopic surgery to the treatment of Crohn's disease with fistulas. Dis Colon Rectum 2002;45:1057–1061.
6 Duepree HJ, et al: Advantages of laparoscopic resection for ileocecal Crohn's disease. Dis Colon Rectum 2002;45:605–610.
7 Benoist S, et al: Laparoscopic ileocecal resection in Crohn's disease: a case-matched comparison with open resection. Surg Endosc 2003;17:814–818.
8a Milsom JW, et al: Prospective, randomized trial comparing laparoscopic vs. conventional surgery for refractory ileocolic Crohn's disease. Dis Colon Rectum 2001;44:1–8; discussion 8–9.
8b Thaler K, Dinnewitzer A, Oberwalder M, Weiss EG, Nogueras JJ, Wexner SD: Assessment of long-term quality of life after laparoscopic and open surgery for Crohn's disease. Colorectal Dis 2005;7:375–381.
9 Young-Fadok TM, et al: Advantages of laparoscopic resection for ileocolic Crohn's disease. Improved outcomes and reduced costs. Surg Endosc 2001;15:450–454.
10 Hamel CT, Pikarsky AJ, Wexner SD: Laparoscopically assisted hemicolectomy for Crohn's disease: are we still getting better? Am Surg 2002;68:83–86.
11 Bach SP, Mortensen NJ: Revolution and evolution: 30 years of ileoanal pouch surgery. Inflamm Bowel Dis 2006;12:131–145.
12 Garbus JE, Potenti F, Wexner SD: Current controversies in pouch surgery. South Med J 2003;96:32–36.
13 Bruch HP, et al: Pouch reconstruction in the pelvis. Langenbecks Arch Surg 2003;388:60–75.
14 Ravitch MM, Sabiston DC: Anal ileostomy with preservation of the sphincter: A proposed operation in patients requiring total colectomy for benign lesions. Surg Gynecol Obstet 1947;8:1095–1099.
15 Parks AG, Nicholls RJ: Proctocolectomy without ileostomy for ulcerative colitis. Br Med J 1978;2:85–88.
16 Dunker MS, et al: Functional outcome, quality of life, body image, and cosmesis in patients after laparoscopic-assisted and conventional restorative proctocolectomy: a comparative study. Dis Colon Rectum 2001;44:1800–1807.
17 Kienle P, et al: Laparoscopically assisted colectomy and ileoanal pouch procedure with and without protective ileostomy. Surg Endosc 2003;17:716–720.
18 Ky AJ, Sonoda T, Milsom JW: One-stage laparoscopic restorative proctocolectomy: an alternative to the conventional approach? Dis Colon Rectum 2002;45:207–211.
19 Larson DW, et al: Safety, feasibility, and short-term outcomes of laparoscopic ileal-pouch-anal anastomosis: a single institutional case-matched experience. Ann Surg 2006;243:667–672.
20 Larson DW, et al: Laparoscopic-assisted vs. open ileal pouch-anal anastomosis: functional outcome in a case-matched series. Dis Colon Rectum 2005;48:1845–1850.
21 Maartense S, et al: Hand-assisted laparoscopic versus open restorative proctocolectomy with ileal pouch anal anastomosis: a randomized trial. Ann Surg 2004;240:984–992.
22 Knight CD, Griffen FD: An improved technique for low anterior resection of the rectum using the EEA stapler. Surgery 1980;88:710–714.
23 Metcalf AM, et al: Ileal pouch-anal anastomosis without temporary, diverting ileostomy. Dis Colon Rectum 1986;29:33–35.
24 Jarvinen HJ, Luukkonen P: Comparison of restorative proctocolectomy with and without covering ileostomy in ulcerative colitis. Br J Surg 1991;78:199–201.
25 Matikainen M, Santavirta J, Hiltunen KM: Ileoanal anastomosis without covering ileostomy. Dis Colon Rectum 1990;33:384–388.
26 Wexner SD, et al: Laparoscopic total abdominal colectomy. A prospective trial. Dis Colon Rectum 1992;35:651–655.
27 Wexner SD, Johansen OB: Laparoscopic bowel resection: advantages and limitations. Ann Med 1992;24:105–110.
28 Schmitt SL, et al: Does laparoscopic-assisted ileal pouch anal anastomosis reduce the length of hospitalization? Int J Colorectal Dis 1994;9:134–137.
29 Hasegawa H, et al: Laparoscopic restorative proctocolectomy for patients with ulcerative colitis. J Laparoendosc Adv Surg Tech A 2002;12:403–406.
30 Hildebrandt U, et al: Laparoscopically-assisted proctocolectomy with ileoanal pouch in ulcerative colitis (in German). Zentralbl Chir 1998;123:403–405.
31 Liu CD, et al: Laparoscopic surgery for inflammatory bowel disease. Am Surg 1995;61:1054–1056.
32 Pace DE, et al: Early experience with laparoscopic ileal pouch-anal anastomosis for ulcerative colitis. Surg Laparosc Endosc Percutan Tech 2002;12:337–341.
33 Santoro E, et al: Laparoscopic total proctocolectomy with ileal J pouch-anal anastomosis. Hepatogastroenterology 1999;46:894–899.
34 Tucker JG, et al: Laparoscopically assisted bowel surgery. Analysis of 114 cases. Surg Endosc 1995;9:297–300.
35 Marcello PW, et al: Laparoscopic restorative proctocolectomy: case-matched comparative study with open restorative proctocolectomy. Dis Colon Rectum 2000;43:604–608.
36 Marcello PW, et al: Laparoscopic total colectomy for acute colitis: a case-control study. Dis Colon Rectum 2001;44:1441–1445.
37 Araki Y, et al: The usefulness of restorative laparoscopic-assisted total colectomy for ulcerative colitis. Kurume Med J 2001;48:99–103.
38 Hashimoto, A, et al: Laparascope-assisted versus conventional restorative proctocolectomy with rectal mucosectomy. Surg Today 2001;31:210–214.

Treatment Algorithms in the Case of Perianal Complications of Crohn's Disease

Y.S. Lozynskyy

Lviv National Medical University, Coloproctology Department, Lviv, Ukraine

Key Words
Crohn's disease · Perianal fistula · Perianal fissure · Diagnostics · Treatment algorithm

Abstract

Aim: To construct an algorithm of the treatment tactics which would include modern conservative and surgical methods. **Materials and Methods:** Endoscopy under anesthesia, endorectal ultrasonography, histological and radiological examinations, MRT. In the last 22 years, 310 patients with Crohn's disease (CD) have been treated in our clinic of which 144 had perianal complications (60 fissure, 52 fistula, 61 perianal abscess). **Results:** The treatment of perianal abscesses is opening and drainage, followed by conservative treatment (local and systemic). Using conservative treatment for patients with fissure, clinical remission was attained in 45 (75%); another 15 patients (25%) were operated using Maslyak's method. We have not conducted surgical treatment of fissures for the last 5 years. 51 patients with fistulas were operated on. When the malignation was confirmed, we conducted extirpation of the rectum or coloproctectomy. Recurrence of CD was observed in 65 patients (45.1%) during the first 2 years after the beginning treatment and in 128 patients (88.9%) during 5 years. CDAI varied from 150 to 450. PCDAI was in the range of 5–20. **Conclusions:** (1) Planned surgical treatment of perianal complications requires complex examination of the gastrointestinal tract; (2) pararectal fistulas should be operated In the period of complete remission; (3) surgical treatment of perianal complications should be microinvasive, using non-cutting seton, fistulotomy and advancement flap, and (4) coloproctectomy is the final stage of treatment of perianal CD in severe cases.

Copyright © 2009 S. Karger AG, Basel

Introduction

The etiology of Crohn's disease (CD) is still poorly understood, so in spite of much progress in diagnostics and pharmacological treatment, we do not have any effective facilities to cure the disease or to prevent its recurrences. Surgical treatment is still the only effective way of managing drug resistance of complicated cases [1, 2].

Perianal lesions that occur in patients with CD include skin tags, hemorrhoids, fissures, anal ulcers, low fistulas, high fistulas, rectovaginal fistulas, perianal abscesses, anorectal strictures, and cancer. Fistulas may originate below or above the dental line, and many colorectal surgeons simply classify them as low or high. Parks' classification, a more anatomically precise classification system, uses the external sphincter as a central point of reference to describe five types of perianal fistulas: superficial (low), intersphincteric (low or high), transsphincteric (low or high), suprasphincteric (high), and extrasphincteric (high) [3]. Perianal fistulas in CD may form from inflamed or infected anal glands and/or penetration of fissures or ulcers in the rectum or anal canal. In clinical practice, an empiric classification that is relatively widely used includes physical examination of the perianal area

Table 1. Clinical approach for treatment of abscesses

Stages	Diagnostic methods	Treatment		
I	EUA EUS MRI	Surgical	Incision, drainage Excision, drainage	± Non-cutting seton, mushroom catheter
II		Conservative	Systemic	Salofalk (3 g) Azathioprine (50 mg) Enterol-250 × 2 Ciprofloxacin 600 mg Metronidazole 1.5 g
			Local	Dioxyzol (emulsion) Povidone-iodine solution 10% (wound lavement) Salofalk (suppl. 1 g) Relief advance, betadine (suppl.), metronidazole gel
		Failure		
III		Surgical		± Colostomy, ± enterostomy, proctectomy

to identify anal skin tags, anal fissures, perianal fistulas, suspected perianal abscesses, anorectal strictures, and rectovaginal fistulas as well as an endoscopic evaluation to determine whether or not there is macroscopically evident inflammation of the rectum.

Fistulas are classified as either 'simple' or 'complex'. A *simple fistula* is low (superficial or low intersphincteric, or low transsphincteric origin of the fistula tract), has a single external opening, no pain or fluctuation to suggest perianal abscess, no evidence of a rectovaginal fistula, and no evidence of anorectal stricture. A *complex fistula* is high (high intersphincteric or high transsphincteric or extrasphincteric or suprasphincteric origin of the fistula tract), it may have multiple external openings, may be associated with the presence of a rectovaginal fistula, an anorectal stricture, and an active rectal disease at endoscopy [4, 5].

Two population-based studies have reported that perianal fistulas occurred in respectively 23 and 21% of the patients. Perianal fistulas occurred in 12% of patients with ileal CD, 15% of patients with ileocolonic disease, 41% of patients with colonic disease with rectal sparing, and in 92% of patients with colonic disease and rectal involvement. Anal fissure or perianal fistula or abscess precedes or presents simultaneously with the diagnosis of intestinal disease in 36–81% of CD patients, who develop perianal disease. Perianal changes are the first sign of CD in 2–4% of patients [6].

Modalities used to diagnose and classify Crohn's perianal disease include examination under anesthesia (EUA), pelvic MRI, endorectal ultrasonography (EUS) and computerized tomography, anal manometry and fistulography [7, 8].

Materials and Methods

Recently, an increasing number of patients operated on in our clinic with the diagnosis of CD have been seen, partly because we have become a reference center for the treatment of patients with non-specific bowel inflammations. During the last 25 years, we have observed 310 CD patients. In our study, 144 (46.4%) patients had perianal complications.

The clinical approach for the treatment of perianal abscesses consists of two parts: surgical treatment and conservative treatment (table 1). Surgical treatment implies incision, revision and drainage of the abscess cavity with obligatory verification of the internal opening. When there are plenty of necrotic tissues, resection is conducted. Incision, revision and excision suggest disconnection of all purulent leakages and complete evacuation with minimal trauma of sphincter. The cavity of the abscess is irrigated with plenty of antiseptic liquid (hydrogen peroxide, betadinum), and then is dried out. Drainage of the cavity is provided by introduction of a mushroom-like catheter and clean gauze tampon with hydrogen peroxide for more reliable hemostasis. In the rectum a gauze strip is inserted with soluble ointment (levomicol or levasin) and a betadinum suppository. Such an approach is more frequently used for ischio- and pelviorectal paraproctitis [9].

In transsphincteric paraproctitis where there is a high probability of injuring the sphincter, incision and drainage of the abscess are performed. The internal opening of the inflammatory crypt is verified and then the ligature is put on the muscle; however, it is not tightened but tied in a bow. A gauze strip with disinfectant solution is placed on the perineum wound. A strip with soluble ointment and betadine suppository is introduced into the rectum. For ligature drainage silk, latex strips and vicryl seton are used.

The tampons are removed from the wound and rectum the next day after the operation. The perineum wound is irrigated through a mushroom catheter beside the ligature with a solution of Dioxizol, which provides an antiseptic effect and local anesthetization. A Salofalk suppository together with metronidazole gel are introduced into the rectum daily. The drainage and washing through a mushroom catheter is conducted for 10–14 days, which follows irrigation of the abscess cavity by antiseptics. Mesalazine is permanently introduced into the rectum (in the form of suppositories, foam, and solution). For the rectum we use a gel (Dioxizol, Categel, Luan, Nefluan) which contains the anesthetic lidocaine. For antisepsis we apply metronidazole gel into the wound and into the rectum.

System infusion therapy with metronidazole and ciprofloxacin is conducted to avoid sepsis at the time of operation and in the early postoperational period. It is advisable to form an enterostomy or colostomy (which may be liquidated later in time of remission of the disease) in patients with septic changes and considerable perianal defect. Ligature drainage is kept until remission or substantial improvement of the clinical picture (the CDAI diminishment for 70–100 points, the PCDAI decline for 6–8 points) [10, 11].

Usually we perform hypodermic paraproctitis using Gabriel's method. We complement incision and drainage of the abscess cavity by incision of the skinning-mucus strip in the opening of the rectum with liquidation of the crypt and without damage to the sphincter. A catheter and ligature are not used. The bottom of the wound and the cavity of the abscess are carefully irrigated by an antiseptic solution. A strip with soluble ointment and metronidazole gel, together with a Salofalk suppository, is entered into the rectum. The drainage by the ligature lasts 4–8 weeks. The antiseptic bandaging is applied to the patients not less than once a week. Ambulatory patients use a rectal Salofalk suppository (500–1,000 mg) with metronidazole gel; Salofalk enemas are used at night.

It is necessary to look after granulation formation during the treatment, preventing premature adhesion of skin edges (the process should be performed from the bottom of the wound). All surgical operations and manipulations are made under general anesthesia, enabling painless rectal sonography and endoscopic examination of the colon for the control of the distribution of the disease and abscess. In some cases, when preoperational verification of location of the abscess is difficult, we use rectal ultrasonography with transcutaneous puncture of the abscess. This enables us to open all purulent leakages less traumatically and more effectively. An X-ray of the abscess was performed with a needle in 3 cases, using soluble contrast if the abscess was connected to the rectum (this pertains to pelviorectal abscesses). It is practical to use MRI, which allows not only a reliable diagnosis of the deeply placed abscesses in cases when endosonography is impossible, but also defines their relation with the anatomic structures of the pelvis, such as the sphincter and levator ani. Moreover, MRI is painless and comparatively accessible.

We have observed 144 patients with perianal changes, and abscesses developed in 61 (42.4%). With the exception of 2 patients with recurrent pelviorectal abscesses, the abscesses were related to the fissure or fistula. Only 6 abscesses (6.4%) developed when patients had a stoma, in comparison with 103 abscesses (93.6%) in patients without a stoma.

At the beginning of our investigation, 8 patients (13.0%) reported partial incontinence of liquid stool. This symptom was related to perianal abscess in 5 of the 8 patients. It disappeared once the abscess was liquidated. Incontinence of stool was present in 5 patients during the last examination (4/5 had patients incontinence of gases, and another patient had liquid excrements).

CDAI during the course of perianal abscess was in the range of 168 ± 101. We had to use glucocorticoids in combination with sulfasalazines and immunosuppressive drugs in 16 of 110 patients (CDAI >250). A mild or moderate course of the disease was observed in the other patients. Moderate CDAI was considerably higher during the formation of the abscesses (168 ± 101) than after abscess liquidation. PCDAI [11] with perianal abscess was 18 ± 2, and it was 9 ± 3 without perianal abscess; after incision of the abscess, the PCDAI was in the range of 61 ± 37.

The primary perianal abscesses developed in the tracts of infected fistulas, when the direct drainage through openings of fistulas was impaired, except two pelviorectal abscesses which had no connection with the rectum. The other cause of origin of abscesses was anal fissures, which were the pathways for infection to reach pararectal cellular tissue spaces. Frequency of the abscesses was higher in patients with deep ischio- and pelviorectal fistulas. Transsphincteric fistulas resulted in abscess formation more frequently than hypodermic fistulas. Ischiorectal and hypodermic abscesses were dominant.

About one-half of patients had a recurrent abscess in the next 14.2 months; about one-quarter had a second relapse. The 2-year relapse rate was 54.0% and the 3-year rate was 70.0%. Recurrent abscesses developed more frequently in patients without a stoma and in those with ischio- and pelviorectal abscesses. We performed proctectomy in 4 patients, of which 3 had recurrent pelviorectal abscesses. However, perianal sepsis was not the only reason for the proctectomy because all 4 patients had chronic proctitis, of which 2 had well-marked anal stenosis.

In order to reduce the risk of relapse, we administered supporting doses of mesalazine (2 g/day orally) in combination with local mesalazine into the rectum (0.5 g suppository and 2 g (30 ml) microenemas at night). According to the literature, perianal fistulas develop in CD patients with a frequency of up to 43% [12]. In our study, perianal fistulas were found in 52 patients (36.0%). Simple fistulas (simple superficial and intersphincteric) occurred in 30 patients. Supra-, trans- and extrasphincteric complex fistulas were found in 15 patients and rectovaginal complex fistulas in 7 patients.

There are two major steps for fistula treatment: the first is to define the activity of the disease, particularly in the rectum, and the second is localization of the internal opening and relationships of the fistula tract to the internal and external sphincter and levators. The diagnostic algorithm implies finger EUA, EUS or MRI (table 2). It is advisable to perform colonoscopy under anesthesia for determination of the disease localization in the colon and terminal part of the small intestine. If necessary, fibrogastroscopy, barium passage in small intestine and capsule endoscopy are performed. A finger EUA is always followed by precise examination of the fistula tract, irrigation of the tract by a disinfectant solution, painting over with methylene blue and fistulography.

Table 2. Clinical approach for treatment of fistulas

Stages	Diagnostic methods		Treatment			
			systemic		local	
I	EUA EUS MRI	Conservative	Salofalk (3 g) Ciprofloxacin (400 mg) Metronidazole (1.5 g) Azathioprine (50 mg) Enterol-250 × 2 Infliximab (5 mg/kg weeks 0, 2, 6)		Salofalk (suppl., enemas, foam, 3 g) Metronidazole (gel) Dioxyzol (emulsion) Povidone-iodine solution 10% (fistula lavement)	
II		Operation	CDAI <150	Non-cutting seton, fistulotomy, advancement flap		PCDAI ≤7
III		Conservative	Salofalk (3 g) Azathioprine (50 mg) Ciprofloxacin (600 mg) Metronidazole (1.5 g) Enterol-250 × 2		Dioxyzol (emulsion) Povidone-iodine solution 10% Posterizan forte (suppl. and liniment) Salofalk (suppl. 1 g) Metronidazole (gel)	
		Failure				
IV		Operation	CDAI >250	Enterostomy, colostomy, proctectomy		PCDAI >12

The principles of medical approaches vary in patients with active colitis and by the stage of remission. Surgical methods in patients with simple and complex fistula also differ. It is possible to perform fistulotomy in patients with superficial hypodermic fistula in the case of minimum activity of the disease (CDAI <150 and PCDAI <6) under antibiotic protection (metronidazole, ciprofloxacin) and azathioprine. Best of all is to perform it at the time of complete remission, when the clinical remission coincides with the endoscopic remission.

Results

In all, we have performed 30 complex operations. 25 (83%) patients recovered and a relapse of the disease was seen in 5 (17%) patients. The insufficiency of the anal sphincter was revealed in the postoperative period in 3 (10%) patients (table 3).

A temporary stoma was formed for 3 patients, because of the relapse of the disease. We made an ileostomy for 1 patient with different parts of colon affected, and a transversostomy was made for the other 2 patients. Proctectomy was performed for 2 (6%) patients because of disease progression, and in 1 case due to formation of the stricture. After the fistulotomy, the bottom of the wound is neatly carried out by the Volkmann spoon and irrigated by antiseptic solutions; the mucous layer in the place of the internal opening is carefully incised. Hemostasis is made by diathermocoagulator. A tampon with soluble ointment (such as metronidazole gel, levamisole and levasin) is introduced into the rectum and downstream of the fistula tract. A daily antiseptic bandaging with replacement of the rectal tampon with Dioxizol, Metrogel and Salofalk suppository are performed. During bandaging we control the edges of postoperational wound to prevent premature conglutination. For the complex (high) fistulas we use the method of Maslyak, which is the modification of the Jadd-Rouble method [13]. It should be noted that the operation can only be performed after careful systematic examination of the patient and in the absence of signs of disease activity (CDAI <150, PCDAI <6), which correlates with the results of histological examination of the rectum (table 4).

The value of the operation lies in the preparation of a trapezius flap with the basis toward the lumen of the rectum. The inner aperture of the fistula with scar margins is excised. The defective area – the proximal, partly separated mucosal-submucosal-muscular (the superficial portion of internal sphincter) flap – is translocated. The advancement flap is fixed to the mucosa and perianal skin with several sutures from three sides. After the fistula is separated and excised (inside the wall of bowel), the wound is tamponated with gauze tampon with solutions of 3%

Table 3. Results of conventional fistulotomy by laying open the tract for low perianal fistulas in CD patients

Study	Patients	Healed (%)	Recurrence (%)	Incontinence (%)	Proctectomy (%)
Hobbis et al., 1982	32	18 (90)	4 (22)	Not stated	3 (15)
Keightly et al., 1986	12	1 (8)	Not stated	6 (50)	Not stated
Williams et al., 1991	41	38 (93)	Not stated	7 patients (21)	3 patients (9)
Halme et al., 1995	10	10 (100)	4 (40)	5 (50)	1 (10)
Scott et al., 1996	27	22 (81)	Not stated	5 (19)	5 (19); 3 proctectomy; 2 stoma
McKee et al., 1996	34	21 (62)	4 (18)	Not stated	10 (29); 7 proctectomy; 3 stoma
Michelassi et al., 2000	33	27 (82)	Not stated	Not stated	Not stated
Lozynskyy et al., 2004	30	25 (83)	5 (17)	3 (10)	3 (10) stoma: (1 ileostomy) (2 colostomy); 2 (7) proctectomy

Table 4. Results of treatment of high or complex fistulas in CD patients

Study	Patients	Treatment	Healed (%)	Recurrence (%)	Incontinence (%)	Proctectomy (%)
Williams et al., 1991	22	Seton	19 (86)	9 (47)	14 (66)	3 (14)
Sangwan et al., 1996	24	Seton	22 (92)	17 (63)	Not stated	7 (33)
Williamson et al., 1995	9	Seton	2 (22)	2 (22)	Not stated	Not stated
Makowiec et al., 1995	20	Transanal advancement flap	16 (80)	4 (20)	0	0
Joo et al., 1998	26	Transanal advancement flap	19 (73)	7 (27)	Not stated	2 (9)
Robertson et al., 1998	6	Transanal advancement flap	3 (50)	3 (50)	Not stated	0
Lozynskyy et al., 2004	11	Transanal advancement flap	5 (45)	6 (55)	3 (27)	2 (18)
	4	Non-cutting seton	2 (50)	2 (50) Cr. recti	0	2 (50)

Table 5. Results of surgical treatment of rectovaginal fistulas in CD patients

Study	Patients	Type of repair	Healed (%)	Proctectomy (%)
Makowiec et al., 1995	12	Transanal advancement flap	10 (83)	0
O'Leary et al., 1998	6	Transanal advancement flap	3 (50)	0
Sher et al., 1998	14	Transvaginal flap	13 (93)	1 ileostomy (7)
Michelassi et al., 2000	16	Transanal advancement flap	4 (25)	11 (69)
Michelassi et al., 2000	1	Seton	0	0
Lozynskyy et al., 2004	2	Transanal advancement flap	0	2 (100)
	2	Transvaginal flap	1 (50)	1 coloproctectomy-ileostomy (50)
	2	Seton	2 (100)	0

hydrogen peroxide and 10% povidone-iodine. Gauze tampon with hydrophylous antiseptic unguent, e.g. levamisole or levasin, is placed into the lumen of the rectum. The tampons are removed the following day and changed every day. We apply metranidazole gel and Dioxizol emulsion on the wound for an antibacterial effect. We then administer Salofalk and Posterizan-Forte suppositories with metranidazole gel and Dioxizol emulsion. The treatment of rectovaginal fistulas deserves special attention. We have observed 7 female patients: in 1 patient under the influence of combined therapy (systemic and local), the fistula closed by itself when a compensative stricture formed. Colostomy was performed because the stricture extended to the ileus. One year later, coloproctectomy was performed. Two patients with superficial fistulas were successfully operated on using cutting seton at the time of remission. Two patients were operated on after the Maslyak method (transanal advancement flap). In early postoperative treatment the retraction of the flap appeared and the patients underwent proctectomy. In another 2 patients, the transvaginal advancement flap operation was performed under the protection of an ileostomy. In spite of preventive stoma in 1 patient, additional fistulas developed later and the patient insisted on coloproctectomy (table 5).

The methods reported in the literature on fistula treatment with collagen plug and fibrin glue have still not been used in our practice [14, 15]. Due to the rather high price and the absence of reimbursement in Ukraine, there is sporadic use of infliximab (Remicade) – the anti-TNF-α medicine for the treatment of perianal complications. We observed 2 patients with rectal cancer as a result of long-standing CD with high fistulas. Histologically they were adenocarcinomas with a middle grade of differentiation. They appeared after 8 and 12 years of perianal disease duration. Initially, fistulas appeared at the inner aperture and afterwards became malignant. They were treated with a course of intensive gamma therapy with a dose of 25 Gy followed by rectum extirpation according to Canew-Miles. One patient died 2 years after the operation because of lung, liver and brain metastases, in spite of adequate adjuvant chemotherapy (irinotecan, leucovorin and 5-FU). One patient had a squamous cell cancer caused by perianal ulcer. Gamma therapy and the following extirpation brought about a positive outcome. The quality of life was determined by the IBDQ questionnaire both before and after the operation [16, 17]. Postoperative quality of life according to IBDQ questionnaire was assessed in 17 patients, and the mean score was 172 (range 129–208). Good results (score >180) were obtained in 9 patients, moderate results in 5, while in 3 patients the score was <140. The mean quality of life score according to IBDQ was 161 (range 129–191) in a subgroup of 10 patients, who were recurrence-free for over 5 years. Good results (score >180) were noted in 2 patients only, while in another 2 the score was <140. In this subgroup, 3 persons did not agree to fill in the questionnaire.

To conclude: (1) planned surgical treatment of the perianal complications requires complex examination of the gastrointestinal tract; (2) the pararectal fistulas should be operated in the period of complete remission (clinical and endoscopic); (3) surgical treatment of perianal complications should be microinvasive, using non-cutting seton, fistulotomy and advancement flap; (4) incontinence and decrease of quality of life appears to be due to aggressive local surgical treatment; (5) colostomy and enterostomy in combination with systemic treatment are an effective method to achieve remission and to decrease the frequency of recurrences of perianal CD, and finally, (6) in severe cases, coloproctectomy is the final stage of treatment of the perianal CD.

Disclosure Statement

The author declares that no financial or other conflict of interest exists in relation to the content of this article.

References

1 Schwartz DA, Pemberton JH, Sandborn WJ: Diagnosis and treatment of perianal fistulas in Crohn's disease. Ann Intern Med 2001; 135:906–918.
2 Travis SPL, Stange EF, Lemann M, et al: European evidence-based consensus on the diagnosis and management of Crohn's disease: current management. Gut 2006;55(suppl 1): i16–i35.
3 Parks AG, Gordon PH, Hardcastle JD: A classification of fistula in ano. Br J Surg 1976; 63:1–12.
4 Buchanan GN, Halligan S, Bartram CI, et al: Clinical examination, endosonography, and MR imaging in preoperative assessment of fistulas in ano: comparison with outcome-based reference standard. Radiology 2004; 233:674–681.
5 Kolodziejczak M, Sudol-Szopinska I: Diagnostic and Treatment Abscess and Perianal Fistula. Warsaw, Borgis, 2008, p 267.
6 American Gastroenterological Association medical position statement: perianal Crohn's disease. Gastroenterology 2003;125:1503–1507.
7 Sandborn WJ, Fazio VW, Feagan BG, Hanauer SB: American Gastroenterological Association Clinical Practice. C. AGA technical review on perianal Crohn's disease. Gastroenterology 2003;125:1508–1530.
8 Lozynskyi Y, Lozynskyi R: The Crohn's diseases. Treatment of perianal complications. Proctologia 2004(suppl N1):40–41.
9 Dulcev Y, Salamov K: Paraproctitis. M Med 1987, p 140.
10 Best WR, Bectel JM, Singleton JW, Kern FJ: Development of a Crohn's disease activity index. National Cooperative Crohn's Disease Study. Gastroenterology 1976;70:439–444.
11 Irvine EJ: Usual therapy improves perianal Crohn's disease as measured by a new disease activity index. McMaster IBD Study Group. J Clin Gastroenterol 1995;20:27–32.
12 Irvine EJ, Feagan B, Rochon J, et al: Quality of life: a valid and reliable measures of therapeutic efficacy in the treatment of inflammatory bowel disease. Canadian Crohn's Relapse Prevention Trial Study Group. Gastroenterology 1994;106:286–296.
13 McLeod RS, Baxter NN: Quality of life of patients with inflammatory bowel disease after surgery. World J Surg 1998;22:375–381.
14 Williams JG, Farrands PA, Williams AB, et al: The treatment of anal fistula. Position statement of the Association of Coloproctology of Great Britain and Ireland. Colorectal Dis 2007;9(suppl 4):18–50.
15 Pavlovskyy M, Maslyak V, Lozynskyi Y, Varivoda I: Practical coloproctology (in Ukrainian). Lviv, Svit, 1993, p 183.
16 O'Connor L, Champagne BJ, Ferguson MA, et al: Efficacy of anal fistula plug in closure of Crohn's anorectal fistulas. Dis Colon Rectum 2006:49:1569–1573.
17 Khaikin M, Chowers Y, Zmora O: Perianal Crohn's disease. Isr Med Assoc J 2007;9:163–168.

Malignant Transformation in Inflammatory Bowel Disease: Prevention, Surveillance and Treatment – New Techniques in Endoscopy

Christian Bojarski

Charité, Campus Benjamin Franklin, Medizinische Klinik I, Gastroenterologie, Rheumatologie, Infektiologie, Berlin, Germany

Key Words

Autofluorescence imaging · Chromoendoscopy · Endoscopy, new techniques · Fluorescence endoscopy · Inflammatory bowel disease, malignant transformation · In-vivo histology techniques · Intraepithelial neoplasia, treatment · Magnification endoscopy · Optical coherence tomography

Abstract

Patients with a long-standing history of ulcerative colitis (UC) or Crohn's disease (CD) with a history of inflammation in the colon have a risk for the development of colon cancer. To these patients at least one colonoscopy per year should be offered according to national surveillance guidelines in patients with inflammatory bowel disease (IBD). Following general recommendations, surveillance colonoscopy should be performed without disease activity and four tissue samples each 10 cm should be taken. Beside high-resolution videoendoscopy and magnification endoscopy, the application of dyes applied via a spraying catheter are of additional diagnostic value with a factor 3–4 higher detection rate of intraepithelial neoplasia (IEN). It is under current evaluation if the use of computerized virtual chromoendoscopy techniques (NBI, FICE, High Line/HD+) has the same diagnostic output compared to classical spraying techniques. The detection rate of IEN can be further improved by using newly developed in-vivo histology techniques. A combination of chromoendoscopy with confocal endomicroscopy (CEM) can detect 5-fold higher rates of IEN compared with random biopsy protocols. An alternative technique to CEM is the miniprobe-based CEM. Autofluorescence imaging is an interesting approach for the surveillance of IBD patients with first clinical data published.

Copyright © 2009 S. Karger AG, Basel

Patients with a long-standing history of ulcerative colitis (UC) (>8 years of pancolitis, >15 years of left-sided colitis) have a significant risk for the development of colon cancer. To these patients at least one colonoscopy per year should be offered according to the national surveillance guidelines in patients with inflammatory bowel disease (IBD). In patients with long-standing Crohn's disease (CD) and a history of inflammatory activity also in the colon, the risk of colon cancer development is less documented. However, following the results of large meta-analysis, these patients should also enter surveillance programs. During a surveillance colonoscopy with no or mild disease activity, four random quadrant biopsies each 10 cm should be taken. The diagnostic precision to detect intraepithelial neoplasia (IEN) is 90% when 33 biopsies were taken [1] and 95% after collection of 56 biopsies [2]. However, these recommendations were not strictly transferred into daily practice and the number of biopsies taken during surveillance colonoscopy is often <25 tissue samples per patient. In The Netherlands only 25% of the gastroenterologists follow the national surveillance guidelines in patients with UC [3], in Great Britain 57% of the gastroenterologists take <10 biopies per patient [4] and in New Zealand 50% of the specialists take <17 biopsies per patient [5]. In Germany, only 9% of the gastroenterologists follow the recommendations of their national guidelines, in 50% of all colonoscopies <10 biopsies [6] were taken for histology. Keeping these discouraging data in mind, there is an unequivocal need for endoscopic techniques with the potential to avoid unnecessary biopsies towards techniques with the potential to obtain targeted biopsies.

Chromoendoscopy

The standard endoscopy should be performed with a high-resolution videoendoscope. The application of contrast dyes applied via a spraying catheter is of additional diagnostic value with a factor 3–4 higher detection rate of IEN [7, 8]. We differentiate absorptive dyes (methylene blue 0.1–0.5%, cresyl violet 0.2%) from contrast dyes (indigo carmine 0.2–0.4%). In daily practice, classical panchromoendoscopy is not widely accepted due to a relatively high time consumption for this procedure.

It is under current evaluation if the use of computerized virtual chromoendoscopy techniques (NBI, FICE, High Line/HD+) has the same diagnostic output compared to classical spraying techniques. However, one has to face the fact that the visual enhancement of classical contrast dyes applied locally via a spraying catheter are completely different from the enhanced effects caused by activation of e.g. narrow band imaging (NBI) which mainly focused on pathological vessel architecture.

First data in a limited number of patients are promising and will potentially recognize a certain comparability of both methods. One study published in this field examined NBI for the detection of IEN in patients with UC. In this prospective randomized crossover study, 42 patients underwent one conventional colonoscopy and a further NBI colonoscopy within 3 weeks. 11 patients with neoplasia were identified, in 4 patients by both techniques, in 4 patients by NBI and in 3 patients by conventional endoscopy alone. The authors conclude that it is still too early to stop taking additional random biopsies [9].

Magnification Endoscopy

Magnification and Zoom endoscopy allows a magnification of the mucosal surface up to 100-fold. Mucosal lesions can be characterized by the Pit Pattern Classification [10]. The largest prospective study compared conventional endoscopy with magnification endoscopy in 300 patients with UC and found a high correlation of magnification with disease activity and histopathological grading [11]. It seems to be of high diagnostic relevance to combine chromoendoscopy with magnification. In 46 patients with UC, 3 with tortuous pattern were identified by magnification and NBI [12].

Autofluorescence Imaging

The autofluorescence technique is considered to act as a real *red flag* technology with encouraging clinical data in e.g. the human respiratory tract. However, transferring this technique into the gastrointestinal tract is hampered by several technical challenges. There is now one comparative randomized trial available which compared 50 patients with UC in an endoscopic tri-model imaging protocol (white light endoscopy vs. autofluorescence imaging and NBI). The authors conclude that autofluorescence imaging improves the detection of neoplasia in patients with UC and that autofluorescence imaging color appears valuable in excluding the presence of neoplasia [13].

In-vivo Histology Techniques

The detection rate of IEN can be further improved by using in-vivo histology techniques. A combination of chromoendoscopy with confocal endomicroscopy (CEM) can detect 5-fold higher rates of IEN compared with random biopsy protocols [14]. CEM is possible after injecting 2.5–5 ml fluorescein 10% intravenously. A confocal miniaturized laser with a defined wavelength of 488 nm generates in-vivo histology images up to a 1,000-fold magnification. During ongoing endoscopy, single cellular and subcellular tissue analysis 0–250 μm in depth are visible (Pentax, Japan). In patients with UC, targeted biopsies of mucosal areas suspicious of IEN can be identified directly while performing the colonoscopy (fig. 1).

An alternative technique to CEM is the miniprobe-based endomicroscopy technique. After the miniprobe is pleaded through a 2.8-mm working channel of any stan-

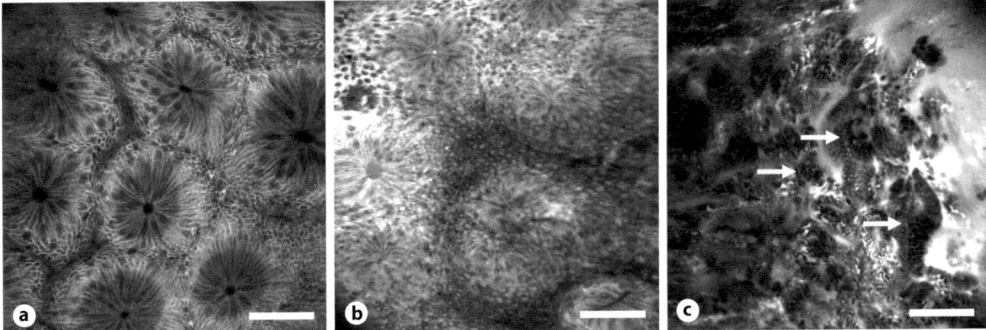

Fig. 1. CEM images in normal sigmoid colon (**a**), active inflammation in a patient with UC (**b**) and in a flat DALM lesion with IEN (**c**). Bar = 100 μm. Active inflammation is characterized by a high density of inflammatory cells around the crypts together with a slight disturbance in crypt architecture (**b**), intraepithelial neoplastic cells (arrows) are recognized as dark irregular-shaped cells in an area with a massive destruction of normal colonic crypt architecture (**c**).

dard videoendoscope, the laser unit generates a confocal image with a high frame rate per second. Special attention towards this technology by Mauna Kea Technologies (Paris, France) has taken place since the company developed a high-resolution miniprobe device. However, comparable studies with other techniques are under current evaluation and no data are available at present in patients with IBD.

Endocytoscopy is a kind of reflecting light microscopy and the device is pleaded through a 3.7-mm working channel of any suitable endoscope. The magnification ranges from 450- to 1,100-fold depending on the device and the in-vivo recognition of superficial surface cells is possible after topically applying acylcysteine for mucolysis and methylene blue for staining. So far, there are no published data of this technique in patients with IBD.

Optical Coherence Tomography and Fluorescence Endoscopy

Some innovative endoscopy imaging techniques are under current evaluation to prove their eligibility for clinical routine endoscopy. Optical coherence tomography is an optical analogue to endoscopic ultrasound with an imaging depth of 2 mm. The device is also used in a 'mother-baby fashion' through the working channel of the endoscope as mentioned above. There are two publications of this technique in patients with IBD [15, 16]. These studies have started to show the feasibility of this method and to differentiate transmural inflammation in CD from patterns of active UC.

Fluorescence endoscopy is a technique which assessed IEN after topical or systemical sensitization with 5-aminolevulinic acid (5-ALA). After the application of 5-ALA, this substance is converted intracellularly into the fluophore protoporphyrin IX which accumulates selectively in neoplastic tissue allowing to detect a reddish spot while illuminated with blue monochromatic light (442 nm). The first report which evaluated fluorescence endoscopy in patients with UC was published in 2003 [17]. This study examined 37 patients with UC and found a sensitivity of 87–100% after local application and 43% after systemical application with 5-ALA. The specificity was lower with 62% after systemic and 51% after local sensitization. However, 3 years later another study could not confirm these results and evaluated 682 biopsies in 42 patients with IBD. The corresponding histology in 2 patients with IEN showed no correlation with the red fluorescent areas during fluorescence endoscopy [18]. However, neither optical coherence tomography nor fluorescence endoscopy is currently suitable for the detection of IEN in patients with IBD.

Future Aspects: Molecular Imaging

In-vivo histology techniques are the basics for further diagnostic improvement on a single cellular level and have opened the door for molecular imaging in the gastrointestinal tract. There is one in vivo animal approach where colonic tissue samples are incubated with FITC-marked antibodies against epithelial growth factor receptor, in this mouse model confocal microscope was able to detect the EGFR on the surface of tissue after inducing a colitis [19]. The first in-vivo detection of dysplastic crypts by confocal microscopy in humans during ongoing endoscopy was possible after topical application of fluorescent-labeled heptapeptides which were identified previously to bind to premalignant tissue as high-affinity ligands [20].

Treatment of Intraepithelial Neoplasia

Following current national guidelines the presence of high-grade IEN, not only in flat lesions but also in macroscopically dubious areas with slightly elevated lesions (dysplasia-associated lesions or mass (DALM)) during surveillance colonoscopy, should directly introduce these patients to surgical treatment after confirmation by a reference pathologist. Low-grade intraepithelial neoplastic lesions should lead to a more strict endoscopic follow-up in 6 months after first diagnosis. Sporadic adenoma in patients with IBD should be removed by polypectomy. The definition of a DALM lesion needs to be redefined since new endoscopic technologies are available which have clearly proven the visibility of such lesions in vivo depending on the technique used for surveillance endoscopy.

Conclusion

Classical high-resolution endoscopy in combination with chromoendoscopy is evidence-based and should be used for routine surveillance colonoscopy in patients with long-lasting UC or Crohn's colitis. It seems that the detection rates of IEN can also be improved by using virtual chromoendoscopy techniques. In the near future, targeted biopsies will replace random biopsy protocols and will lead to a more accepted diagnostic approach in surveillance colonoscopy. In-vivo histology has become a fundamental step forward in the diagnosis of malignant transformation in IBD and will open the door for the realization of molecular imaging.

Disclosure Statement

The author declares that no financial or other conflict of interest exists in relation to the content of this article.

References

1 Rubin C, Haggitt R, Burmer G: DNA aneuploidy in colonic biopsies predicts future development of dysplasia in ulcerative colitis. Gastroenterology 1992;103:1611–1620.
2 Connell WR, Lennard-Jones JE, Williams CB, Talbot IC, Price AB, Wilkinson KH: Factors affecting the outcome of endoscopic surveillance for cancer in ulcerative colitis. Gastroenterology 1994;107:934–944.
3 Obrador A, Ginard D, Barranco L: Colorectal cancer surveillance in ulcerative colitis – what should we be doing? Aliment Pharmacol Ther 2006;24:56–63.
4 Eaden JA, Ward BA, Mayberry JF: How gastroenterologists screen for colonic cancer in ulcerative colitis: an analysis of performance. Gastrointest Endosc 2000;51:123–128.
5 Gearry RB, Wakeman CJ, Barclay ML, Chapman BA, Collett JA, Burt MJ, Frizelle FA: Surveillance for dysplasia in patients with inflammatory bowel disease: a national survery of colonoscopic practice in New Zealand. Dis Colon Rectum 2004;47:314–322.
6 Kaltz B, Bokemeyer B, Hoffmann J, Porschen R, Rogler G, Schmiegel W: Surveillance colonoscopy in ulcerative colitis patients in Germany. Z. Gastroenterol 2007;45:325–331.
7 Kiesslich R, Fritsch J, Holtmann M, Koehler HH, Stolte M, Kanzler S, Nafe B, Jung M, Galle PR, Neurath MF: Methylene blue-aided chromoendoscopy for the detection of intraepithelial neoplasia and colon cancer in ulcerative colitis. Gastroenterology 2003;124:880–888.
8 Hurlstone DP, McAlindon ME, Sanders DS, Koegh R, Lobo AJ, Cross SS: Further validation of high-magnification chromoscopic colonoscopy for the detection of intraepithelial neoplasia and colon cancer in ulcerative colitis. Gastroenterology 2004;126:376–378.
9 Dekker E, van den Broek FJ, Reitsma JB, Hardwick JC, Offerhaus GJ, van Deventer SJ, Hommes DW, Fockens P: Narrow-band imaging compared with conventional colonoscopy for the detection of dysplasia in patients with long-standing ulcerative colitis. Endoscopy 2007;39:216–221.
10 Kudo S, Tamura S, Nakajima T, et al: Diagnosis of colorectal tumorous lesions by magnifying colonoscopy. Gastrointest Endosc 1996;44:8–14.
11 Hurlstone DP, Sanders DS, McAlindon ME, Thomson M, Cross SS: High-magnification chromoscopic colonoscopy in ulcerative colitis: a valid tool for in vivo optical biopsy and assessment of disease extent. Endoscopy 2006;38:1213–1217.
12 Matsumoto T, Kudo T, Jo Y, Esaki M, Yao T, Iida M: Magnifying colonoscopy with narrow band imaging system for the diagnosis of dysplasia in ulcerative colitis: a pilot study. Gastrointest Endosc 2007;66:957–965.
13 Van den Broek FJ, Fockens P, van Eeden S, Reitsma JB, Hardwick JC, Stokkers PC, Dekker E: Endoscopic tri-modal imaging for surveillance in ulcerative colitis: randomised comparison of high-resolution endoscopy and autofluorescence imaging for neoplasia detection, and evaluation of narrow-band imaging for classification of lesions. Gut 2008;57:1083–1089.

14 Kiesslich R, Goetz M, Lammersdorf K, Schneider C, Burg J, Stolte M, Vieth M, Nafe B, Galle PR, Neurath MF: Chromoscopy-guided endomicroscopy increases the diagnostic yield of intraepithelial neoplasia in ulcerative colitis. Gastroenterology 2007;132: 874–882.

15 Shen B, Zuccaro G Jr, Gramlich TL, Gladkova N, Trolli P, Kareta M, Delaney CP, Connor JT, Lashner BA, Bevins CL, Feldchtein F, Remzi FH, Bambrick ML, Fazio VW: In vivo colonoscopic optical coherence tomography for transmural inflammation in inflammatory bowel disease. Clin Gastroenterol Hepatol 2004;2:1080–1087.

16 Consolo P, Strangio G, Luigiano C, Giacobbe G, Pallio S, Familiari L: Optical coherence tomography in inflammatory bowel disease: prospective evaluation of 35 patients. Dis Colon Rectum 2008;51:1374–1380.

17 Messmann H, Endlicher E, Freunek G, Rümmele P, Schölmerich J, Knüchel R: Fluorescence endoscopy for the detection of low and high grade dysplasia in ulcerative colitis using systemic or local 5-aminolaevulinic acid sensitisation. Gut 2003;52:1003–1007.

18 Ochsenkühn T, Tillack C, Stepp H, Diebold J, Ott SJ, Baumgartner R, Brand S, Göke B, Sackmann M: Low frequency of colorectal dysplasia in patients with long-standing inflammatory bowel disease colitis: detection by fluorescence endoscopy. Endoscopy 2006; 38:477–482.

19 Goetz M, Ziebart A, Vieth M, Delaney P, Galle PR, Neurath MF, Kiesslich R: In vivo molecular imaging of colorectal cancer by confocal endomicroscopy. Gastroenterology 2008;134:A48.

20 Hsiung PL, Hardy J, Friedland S, Soetikno R, Du CB, Wu AP, Sahbaie P, Crawford JM, Lowe AW, Contag CH, Wang TD: Detection of colonic dysplasia in vivo using a targeted heptapeptide and confocal microendoscopy. Nat Med 2008;14:454–458.

Diagnostic Standards in the Pathology of Inflammatory Bowel Disease

Christoph Loddenkemper

Institute of Pathology/Research Center ImmunoSciences, Charité – Universitätsmedizin Berlin, Campus Benjamin Franklin, Berlin, Germany

Key Words

Carcinoma in inflammatory bowel disease · Dysplasia-associated lesion or mass · Inflammatory bowel disease, diagnostic standards in pathology · Inflammatory bowel disease, differential diagnosis · Intraepithelial neoplasia · Iatrogenic lymphoproliferative disorders

Abstract

Inflammatory bowel disease (IBD) includes Crohn's disease (CD) and ulcerative colitis (UC). The recognition of typical morphological features usually allows to distinguish CD from UC. Several infectious diseases like tuberculosis as well as other disorders can mimic IBD and need to be excluded before immunosuppressive treatment is started or surgical intervention planned. IBD is associated with an increased risk for the development of colorectal adenocarcinoma. There is a strong relationship between the presence of intraepithelial neoplasia (IEN) in patients with CD or UC and colon cancer. Thus, the differentiation between biopsies with reactive atypia, low-grade IEN and high-grade IEN is of great importance. Furthermore, distinction between dysplasia-associated lesions or masses (DALM) and sporadic adenoma-like masses (ALM) is crucial as prophylactic colectomy is usually recommended for DALM and polypectomy may be sufficient for ALM. Various features like localization of the lesion, architecture, inflammation and immunohistochemical evaluation of additional markers, e.g. p53 and β-catenin, may be helpful in the distinction of DALM versus ALM. Finally, the use of modern immunosuppressive therapies may go along with an increased susceptibility towards infections, e.g. cytomegalovirus colitis or Epstein-Barr virus-induced lymphoproliferative disorders, and a high degree of awareness by clinicians and pathologists is required in order not to miss these life-threatening complications of IBD.

Copyright © 2009 S. Karger AG, Basel

Introduction

Inflammatory bowel disease (IBD) includes two chronic gastrointestinal disorders – Crohn's disease (CD) and ulcerative colitis (UC). CD (fig. 1a) and UC (fig. 1b) can usually be distinguished based on clinical information, an adequate number and size of biopsies and the recognition of characteristic pathological changes. A small proportion of cases initially has to be labeled 'indeterminate colitis' due to overlapping features of both CD and UC [1]. Biopsies and resection specimens should be evaluated in a systematic approach including epithelial alterations, lamina propria changes and the distribution of inflammation together with other morphological signs like presence of granulomas or lymphoid follicles (table 1).

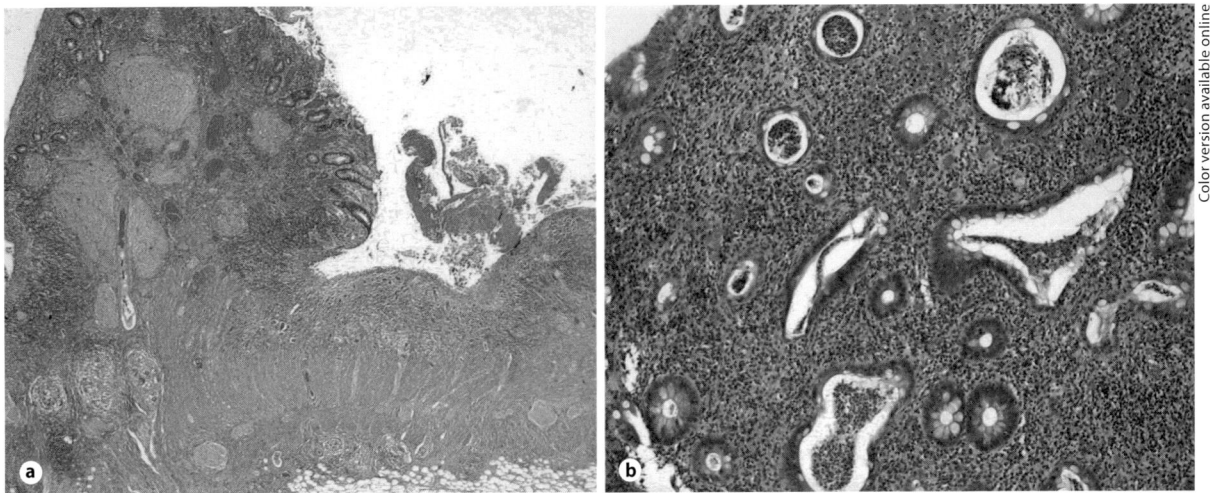

Fig. 1. Histopathology of IBD. CD with an aphthous ulcer, numerous epithelioid granulomas and prominent lymphoid aggregates (**a**). UC with a dense infiltrate of lymphocytes and plasma cells in the lamina propria and crypt abscess formation (**b**).

Differential Diagnosis of IBD

Several infectious diseases and other disorders can clinically mimic IBD and need to be considered before immunosuppressive treatment is started or surgical intervention performed. Among the infectious diseases included in the differential diagnosis are bacterial infections (e.g. tuberculosis (fig. 2a), *Clostridium*, *Yersinia*, *Salmonella*, Whipple's disease), viral infections (cytomegalovirus (CMV) (fig. 2b), herpes simplex), protozoan infections (amebiasis, schistosomiasis) and fungal infections (histoplasmosis) [2–4]. Among other disorders that need to be excluded are pseudomembranous colitis (fig. 2c), ischemic colitis (fig. 2d), eosinophilic gastroenteritis, collagenous colitis, celiac disease, diverticulitis and drug-induced colitis [5].

Intraepithelial Neoplasia

IBD is associated with an increased risk for the development of colorectal adenocarcinoma. Precursor lesions of carcinoma have in the past been referred to as 'dysplasia', but according to the WHO Classification of Tumours of the Digestive System, the term 'intraepithelial neoplasia (IEN)' should now be applied [6]. IEN is classified according to histological criteria (i.e. degree of nuclear hyperchromatism and pleomorphism, stratification,

Table 1. Microscopic features of CD versus UC

	CD	UC
Distribution of inflammation	Segmental, transmural	Diffuse, (sub)mucosal
Ileal inflammation	Common	Minimal
Crypt abscesses	Rare	Common
Crypt distortion	Minimal	Common
Paneth cell metaplasia	Rare	Common
Granulomas	Common	Absent
Lymphoid hyperplasia	Common	Rare
Fissures	Common	Absent
Neural hyperplasia	Common	Rare

loss of polarity, absence of mucin) into 'low-grade IEN' and 'high-grade IEN'. As there is a certain degree of subjectivity in the diagnosis and grading of IEN, there is consensus that a second opinion should be obtained from a reference pathologist specialized in gastrointestinal pathology [7] (fig. 3).

Dysplasia-Associated Lesion or Mass

Macroscopically polypoid areas occurring in association with IBD are diagnosed as dysplasia-associated lesion or mass (DALM) and carry a high risk of progres-

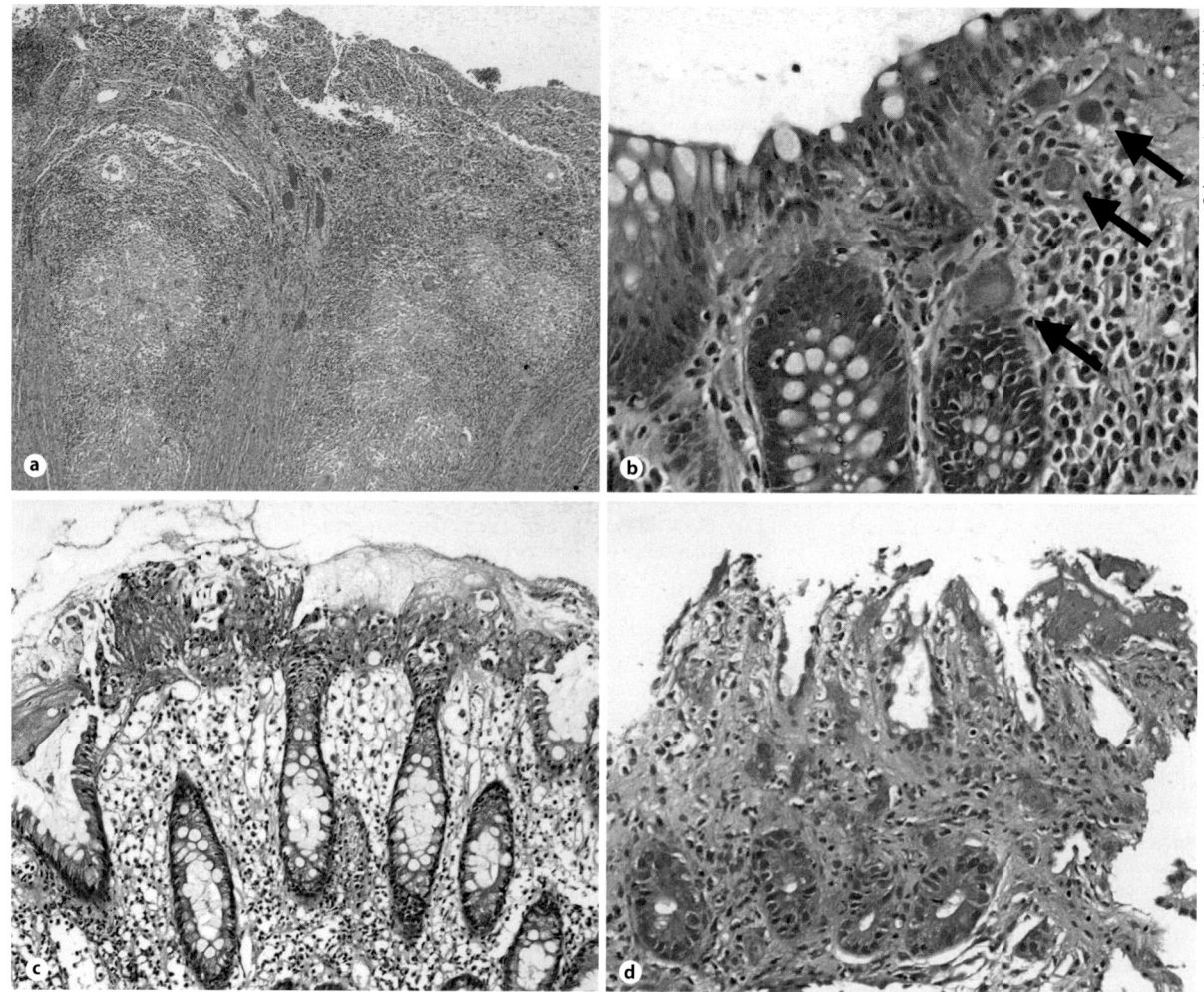

Fig. 2. Differential diagnosis of IBD. Tuberculosis with ulceration, epithelioid granulomas and giant cells of Langhans' type (**a**). CMV colitis with typical owl's eye cells (arrows) (**b**). Pseudomembranous colitis due to *Clostridium difficile* toxin with volcano-like crypt eruptions and a band-like fibrin deposition covering the surface (**c**). Ischemic colitis with necrosis of the upper part of the mucosa, edema, vascular congestion and microthrombi (**d**).

sion to colorectal carcinoma [8]. As patients with DALM are encouraged to undergo prophylactic total proctocolectomy, DALM must be distinguished from sporadic adenomas ('adenoma-like mass'(ALM)) which are similar to those observed in non-IBD patients and may be treated by polypectomy [9]. Several features may aid in the differential diagnosis of DALM versus ALM (table 2).

DALM and ALM may present as various types of polypoid masses, resembling tubular adenomas (fig. 4a, b), flat adenomas (fig. 4c) or serrated adenomas (fig. 4d). The use of immunohistochemistry can aid in the differential diagnosis of DALM versus ALM as strong p53 expression and absence of nuclear β-catenin are usually observed in colitis-associated DALM (fig. 5a, c) as opposed to weak expression of p53 and often nuclear β-catenin in sporadic ALM [10].

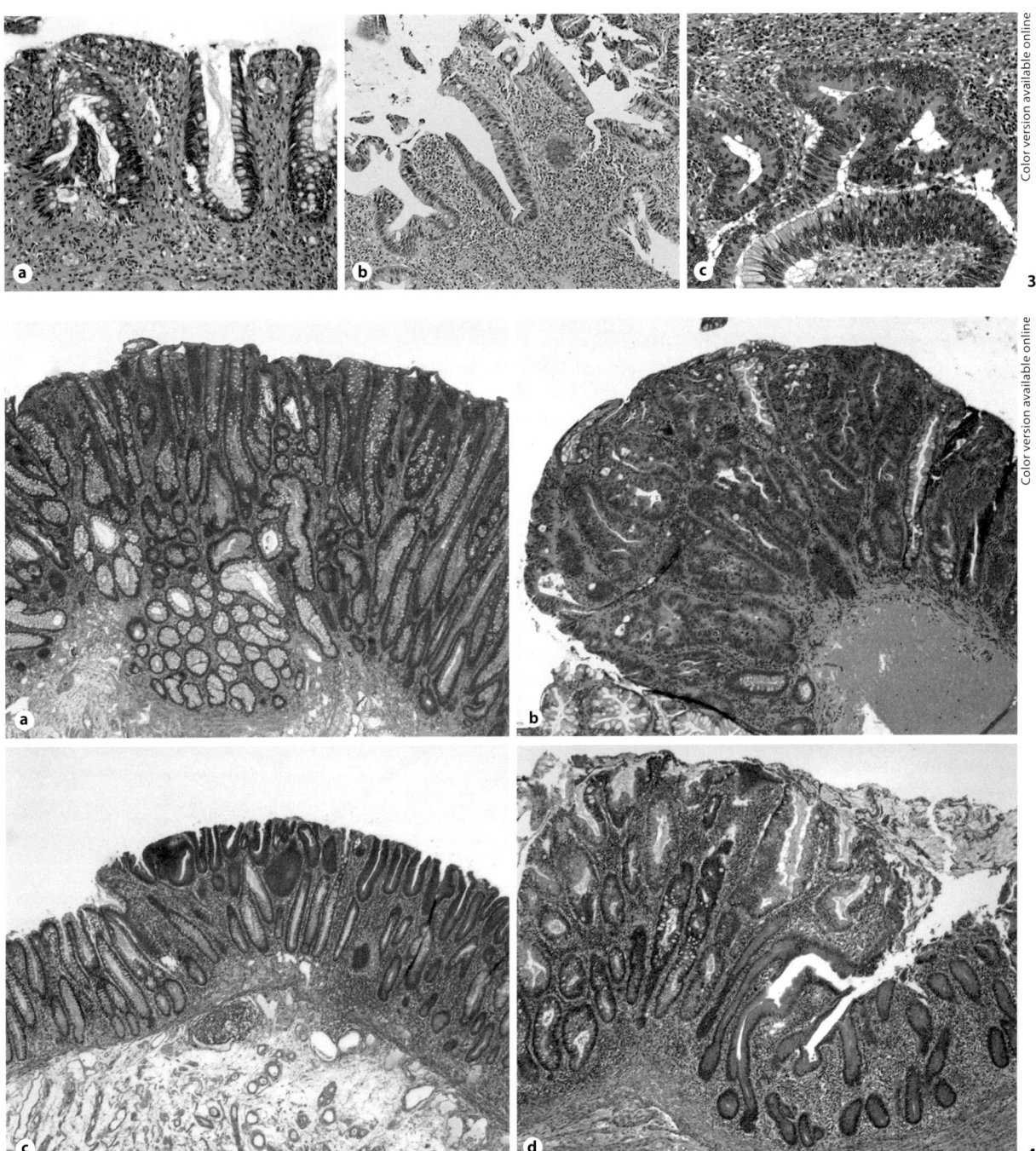

Fig. 3. IEN in IBD. Colonic mucosa with mild mucin depletion, slight nuclear stratification and signs of epithelial regeneration diagnosed as 'indefinite for dysplasia' (**a**). Low-grade IEN with some basal polarity maintained in the dysplastic epithelium (**b**). High-grade IEN with severe nuclear hyperchromatism, true stratification and elongated nuclei extending to the luminal surface (**c**).

Fig. 4. DALM with a mixture of dysplastic and benign crypts (**a**) as opposed to an ALM (**b**). DALM can also occur as a relatively flat lesion (**c**) or a polypoid mass resembling a serrated adenoma with irregular indentation of the neoplastic epithelium (**d**).

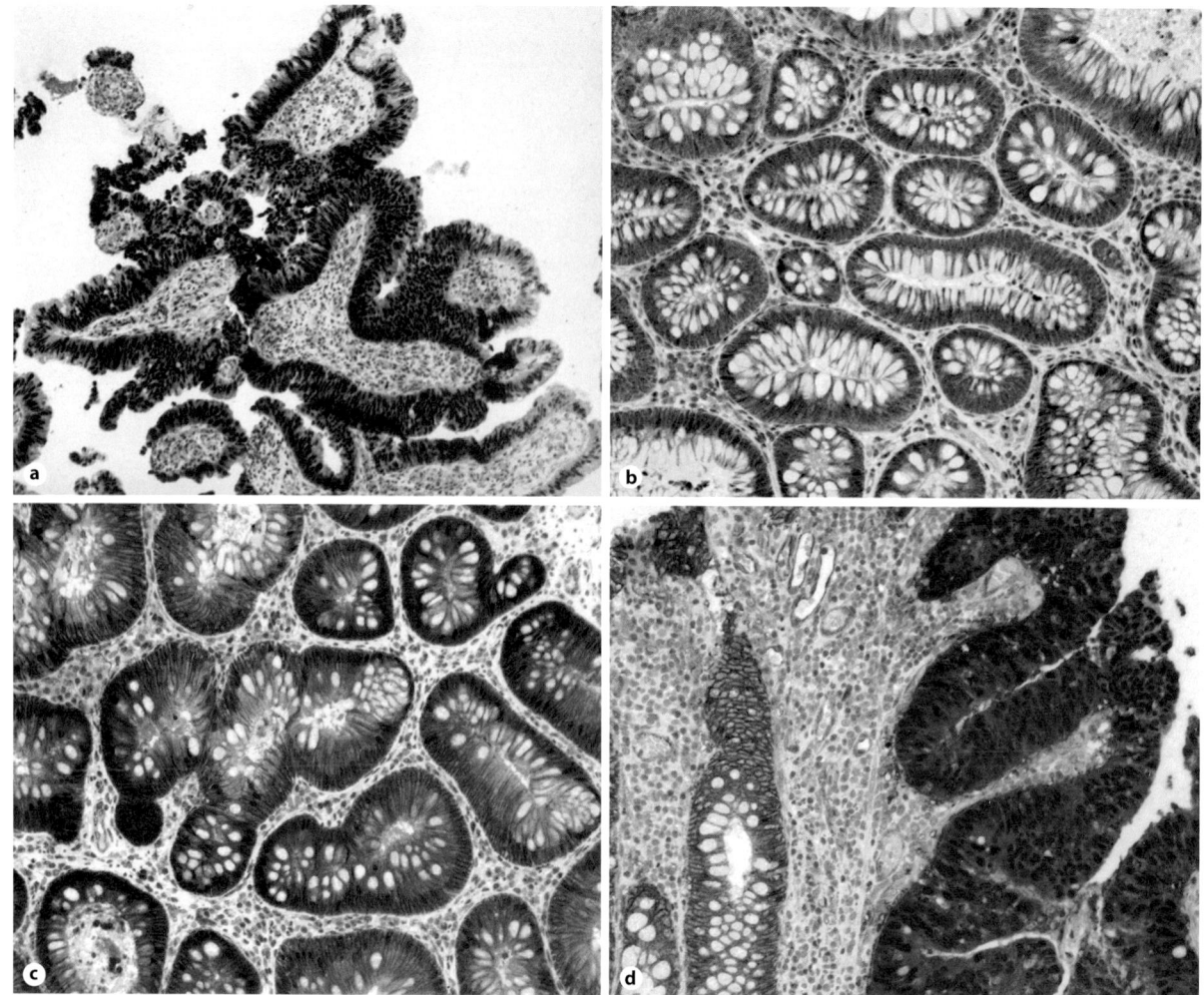

Fig. 5. Immunohistochemistry in DALM versus ALM. DALM with strong expression of p53 (**a**) as compared to low expression of p53 in an ALM (**b**). Predominantly cytoplasmic β-catenin expression in DALM (**c**) as opposed to nuclear β-catenin expression in the dysplastic epithelium of ALM (**d**, right side) and membranous β-catenin expression in the normal colonic crypts for comparison (**d**, left side).

Table 2. Features that may aid in the differential diagnosis of DALM versus ALM

DALM	ALM
Left-sided	Right-sided
Flat dysplasia/IEN	Absent
Mixture of benign/dysplastic crypts at surface	Rare
Inflammation of mucosa/stroma polyp	Rare
p53 strong	p53 weak
β-Catenin cytoplasmic	β-Catenin nuclear

Carcinoma in IBD

Adenocarcinomas arising in IBD patients have a higher proportion of poorly differentiated and mucinous tumors (fig. 6) [11]. Differences in the frequency and order of genetic alterations detected in colitis-associated carcinomas compared to sporadic colorectal cancer may indicate that progression to cancer involves distinct pathways in patients with IBD [12]. In patients with UC and primary sclerosing cholangitis, treatment with ursodeoxy-

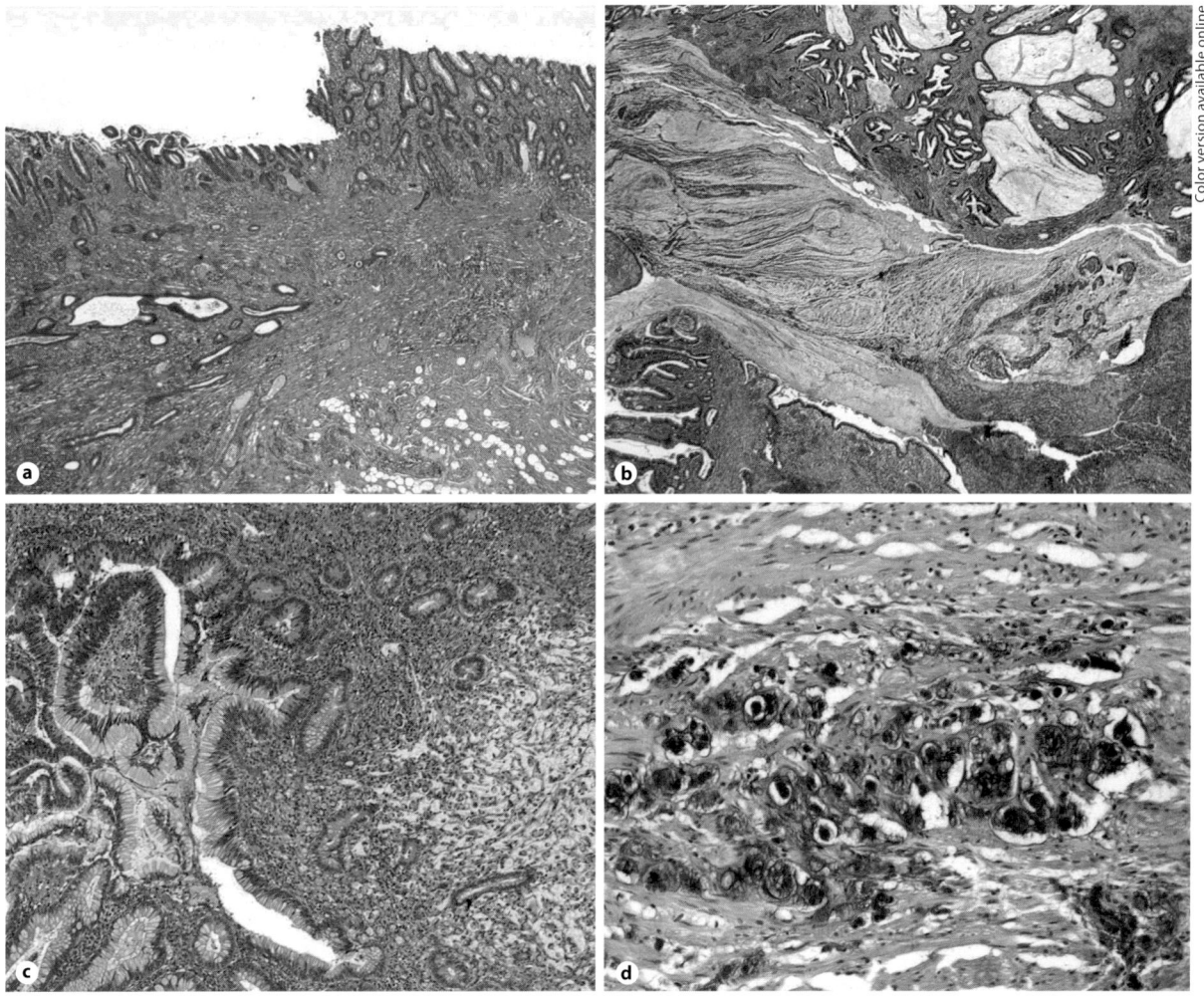

Fig. 6. Adenocarcinoma in IBD. Well-differentiated adenocarcinoma arising in CD with glandular tumor growth in the submucosa (**a**) and a poorly differentiated mucinous component (**b**). High-grade IEN (**c**, left side) in a patient with UC and adjacent invasive adenocarcinoma of signet-ring type (**c**, right side). Larger magnification of the signet-ring cells (**d**), PAS stain.

cholic acid was associated with a lower risk of colitis-associated cancer, and in an animal model, ursodeoxycholic acid has been shown to suppress colitis-associated carcinogenesis [13].

Iatrogenic Lymphoproliferative Disorders

Various immunosuppressive drugs are used for the treatment of IBD and carry an increased risk of developing an iatrogenic lymphoproliferative disorder (LPD). These LPDs can resemble polymorphic proliferations, diffuse large B-cell lymphoma, peripheral T-cell lymphomas or classical Hodgkin lymphoma [14]. A significant proportion of LPD is associated with Epstein-Barr virus (EBV) infection and may show at least partial regression after withdrawal of the immunosuppressive therapy (fig. 7). Recently, a strong association between patients with CD receiving the TNF-α-antagonist infliximab in combination with other immunomodulators like azathioprine or 6-mercaptopurine and the development of hepatosplenic T-cell lymphoma has been described [15, 16].

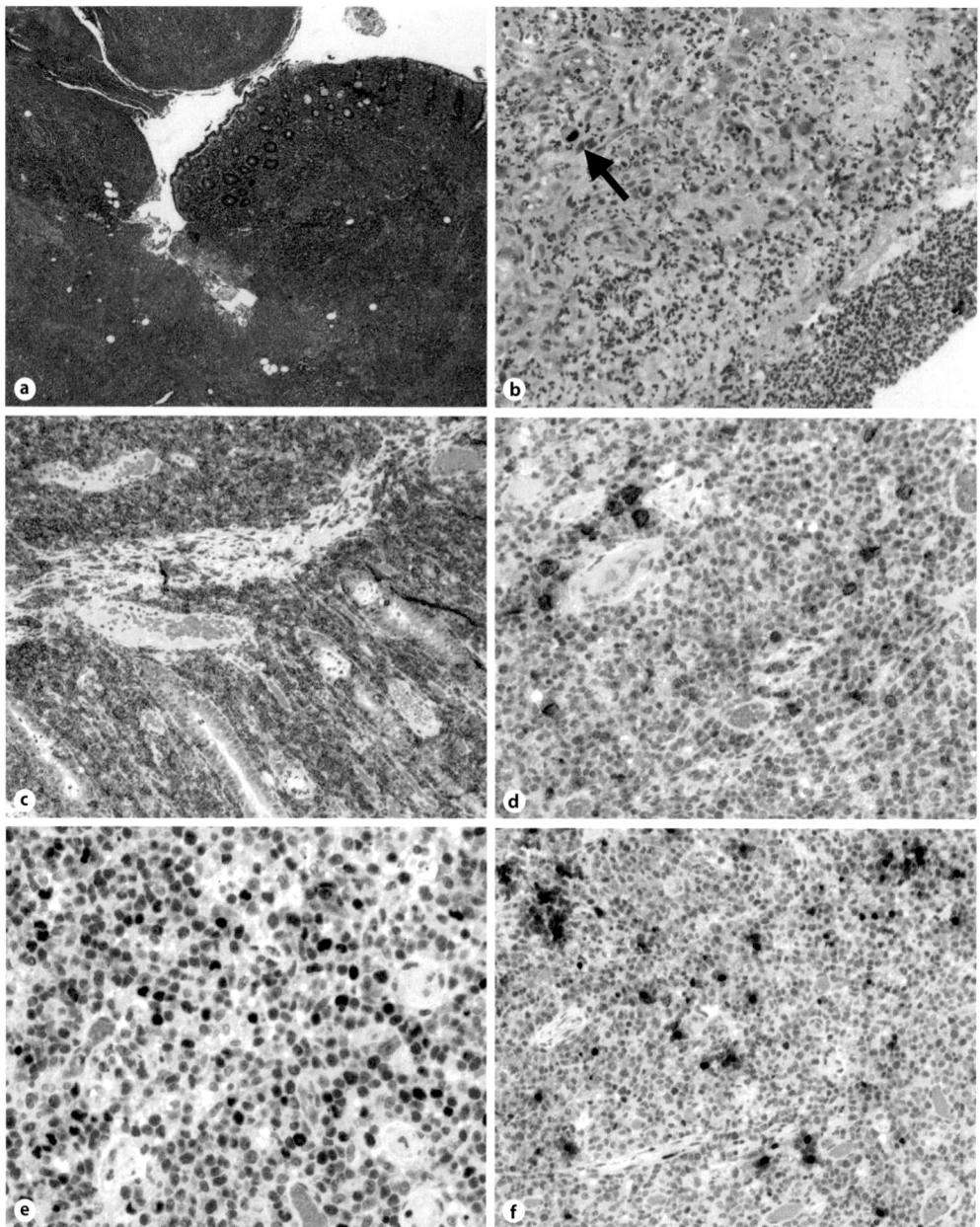

Fig. 7. Iatrogenic immunodeficiency-associated LPD. Specimen of a perforated sigmoid colon with a deep ulcer and a dense infiltrate of lymphoid cells in the bowel wall (**a**). Granulation tissue with detection of few CMV-infected cells using immunohistochemical staining against the pp65 antigen (**b**, arrow). The dense lymphoid infiltrate consists of CD20-positive B cells (**c**) and a significant proportion of these cells express the EBV-encoded latent membrane protein (**d**) as well as the nuclear antigen of the EBV (EBNA2) (**e**) and the zebra antigen (BZ1) indicating active EBV replication (**f**).

In summary, pathology plays an important role in the diagnosis and surveillance of patients with CD or UC, and a close interdisciplinary approach will improve the outcome of patients with these chronic gastrointestinal diseases.

Disclosure Statement

The author declares that no financial or other conflict of interest exists in relation to the content of this article.

References

1 Fenoglio-Preiser CM: Gastrointestinal Pathology: An Atlas and Text, ed 3. Philadelphia, Lippincott Williams & Wilkins, 2008.
2 Schneider T, Ulrichs T, Loddenkemper C, Lode H, Zeitz M, Scherubl H: Intestinal tuberculosis: a clinical and diagnostic challenge. Dtsch Med Wochenschr 2004;129: 1747–1752.
3 Schneider T, Moos V, Loddenkemper C, Marth T, Fenollar F, Raoult D: 100th anniversary of Whipple's disease: new aspects on pathogenesis and treatment of this enigmatic multisystemic infection. Lancet Infect Dis 2008;8:179–190.
4 Karcher H, Loddenkemper C, Zeitz M, Schneider T: Intestinal schistosomiasis in a traveller returning from Rwanda and Burundi. Int J Colorectal Dis 2008;23:1021–1022.
5 Schellhaas E, Loddenkemper C, Schmittel A, Buhr HJ, Pohlen U: Bowel perforation in non-small cell lung cancer after bevacizumab therapy. Invest New Drugs 2009;27: 184–187.
6 Hamilton SR, Aaltonen LA: World Health Organization Classification of Tumours. Pathology and Genetics of Tumours of the Digestive System. Lyon, ARC Press, 2000.
7 Hoffmann JC, Preiss JC, Autschbach F, Buhr HJ, Häuser W, Herrlinger K, Höhne W, Koletzko S, Krieglstein CF, Kruis W, Matthes H, Moser G, Reinshagen M, Rogler G, Schreiber S, Schreyer AG, Sido B, Siegmund B, Stallmach A, Bokemeyer B, Stange EF, Zeitz M: Clinical practice guideline on diagnosis and treatment of Crohn's disease. Z Gastroenterol 2008;46:1094–1146.
8 Blackstone MO, Riddell RH, Rogers BH, Levin B: Dysplasia-associated lesion or mass detected by colonoscopy in long-standing ulcerative colitis: an indication for colectomy. Gastroenterology 1981;80:366–374.
9 Engelsgjerd M, Farraye FA, Odze RD: Polypectomy may be adequate treatment for adenoma-like dysplastic lesions in chronic ulcerative colitis. Gastroenterology 1999;117: 1288–1294.
10 Walsh SV, Loda M, Torres CM, Antonioli D, Odze RD: P53 and β-catenin expression in chronic ulcerative colitis-associated polypoid dysplasia and sporadic adenomas: an immunohistochemical study. Am J Surg Pathol 1999;23:963–969.
11 Heimann TM, Oh SC, Martinelli G, Szporn A, Luppescu N, Lembo CA, Kurtz RJ, Fasy TM, Greenstein AJ: Colorectal carcinoma associated with ulcerative colitis: a study of prognostic indicators. Am J Surg 1992;164: 13–17.
12 Aust DE, Terdiman JP, Willenbucher RF, Chang CG, Molinaro-Clark A, Baretton GB, Loehrs U, Waldman FM: The APC/β-catenin pathway in ulcerative colitis-related colorectal carcinomas: a mutational analysis. Cancer 2002;94:1421–1427.
13 Loddenkemper C, Keller S, Hanski ML, Cao M, Jahreis G, Stein H, Zeitz M, Hanski C: Prevention of colitis-associated carcinogenesis in a mouse model by diet supplementation with ursodeoxycholic acid. Int J Cancer 2006;118:2750–2757.
14 Swerdlow SH, Campo E, Harris NL, Jaffe ES, Pileri SA, Stein H, Thiele J, Vardiman JW: WHO Classification of Tumours of Haematopoietic and Lymphoid Tissues. Lyon, IARC, 2008.
15 Mackey AC, Green L, Liang LC, Dinndorf P, Avigan M: Hepatosplenic T-cell lymphoma associated with infliximab use in young patients treated for inflammatory bowel disease. J Pediatr Gastroenterol Nutr 2007;44: 265–267.
16 Rosh JR, Gross T, Mamula P, Griffiths A, Hyams J: Hepatosplenic T-cell lymphoma in adolescents and young adults with Crohn's disease: a cautionary tale? Inflamm Bowel Dis 2007;13:1024–1030.

Malignant Transformation in Inflammatory Bowel Disease – Surveillance Guide

Andreas Stallmach   Christiane Bielecki   Carsten Schmidt

Department of Gastroenterology, Hepatology and Infectiology, Friedrich Schiller University, Jena, Germany

Key Words

Colorectal cancer in Crohn's disease · Colorectal cancer in ulcerative colitis · Inflammatory bowel disease, malignant transformation · Surveillance in Crohn's disease · Surveillance programs and guidelines · Surveillance strategies, problems

Abstract

Nowadays, it is considered as an established fact that patients with long-standing ulcerative colitis (UC) are at an increased risk of developing colorectal cancer (CRC). Although data for CRC risk in Crohn's disease (CD) are not as extensive, it has been suggested that the risks are comparable to UC. Current strategies for the prevention and early detection of cancer in this high-risk population are grounded in the concept of an inflammation-neoplasia-carcinoma sequence. To reduce CRC mortality in inflammatory bowel disease, colonoscopic surveillance with random and targeted biopsies were recommended to detect early neoplasia. The introduction of novel endoscopic techniques such as chromoendoscopy, narrow band imaging or confocal endomicroscopy to facilitate targeted biopsy has become increasingly associated with enhanced neoplasia detection. However, there is only indirect evidence that such surveillance strategies are likely to be effective at reducing the risk of death from inflammatory bowel disease-associated CRC. Further, new data revealed that surveillance strategies largely based upon disease duration delayed or missed a substantial number of patients with early CRC. Therefore, actual surveillance guidelines seem to be insufficient and need to be restructured.

Copyright © 2009 S. Karger AG, Basel

Colorectal Cancer in Ulcerative Colitis

In 1927, Yeomans [1] reported the first case of malignant transformation complicating chronic ulcerative colitis (UC), and, subsequently in 1928, Bargen [2] described 20 cases of colorectal cancer (CRC) resulting from UC. A comprehensive meta-analysis from 2001 presented data regarding all published studies estimating the risk for CRC in UC (cumulative incidence) to be 1.6% after 10 years, 8.3% after 20 years and 18.4% after 30 years of disease duration for all patients with colitis with an overall prevalence of 3.7% [3]. However, these data may overestimate the real incidence and prevalence of UC-associated carcinoma, as data were collected from tertiary care centers for inflammatory bowel disease (IBD), where particularly patients with a severe disease process are treated. Prospectively collected data from a surveillance program over a 30-year period showed a lower cumulative incidence of CRC: 2.5% after 20 years, 7.6% after 30 years, and 10.8% after 40 years of UC [4]. Other investigators described CRC incidences in IBD in between 1.9 and 2.1% [5, 6].

However, not only the duration of the disease, but also the anatomic extent of the disease is an important risk factor for UC-associated CRC. To be more specific, patients with proctitis showed a 1.7-fold increased risk of CRC compared to the general population, patients with left-sided colitis were found to have a 2.8-fold risk, whereas patients suffering from pancolitis were at a 14.8-fold risk of developing CRC [7]. Data to specify CRC risk in greater detail point out that patients with backwash ileitis as compared to left-sided colitis have a 10-fold higher risk to develop CRC [8].

Primary sclerosing cholangitis (PSC) has been associated with up to 5% of UC patients. A meta-analysis revealed that patients with UC and PSC had a significantly higher risk for the development of colorectal neoplasia than patients with UC without PSC [9]. Another important point is that familial occurrence of CRC was associated with a more than 2-fold risk of CRC in IBD patients [10]. Patients with a first-degree relative diagnosed with CRC before 50 years of age had the highest absolute risk for CRC, whereas first-degree relatives of patients with Crohn's disease (CD) or UC were not at increased risk of cancer. Relatives of patients with both IBD and CRC had an 80% increased risk of CRC [11]. Therefore, taking family history in account is an important issue in evaluating the specific cancer risk in a patient with IBD.

According to the severity of the disease, in 2004, Rutter et al. [12] presented data that showed a highly significant correlation between the colonoscopic (odds ratio 2.5; p = 0.001) and histological (odds ratio 5.1; p < 0.001) inflammation scores and the risk of colorectal neoplasia. In a cohort of 418 patients undergoing regular endoscopic surveillance for dysplasia, 65 patients progressed to any neoplasia (low-grade dysplasia, high-grade dysplasia, or CRC). Univariate analysis demonstrated a significant relationship between histologic inflammation over time and progression to advanced neoplasia [13]. Subsequently, another retrospective study revealed that many macroscopic colonoscopic features (post-inflammatory polyps, colonic strictures, segments of severe inflammation) correlate with the risk of developing CRC [14].

Importantly, it must be noted that there might be a decreased incidence of CRC in UC in the last decades. A Swedish review indicated that the risk of CRC in Scandinavian countries is decreasing [15]. A trend towards lower incidence rates over the last 30 years was also seen in a study of Rutter et al. [4]. The reasons for this observed decline in incidence may be the more widespread use of surveillance colonoscopy, a chemoprotective effect attributable to the more widespread use of 5-ASA therapies,

Table 1. Risk factors for development of colorectal cancer in IBD

Younger age at diagnosis
Greater extent and duration of disease
Increased severity of inflammation
Family history of colorectal cancer
Coexisting primary sclerosing cholangitis

more aggressive surgical intervention, dietary or environmental factors. Despite the encouraging finding that CRC in UC appears to be less common than previously believed, one should take caution in interpreting the results of these studies as evidence to relax the practice of routine screening and surveillance.

Colorectal Cancer in Crohn's Disease

Difficulties exist in defining CD association with CRC because of an often more complicating disease course including stenoses, fistulas and a need for surgical interventions, resulting in difficulties to clearly define adequate study groups. Patients with long-lasting CD seem to have a similar risk as patients with CU to develop CRC [16]. Patients with isolated small bowel CD do not have an increased risk for CRC but for adenocarcinoma of the small bowel. In 1990, Ekbom et al. [17] reported a relative risk for CRC in CD of the terminal ileum of 1.0; in ileocolonic CD the relative risk for CRC was 3.2, in colonic CD the relative risk was 5.6. A recent study by Canavan et al. [18] showed comparable results: a 2.5-fold risk in colonic disease and a 1.1-fold risk in ileal disease were shown; interestingly, a reduction in the relative risk over the past 30 years was pointed out. However, the background of these data consists of a limited number of case groups due to the low overall incidence of CRC. But in the end, whatever you choose to do for your patients with UC, do no differently for those with Crohn's colitis of similar duration and extent (table 1) [19].

Basics and Molecular Features to Be Known in the Pathogenesis of CRC

Dysplasia is histologically defined as an unequivocal neoplastic change in the intestinal mucosa. 90% of all CRC develop on the basis of an adenoma (adenoma-carcinoma sequence). Not so in pathogenesis of colitis-associated colorectal cancer (CAC). The molecular pathway of sporadic colorectal cancer (SCC) can be differentiated from CAC. CAC usually progresses to invasive adenocarcinoma from flat, depressed and nonpolypoid dysplasia more frequently than SCC. Genomic instability is a major feature of CRC. 85% of SCC and CAC develop of the basis of chromosomal instability, 15% are based on microsatellite instability that usually result in loss of function of mismatch repair system proteins (e.g. hMLH1). However, the molecular development of CAC and SCC seems to be different in timing and frequency [20].

A result of chromosomal instability is loss of function of chromosomal material such as APC. Loss of function in APC (chromosome 5q21–q22) has been proposed as an early event in the origination of SCC but occurs late in CAC pathogenesis [21, 22]. On the other hand, loss of p53 gene function that is known to be a causative factor in CRC pathogenesis occurs early in CAC, but late in SCC development [23]. Progress has been made in recent times in the identification of novel signal transduction pathways of the immunopathogenesis of IBD and CRC. IBD is characterized by cytokine-driven mixed inflammation. Cytokine signal transduction pathway involves transcription factors called STATs (signal transducers and activators of transcription). IL-6/STAT-3 trans-signaling pathway with STAT-3 activation has been implicated in the pathogenesis of CRC because of its ability to inhibit apoptosis and induce cell proliferation [24, 25]. On the other hand, studies suggest that STAT3 may have anti-inflammatory effects on macrophages and dendritic cells, so that therapeutic approaches targeting this pathway have to be done carefully [26].

NF-κB as a 'rapid-acting' primary transcription factor for proinflammatory cytokines can also work as a tumor promoter. Within the proinflammatory pathway, NF-κB upregulation may increase inflammation-related cancer, as seen in animal models by Pikarsky et al. [27].

Surveillance Programs and Guidelines

Periodic surveillance colonoscopy is our current approach to prevent cancer development in IBD. This strategy relies on the ability to detect CRC at a preclinical phase of neoplasia during which intervention can avert the adverse consequences of invasive cancer. Different national and international gastroenterological societies have published similar surveillance guidelines in order to prevent CRC in IBD patients. According to these guidelines, patients should undergo a surveillance program to detect pre-neoplastic lesions at a curable stage to prevent malignant transformation. All surveillance guidelines are based on two central suggestions: (1) regular surveillance should begin after 8–10 years from onset of symptoms for pancolitis and after 15–20 years for left-sided disease, and (2) surveillance colonoscopy includes the directive to take 2–4 random biopsy specimens every 10 cm from the entire colon with additional samples of suspicious areas.

Beginning Surveillance

Surveillance guidelines currently most often follow recommendations to start surveillance after 8–10 years of disease in case of extensive UC, and after 15 years of disease in case of left-sided UC. Starting surveillance before these time intervals is not recommended. The evidence for this restriction, however, on which this is based, is poor. In an important topical study, Lutgens et al. [28] identified 149 patients with IBD-associated CRCs in a nationwide network and registry of histo- and cytopathology containing pathology reports generated in The Netherlands. Of the patients, 22% developed cancer before the 8- or 15-year starting points of surveillance taking the date of diagnosis as the entry point. Further, 28% developed CRC if surveillance would start 10 or 20 years after diagnosis for extensive or left-sided disease, respectively. Using the onset of symptoms to calculate the time interval, 17–22% of patients would present with cancer prior to surveillance starting points. The implementation of the current starting points for surveillance may lead to a delay in diagnosing CRC in approximately 20% of patients in this study. The trouble is that most guidelines based on the results of a meta-analysis were performed by Eaden et al. [3]. This meta-analysis included data of 19 studies and described IBD-associated cumulative CRC risks of 2, 8 and 18% for the respective disease durations of 10, 20 and 30 years. Furthermore, Eaden and Mayberry [29] state in the surveillance guidelines for the British that CRC is rarely encountered when disease duration is <8–10 years. However, 3 of 19 studies [12, 18, 23] excluded explicitly those patients who developed CRC within 5, 7 or 10 years of IBD duration. Despite these drawbacks, which artificially reduce the risk of CRC in the first 10 years after the onset of IBD, 73 of 394 CRCs (19%) found in 16 of the 19 aforementioned studies [8, 11, 12, 14, 16–18, 21–27] occurred within an IBD duration of <10 years. It is tempting to speculate that IBD patients with early cancer reflect a subset of all patients; however, since we could not identify the patients at risk, early colonoscopies in the whole group were necessary to detect more curable lesions.

Random Biopsies

Nearly all consensus guidelines recommend taking 2–4 random biopsy specimens every 10 cm from the entire colon resulting in 40–50 biopsies. Some experts suggest taking more biopsies in the distal rectosigmoid (e.g. approx. every 5 cm) since the distribution of neoplasia in UC still shows a distal predominance [30]. However, many gastroenterologists are either not fully aware of these recommendations or intentionally do not adhere to them. Recently, it has been shown that in more than 50% of the cases <10 biopsies were taken [31]; therefore, the question arises why random biopsies were not generally accepted. In this context it is important to note that the rationale for this suggestion was based only on a mathematical model. A typical biopsy sample represents less than 0.05% of the colon; therefore, 33 biopsies are required to detect neoplasia with 90% sensitivity, and 64 biopsies are needed to achieve 95% sensitivity [32]. Taylor et al. [33] mimic standard colonoscopy with random biopsies from mucosa from macroscopically unsuspicious areas in 100 colectomy specimens. They demonstrated that 26% of colons with an established cancer harbored no dysplasia in any biopsy from any region in the colon. The sensitivity of random colonic biopsies to detect concomitant carcinoma was only 0.74. Further, Blonski et al. [34] identified a group of 49 UC patients who underwent colonoscopic evaluation for neoplasia detection. Overall, 58 dysplastic sites were detected; 51 were macroscopically visible (87.9%) and only 7 were macroscopically invisible. Thus, one key question resulting from these studies is whether there is still a need for random biopsies in unsuspicious mucosa in UC patients. In the first randomized trial, dysplastic tissue was seen only in conjunction with mucosal alterations [35]. In a large follow-up study with magnifying endoscopy in 886 patients with UC, Sada et al. [36] found that dysplasia and early cancer were best characterized by granular or nodular protruding mucosa seen best after chromoendoscopy. Dysplasia was never found in normal-appearing mucosa after staining. Furthermore, Rutter et al. [37] found no dysplastic tissue in 2,904 nontargeted biopsies. Taken together, multiple random biopsies should be discontinued as a surveillance technique in patients with long-standing UC.

In general, surveillance colonoscopies should be done in a phase of remission because otherwise in the presence of inflammation, dysplastic areas are more difficult or even impossible to discover. If active inflammation of the bowel is present, medical therapy should be started in order to reduce these inflammatory alterations and to perform short-term control colonoscopy afterwards.

Surveillance in Crohn's Disease

Surveillance guidelines for UC patients have been elaborated in greater detail than for CD patients. Crohn's colitis patients are thought to have a comparable risk of CRC as UC patients if there is comparable surface involvement and disease duration [16]. Therefore, screening and surveillance recommendations are similar [41]. However, there are only a few reports on the efficacy of surveillance colonoscopy in patients with chronic Crohn's colitis. Friedman et al. [42] published a study involving 259 patients. Biopsies were performed at 10-cm intervals and from strictures and polypoid masses. The median interval between examinations was 24 months, examinations were performed more frequently (1–6 months) in patients with dysplasia on biopsy. The screening and surveillance program detected dysplasia or cancer in 16% of patients (10 indefinite dysplasia, 23 low-grade dysplasia, 4 high-grade dysplasia and 5 cancers, respectively). It has been concluded that colonoscopic surveillance should also be strongly considered in chronic extensive Crohn's colitis. Beginning after 8–10 years from onset of symptoms and in case no dysplasia was found, the next surveillance endoscopy was recommended within 2 years. If dysplasia was found, the same management as described above in detail concerning UC was suggested. Moreover, after 20 years of disease duration the same management as described in UC should be followed. Patients who have solely small intestinal CD should be managed according to the general population in terms of CRC screening [43]. Strictures in CD will demand repeated endoscopy within 1 year if an endoscopic passage is possible. In case no passage can be performed, barium enema or computed tomography, and with >20 years of disease duration (12% rate of concomitant CRC), surgery should be considered [42]. However, balloon dilatation works best for strictures <6 cm [44]. Anal stricture gives rise to a high risk of cancer development (6.8 vs. 0.7% in 980 patients with CD seen by Yamazaki et al. [45]); therefore, annual examinations are recommended [46].

Problems Existing in Surveillance Strategies

Surveillance colonoscopy has its limitations in detecting neoplastic lesion as shown by Connell et al. [47]. Colonoscopy and biopsy every 10 cm throughout the colon was performed every 2 years or more often if dysplasia was found. Therefore, the detection of 11 symptomless carcinomas (8 Dukes A, 1 Dukes B, and 2 Dukes C) and 6 symptomatic tumors (4 Dukes C and 2 disseminated) were presented 10–43 months after a negative colonoscopy.

Limiting factors have been reported in terms of histopathological identification and grading of dysplasia; therefore, it is mandatory that all pathologists involved are familiar with the terms recommended in 1983 by Riddell et al. [48], and later modified by Schlemper et al. [49]. Consulting a second pathologist is recommended if a probe is indefinite or positive for dysplasia, or if uncertainties remain. A re-colonoscopy by trying to take biopsies from the same area is not recommended as the risk for a so-called 'sampling error' is high [16]. Tissue handling recommends that no more than 4 biopsies should be placed in any one tube, and specimens of suspicious lesions should be placed in separately labeled tubes [16]. Another problem is that a dysplasia-associated lesion or mass [50] can appear in the form of polyps, bumps, plaques and velvety patches that can easily be confused with the typical image of an IBD intestine. Therefore, as stated above, it is mandatory to perform surveillance endoscopy in remission.

The number of samples that have to be taken during colonoscopy is another matter of discussion. According to the guidelines, 4-quadrant biopsies every 10 cm are recommended throughout the colon; probes from arbitrary areas (without dyeing) can exclude dysplasia with 90% guaranty, to reach 95% already twice this amount of probes had to be taken [32]. In UC it has been suggested to take 4-quadrant biopsies every 5 cm in the lower sigmoid and rectum because of a higher CRC risk in this area [30]. But given the fact that only 9.2% of patients in the risk group received a colonoscopy according to the guidelines, this approach seems to be unrealistic. Recently, it has been shown that in more than 50% of the cases, <10 biopsies were taken [31].

The time that is needed for endoscopy obviously plays an important role because there seems to be a correlation between median surveillance coloscopy duration per endoscopist and flat dysplasia detection rate. Toruner et al. [38] reviewed the Mayo Clinic endoscopic database and medical records of patients with IBD who underwent surveillance colonoscopy between 2002 and 2003. There was a significant correlation between median surveillance colonoscopy duration per endoscopist and flat dysplasia detection rate ($p = 0.0066$). Higher rates of detecting adenomas were observed among endoscopists who had longer mean times for withdrawal during colonoscopy (at least 7 min). The effect of variation in withdrawal times on lesion detection and the prevention of CRC in the context of widespread colonoscopic screening are not known [39].

Another issue of importance is bowel preparation. Data from a recent study showed a good correlation between colon cleanliness and the detection rate of adenomas [40]. Therefore, a sufficiently cleaned colon using standard preparation techniques is the basis of an informative endoscopy [16].

The skills of the endoscopist are also an important issue. A study with members of two regional gastroenterology associations in the USA, including both academic and private practice-based gastroenterologists, has shown that only 19% of respondents correctly identified the definition of dysplasia (defined as a neoplastic change of the epithelium without invasion into the lamina propria) and nearly one-third of respondents pursued continued surveillance in case of high-grade dysplasia diagnosis. Some endoscopists took only 3 samples from 8 different regions of the complete bowel during surveillance colonoscopy [51].

All of the above-mentioned facts are thought to have an influence on the outcome of surveillance colonoscopy in IBD and impact the effectiveness. As a matter of fact, continuing the education of gastroenterologist may be the key to a better surveillance of IBD patients.

Choi et al. [52] did an outcome analysis with a total of 41 patients who developed carcinoma-associated UC – 19 patients were under colonoscopic surveillance and 22 patients were not. They found that carcinomas were detected at a significantly earlier Dukes' stage in the surveillance group and the 5-year survival rate was higher in the surveillance group (77.2 and 36.3%, respectively).

To allow critical analysis it is important to define what is 'success' and what is 'failure' in a surveillance program, as done by Lynch et al. [53]. Failure for them is defined as detecting CRC in stage Dukes C, cancer found at colonoscopy performed for any reason other than surveillance, or cancer found at surgery performed for reasons other than dysplasia. Applying these criteria, only 1 of 9 CRC was detected by the surveillance program analyzing 12 published studies of colonoscopic surveillance program. So does colonoscopy surveillance fail to reduce CRC? Lynch et al. [53] also mentioned cases where cancers found earlier than 8 years from onset of disease were defined as failures, as discussed above and in the data of Lutgens et al. [28].

A retrospective study of 1,339 surveillance examinations (including both random biopsies at approximately 10-cm intervals throughout the involved colon and directed biopsies of polypoid lesions, masses, strictures, or irregular mucosa distinct from surrounding inflamed tissue) in 622 patients with UC showed that per-patient sensitivities for dysplasia and cancer was 71.8 and 100%, respectively, so that it can be summarized that dysplasia and cancer in UC are endoscopically visible in most patients and may be reliably identified during scheduled examinations [54]. However, until today, there is no clear evidence that survival is prolonged with periodic surveillance colonoscopy in this group of patients.

Conclusion

Although it is well known that the risk of developing CRC is increased in patients with UC and CD, new data suggest that the risk seems to have decreased during the last years. This might be an effect of surveillance, but perhaps studies which have been done differ from each other and sourced to differences in cohort selection (high-risk patients, patients treated in centers and having a complicated, severe process in disease, geographic varieties). And what also differs today is that we know a lot more risk factors having an influence on disease development and therefore being perhaps an underestimated determining factor. Concerning the effectiveness of surveillance, major problems remain: physicians do not follow practice guidelines sufficiently. More teaching, more awareness and more capacity have to be aimed for [55]. Guidelines are not sufficient enough in detecting CRC, concerning the starting point, recommended biopsy samples (especially random biopsies) and withdrawal time. But, as more biopsies are taken (more sensitivity was described recovering dysplasia), more costs arise – costs for the procedure, the time and pathologist. We think that targeted biopsies with new techniques, pointing out chromoendoscopy as the current most successful method detecting dysplasia, should be done more often. Discussion should begin about development in the existing guidelines to give more effective strategies an integral part, so that patients can hope to receive more sufficient surveillance in the future.

Disclosure Statement

The authors declare that no financial or other conflict of interest exists in relation to the content of this article.

References

1 Yeomans FC: Carcinomatous degeneration of rectal adenomas. JAMA 1927;89:862.
2 Bargen JA: Chronic ulcerative colitis associated with malignant metaplasia. Arch Surg 1928;17:561.
3 Eaden JA, Abrams KR, Mayberry JF: The risk of colorectal cancer in ulcerative colitis: a meta-analysis. Gut 2001;48:526–535.
4 Rutter MD, Saunders BP, Wilkinson KH, et al: Thirty-year analysis of a colonoscopic surveillance program for neoplasia in ulcerative colitis. Gastroenterology 2006;130: 1030–1038.
5 Jess T, Loftus EV Jr, Velayos FS, et al: Risk of intestinal cancer in inflammatory bowel disease: a population-based study from Olmsted County, Minnesota. Gastroenterology 2006;130:1039–1046.
6 Jess T, Gamborg M, Matzen P, et al: Increased risk of intestinal cancer in Crohn's disease: a meta-analysis of population-based cohort studies. Am J Gastroenterol 2005;100:2724–2729.
7 Ekbom A, Helmick C, Zack M, et al: Ulcerative colitis and colorectal cancer. A population-based study. N Engl J Med 1990;323: 1228–1233.
8 Heuschen UA, Hinz U, Allemeyer EH, et al: Backwash ileitis is strongly associated with colorectal carcinoma in ulcerative colitis. Gastroenterology 2001;120:841–847.
9 Soetikno RM, Lin OS, Heidenreich PA, et al: Increased risk of colorectal neoplasia in patients with primary sclerosing cholangitis and ulcerative colitis: a meta-analysis. Gastrointest Endosc 2002;56:48–54.
10 Askling J, Dickman PW, Karlen P, et al: Family history as a risk factor for colorectal cancer in inflammatory bowel disease. Gastroenterology 2001;120:1356–1362.
11 Askling J, Dickman PW, Karlen P, et al: Colorectal cancer rates among first-degree relatives of patients with inflammatory bowel disease: a population-based cohort study. Lancet 2001;357:262–266.
12 Rutter M, Saunders B, Wilkinson K, et al: Severity of inflammation is a risk factor for colorectal neoplasia in ulcerative colitis. Gastroenterology 2004;126:451–459.
13 Gupta RB, Harpaz N, Itzkowitz S, et al: Histologic inflammation is a risk factor for progression to colorectal neoplasia in ulcerative colitis: a cohort study. Gastroenterology 2007;133:1099–1105.
14 Rutter MD, Saunders BP, Wilkinson KH, et al: Cancer surveillance in longstanding ulcerative colitis: endoscopic appearances help predict cancer risk. Gut 2004;53:1813–1816.
15 Rubio CA, Befrits R, Ljung T, et al: Colorectal carcinoma in ulcerative colitis is decreasing in Scandinavian countries. Anticancer Res 2001;21:2921–2924.
16 Itzkowitz SH, Present DH: Consensus conference: colorectal cancer screening and surveillance in inflammatory bowel disease. Inflamm Bowel Dis 2005;11:314–321.
17 Ekbom A, Helmick C, Zack M, et al: Increased risk of large-bowel cancer in Crohn's disease with colonic involvement. Lancet 1990;336:357–359.
18 Canavan C, Abrams KR, Mayberry J: Meta-analysis: colorectal and small bowel cancer risk in patients with Crohn's disease. Aliment Pharmacol Ther 2006;23:1097–1104.
19 Sachar DB: Cancer in Crohn's disease: dispelling the myths. Gut 1994;35:1507–1508.
20 Xie J, Itzkowitz SH: Cancer in inflammatory bowel disease. World J Gastroenterol 2008; 14:378–389.
21 Fearnhead NS, Britton MP, Bodmer WF: The ABC of APC. Hum Mol Genet 2001;10:721–733.

22 Morin PJ, Sparks AB, Korinek V, et al: Activation of β-catenin-TCF signaling in colon cancer by mutations in β-catenin or APC. Science 1997;275:1787–1790.
23 Itzkowitz SH, Harpaz N: Diagnosis and management of dysplasia in patients with inflammatory bowel diseases. Gastroenterology 2004;126:1634–1648.
24 Kusaba T, Nakayama T, Yamazumi K, et al: Expression of p-STAT3 in human colorectal adenocarcinoma and adenoma; correlation with clinicopathological factors. J Clin Pathol 2005;58:833–838.
25 Atreya R, Neurath MF: Signaling molecules: the pathogenic role of the IL-6/STAT-3 trans signaling pathway in intestinal inflammation and in colonic cancer. Curr Drug Targets 2008;9:369–374.
26 Carey R, Jurickova I, Ballard E, et al: Activation of an IL-6:STAT3-dependent transcriptome in pediatric-onset inflammatory bowel disease. Inflamm Bowel Dis 2008;14:446–457.
27 Pikarsky E, Porat RM, Stein I, et al: NF-κB functions as a tumour promoter in inflammation-associated cancer. Nature 2004;431:461–466.
28 Lutgens MW, Vleggaar FP, Schipper ME, et al: High frequency of early colorectal cancer in inflammatory bowel disease. Gut 2008;57:1246–1251.
29 Eaden JA, Mayberry JF: Guidelines for screening and surveillance of asymptomatic colorectal cancer in patients with inflammatory bowel disease. Gut 2002;51(suppl 5):V10–V12.
30 Woolrich AJ, DaSilva MD, Korelitz BI: Surveillance in the routine management of ulcerative colitis: the predictive value of low-grade dysplasia. Gastroenterology 1992;103:431–438.
31 Kaltz B, Bokemeyer B, Hoffmann J, et al: Surveillance colonoscopy in ulcerative colitis patients in Germany (in German). Z Gastroenterol 2007;45:325–331.
32 Rubin CE, Haggitt RC, Burmer GC, et al: DNA aneuploidy in colonic biopsies predicts future development of dysplasia in ulcerative colitis. Gastroenterology 1992;103:1611–1620.
33 Taylor BA, Pemberton JH, Carpenter HA, et al: Dysplasia in chronic ulcerative colitis: implications for colonoscopic surveillance. Dis Colon Rectum 1992;35:950–956.
34 Blonski W, Kundu R, Lewis J, et al: Is dysplasia visible during surveillance colonoscopy in patients with ulcerative colitis? Scand J Gastroenterol 2008;43:698–703.
35 Kiesslich R, Fritsch J, Holtmann M, et al: Methylene blue-aided chromoendoscopy for the detection of intraepithelial neoplasia and colon cancer in ulcerative colitis. Gastroenterology 2003;124:880–888.
36 Sada M, Igarashi M, Yoshizawa S, et al: Dye spraying and magnifying endoscopy for dysplasia and cancer surveillance in ulcerative colitis. Dis Colon Rectum 2004;47:1816–1823.
37 Rutter MD, Saunders BP, Schofield G, et al: Pancolonic indigo carmine dye spraying for the detection of dysplasia in ulcerative colitis. Gut 2004;53:256–260.
38 Toruner M, Harewood GC, Loftus EV Jr, et al: Endoscopic factors in the diagnosis of colorectal dysplasia in chronic inflammatory bowel disease. Inflamm Bowel Dis 2005;11:428–434.
39 Barclay RL, Vicari JJ, Doughty AS, et al: Colonoscopic withdrawal times and adenoma detection during screening colonoscopy. N Engl J Med 2006;355:2533–2541.
40 Thomas-Gibson S, Rogers P, Cooper S, et al: Judgement of the quality of bowel preparation at screening flexible sigmoidoscopy is associated with variability in adenoma detection rates. Endoscopy 2006;38:456–460.
41 Sachar DB: Cancer in Crohn's disease: dispelling the myths. Gut 1994;35:1507–1508.
42 Friedman S, Rubin PH, Bodian C, et al: Screening and surveillance colonoscopy in chronic Crohn's colitis. Gastroenterology 2001;120:820–826.
43 Winawer S, Fletcher R, Rex D, et al: Colorectal cancer screening and surveillance: clinical guidelines and rationale – update based on new evidence. Gastroenterology 2003;124:544–560.
44 Saunders BP, Brown GJ, Lemann M, et al: Balloon dilation of ileocolonic strictures in Crohn's disease. Endoscopy 2004;36:1001–1007.
45 Yamazaki Y, Ribeiro MB, Sachar DB, et al: Malignant colorectal strictures in Crohn's disease. Am J Gastroenterol 1991;86:882–885.
46 Connell WR, Sheffield JP, Kamm MA, et al: Lower gastrointestinal malignancy in Crohn's disease. Gut 1994;35:347–352.
47 Connell WR, Lennard-Jones JE, Williams CB, et al: Factors affecting the outcome of endoscopic surveillance for cancer in ulcerative colitis. Gastroenterology 1994;107:934–944.
48 Riddell RH, Goldman H, Ransohoff DF, et al: Dysplasia in inflammatory bowel disease: standardized classification with provisional clinical applications. Hum Pathol 1983;14:931–968.
49 Schlemper RJ, Riddell RH, Kato Y, et al: The Vienna classification of gastrointestinal epithelial neoplasia. Gut 2000;47:251–255.
50 Kuismanen SA, Holmberg MT, Salovaara R, et al: Genetic and epigenetic modification of MLH1 accounts for a major share of microsatellite-unstable colorectal cancers. Am J Pathol 2000;156:1773–1779.
51 Bernstein CN, Weinstein WM, Levine DS, et al: Physicians' perceptions of dysplasia and approaches to surveillance colonoscopy in ulcerative colitis. Am J Gastroenterol 1995;90:2106–2114.
52 Choi PM, Nugent FW, Schoetz DJ Jr, et al: Colonoscopic surveillance reduces mortality from colorectal cancer in ulcerative colitis. Gastroenterology 1993;105:418–424.
53 Lynch DA, Lobo AJ, Sobala GM, et al: Failure of colonoscopic surveillance in ulcerative colitis. Gut 1993;34:1075–1080.
54 Rubin DT, Rothe JA, Hetzel JT, et al: Are dysplasia and colorectal cancer endoscopically visible in patients with ulcerative colitis? Gastrointest Endosc 2007;65:998–1004.
55 Obrador A, Ginard D, Barranco L: Review article: colorectal cancer surveillance in ulcerative colitis – what should we be doing? Aliment Pharmacol Ther 2006;24(suppl 3):56–63.

Falk Symposium Series

130. Holtmann G, Talley NJ, eds. Gastrointestinal Inflammation and Disturbed Gut Function: The Challenge of New Concepts. Falk Symposium 130. 2003
    ISBN 0-7923-8783-X
131. Herfarth H, Feagan BJ, Folsch UR, Schölmerich J, Vatn MH, Zeitz M, eds. Targets of Treatment in Chronic Inflammatory Bowel Diseases. Falk Symposium 131. 2003   ISBN 0-7923-8784-8
132. Galle PR, Gerken G, Schmidt WE, Wiedenmann B, eds. Disease Progression and Carcinogenesis in the Gastrointestinal Tract. Falk Symposium 132. 2003
    ISBN 0-7923-8785-6
132A. Staritz M, Adler G, Knuth A, Schmiegel W, Schmoll HJ, eds. Side-effects of Chemotherapy on the Gastrointestinal Tract. Falk Workshop. 2003
    ISBN 0-7923-8791-0
132B. Reutter W, Schuppan D, Tauber R, Zeitz M, eds. Cell Adhesion Molecules in Health and Disease. Falk Workshop. 2003   ISBN 0-7923-8786-4
133. Duchmann R, Blumberg R, Neurath M, Schölmerich J, Strober W, Zeitz M. Mechanisms of Intestinal Inflammation: Implications for Therapeutic Intervention in IBD. Falk Symposium 133. 2004   ISBN 0-7923-8787-2
134. Dignass A, Lochs H, Stange E. Trends and Controversies in IBD – Evidence-Based Approach or Individual Management? Falk Symposium 134. 2004
    ISBN 0-7923-8788-0
134A. Dignass A, Gross HJ, Buhr V, James OFW. Topical Steroids in Gastroenterology and Hepatology. Falk Workshop. 2004   ISBN 0-7923-8789-9
135. Lukáš M, Manns MP, Špiccák J, Stange EF, eds. Immunological Diseases of Liver and Gut. Falk Symposium 135. 2004   ISBN 0-7923-8792-9
136. Leuschner U, Broomé U, Stiehl A, eds. Cholestatic Liver Diseases: Therapeutic Options and Perspectives. Falk Symposium 136. 2004   ISBN 0-7923-8793-7
137. Blum HE, Maier KP, Rodés J, Sauerbruch T, eds. Liver Diseases: Advances in Treatment and Prevention. Falk Symposium 137. 2004   ISBN 0-7923-8794-5
138. Blum HE, Manns MP, eds. State of the Art of Hepatology: Molecular and Cell Biology. Falk Symposium 138. 2004   ISBN 0-7923-8795-3
138A. Hayashi N, Manns MP, eds. Prevention of Progression in Chronic Liver Disease: An Update on SNMC (Stronger Neo-Minophagen C). Falk Workshop. 2004
    ISBN 0-7923-8796-1
139. Adler G, Blum HE, Fuchs M, Stange EF, eds. Gallstones: Pathogenesis and Treatment. Falk Symposium 139. 2004   ISBN 0-7923-8798-8

140. Colombel JF, Gasché C, Schölmerich J, Vucelic C, eds. Inflammatory Bowel Disease: Translation from Basic Research to Clinical Practice. Falk Symposium 140. 2005. ISBN 1-4020-2847-4
141. Paumgartner G, Keppler D, Leuschner U, Stiehl A, eds. Bile Acid Biology and Its Therapeutic Implications. Falk Symposium 141. 2005 ISBN 1-4020-2893-8
142. Dienes HP, Leuschner U, Lohse AW, Manns MP, eds. Autoimmune Liver Disease. Falk Symposium 142. 2005 ISBN 1-4020-2894-6
143. Ammann RW, Büchler MW, Adler G, DiMagno EP, Sarner M, eds. Pancreatitis: Advances in Pathobiology, Diagnosis and Treatment. Falk Symposium 143. 2005 ISBN 1-4020-2895-4
144. Adler G, Blum AL, Blum HE, Leuschner U, Manns MP, Mössner J, Sartor RB, Schölmerich J, eds. Gastroenterology Yesterday – Today – Tomorrow: A Review and Preview. Falk Symposium 144. 2005 ISBN 1-4020-2896-2
145. Henne-Bruns D, Buttenschön K, Fuchs M, Lohse AW, eds. Artificial Liver Support. Falk Symposium 145. 2005 ISBN 1-4020-3239-0
146. Blumberg RS, Gangl A, Manns MP, Tilg H, Zeitz M, eds. Gut–Liver Interactions: Basic and Clinical Concepts. Falk Symposium 146. 2005 ISBN 1-4020-4143-8
147. Jewell DP, Colombel JF, Peña AS, Tromm A, Warren BS, eds. Colitis: Diagnosis and Therapeutic Strategies. Falk Symposium 147. 2006 ISBN 1-4020-4315-5
148. Kruis W, Forbes A, Jauch KW, Kreis ME, Wexner SD, eds. Diverticular Disease: Emerging Evidence in a Common Condition. Falk Symposium 148. 2006 ISBN 1-4020- 4317-1
149. van Cutsem E, Rustgi AK, Schmiegel W, Zeitz M, eds. Highlights in Gastrointestinal Oncology. Falk Symposium 149. 2006 ISBN 1-4020-5108-5
150. Galle PR, Gerken G, Schmidt WE, Wiedenmann B, eds. Disease Progression and Disease Prevention in Hepatology and Gastroenterology. Falk Symposium 150. 2006 ISBN 1-4020-5109-3
151. Fraser A, Gibson PR, Hibi T, Qian JM, Schölmerich J, eds. Emerging Issues in Inflammatory Bowel Disease. Falk Symposium 151. 2006 ISBN 978-1-4020-5701-4
152. Fockens P, Schulz H-J, Rösch T, Špicčák J, eds. Endoscopy 2006 – Update and Live Demonstration. Falk Symposium 152. 2008 ISBN 978-1-4020-9147-6
153. Dignass A, Rachmilewitz D, Stange E-F, Weinstock JV, eds. Immunoregulation in Inflammatory Bowel Diseases – Current Understanding and Innovation. Falk Symposium 153. 2007 ISBN 978-1-4020-5888-2
154. Adler G, Fiocchi C, Lazebnik LB, Vorobiev GI, eds. Inflammatory Bowel Disease – Diagnostic and Therapeutic Strategies. Falk Symposium 154. 2007 ISBN 978-1-4020-6115-8
155. Keppler D, Beuers U, Leuschner U, Stiehl A, Trauner M, Paumgartner G, eds. Bile Acids: Biological Actions and Clinical Relevance. Falk Symposium 155. 2007 ISBN 978-1-4020-6251-3
156. Blum HE, Cox DW, Häussinger D, Jansen PLM, Kullak-Ublick GA, eds. Genetics in Liver Diseases. Falk Symposium 156. 2007 ISBN 978-1-4020-6393-0
157. Diehl AM, Hayashi N, Manns MP, Sauerbruch T, eds. Chronic Hepatitis: Metabolic, Cholestatic, Viral and Autoimmune. Falk Symposium 157. 2007 ISBN 978-1-4020-6522-4
158. Gasche G, Herrerías Gutiérrez JM, Gassull M, Monterio E, eds. Intestinal Inflammation and Colorectal Cancer. Falk Symposium 158. 2007 ISBN 978-1-4020-6825-6
159. Tözün N, Mantzaris G, Dağlı, Schölmerich J, eds. IBD 2007 – Achievements in Research and Clinical Practice. Falk Symposium 159. 2008 ISBN 978-1-4020-6986-4

160. Ferkolj I, Gangl A, Galle PR, Vucelic B, eds. Pathogenesis and Clinical Practice in Gastroenterology. Falk Symposium 160. 2008   ISBN 978-1-4020-8766-0

161. Carey MC, Gabryelewicz A, Díte P, Keim V, Mössner J, eds. Future Perspectives in Gastroenterology. Falk Symposium 161. 2008   ISBN 978-1-4020-8832-2

162. Bosch J, Lammert F, Burroughs AK, Lebrec D, Sauerbruch T, eds. Liver Cirrhosis: From Pathophysiology to Disease Management. Falk Symposium 162. 2008
    ISBN 978-1-4020-8655-7

163. Adler G, Fan DM, Jia JD, LaRusso NF, Owyang, C, eds. Chronic Inflammation of Liver and Gut. Falk Symposium 163. 2008   ISBN 978-1-4020-9352-4

164. Tulassay Z, Dítě P, Krejs GJ, Schölmerich J, Schultz HJ, eds. Intestinal Disorders. Falk Symposium 164. 2009   ISBN 978-1-4020-9590-0

165. Keppler D, Beuers U, Stiehl A, Trauner M, eds. Bile Acid Biology and Therapeutic Actions. Falk Symposium 165. 2009   ISBN 978-1-4020-9643-3

165A. Lieberman DA, Malfertheiner P, Riemann JF, Spechler SJ, eds. Strategies of Cancer Prevention in Gastroenterology. Falk Workshop. 2009
    ISBN 978-90-481-2628-6

166. Ell C, Ponchon T, Riemann JF, Sakai P, Yamamoto H, eds. GI Endoscopy – Standards and Innovations. Falk Symposium 166. 2009   ISBN 978-90-481-2748-1

167. Day CP, Galle PR, Lohse AW, Thorgeirsson SS, eds. Liver under Constant Attack – From Fat to Viruses. Falk Symposium 167. 2009
    ISBN 978-90-481-2758-0

168. Rogler G, Gassul M, Levine A, López San Román A, eds. IBD in Different Age Groups. Falk Symposium 168. 2009   ISBN 978-3-8055-9273-4

Author Index

Bashankaev, B. 560
Bielecki, C. 584
Blumberg, R.S. 455
Bojarski, C. 571

Cooney, R. 428
Cosnes, J. 516

Dêchene, A. 526
De Vos, M. 511
Dietrich, C.F. 482
Dorofeyev, A.E. 502

El Fouly, A. 526
Epple, H.-J. 555

Gerken, G. 526
Gubergrits, N.B. 522

Hanauer, S.B. 536
Hering, N.A. 450

Jewell, D. 428

Loddenkemper, C. 576
Lozynskyy, Y.S. 565

Marth, T. 494

Papadakis, K.A. 476

Rassokhina, O.A. 502
Rogler, G. 542
Rosenthal, R.J. 560

Schmidt, C. 584
Schulzke, J.-D. 450
Shen, L. 443
Siegmund, B. 465
Skrypnyk, I.N. 550
Stallmach, A. 584
Su, L. 443

Turner, J.R. 443

Vasilenko, I.V. 502
Vatn, M.H. 470

Wexner, S.D. 560

Zeitz, M. 427

Subject Index

Abdominal ultrasound in inflammatory bowel disease 482
Adaptive immunity 455
Aminosalicylates 542
Angiogenesis 511
Antibiotic-associated colitis 482
Anti-TNF 516
Apoptosis 450
Arthritis 511
Autofluorescence imaging 571
Autophagy 428

Balloon-assisted enteroscopy 476
Barrier function 450

Carcinoma in inflammatory bowel disease 576
Cholangiocarcinoma, imaging techniques 526
Cholangioscopy, ERC brush cytology 526
Chromoendoscopy 571
Claudin 443
Colon mucosal barrier 502
Colorectal cancer in Crohn's disease 584
– – – ulcerative colitis 584
Contrast-enhanced ultrasound 482
Crohn's disease 443, 450, 565
– –, goals 536
– –, medical management 536
Cytokine disturbances 502

Diagnostic algorithms 550
Diagnostics 565
Double-balloon enteroscopy 476
Dysplasia-associated lesion or mass 576

Endoscopy, new techniques 571
EUS fine-needle biopsy 526
Extraintestinal manifestations 502
– –, pathogenic mechanisms 502

Flavonoids 450
Fluorescence endoscopy 571

Genetics 511
Genome-wide association studies 428, 465
Glutamine 450

Iatrogenic lymphoproliferative disorders 576
IL-23R 428
Immunosuppressive therapy, infection prevention 555
Inflammation 455
Inflammatory bowel disease 443, 450, 455, 511, 542, 560
– – –, clinical course 516
– – –, diagnostic standards in pathology 576
– – –, differential diagnosis 576
– – –, infectious complications 555
– – –, malignant transformation 571, 584
– – –, mucosal healing 470
– – –, natural course 470
– – –, natural history 516
– – –, pathogenesis 465
– – –, small bowel involvement 476
Innate immunity 455
Intestines 455
Intraepithelial neoplasia 576
– –, treatment 571
Intraoperative enteroscopy 476
In-vivo histology techniques 571

Joint manifestations 502

Laparoscopy 560
Linkage regions 428

Magnification endoscopy 571
Medical management 542
Monozygotic twins 522
Mucosal healing 470
Myosin light chain kinase 443

Neutropenic enterocolitis 482
NOD2 428
Non-specific ulcerative colitis 522
Non-therapy-dependent infections 555

Occludin 443
Optical coherence tomography 571

Penicillin-induced segmental hemorrhagic colitis 482
Perianal fissure 565
– fistula 565
Primary sclerosing cholangitis 522
– – –, surveillance 526
Probiotics 450
PSC, first-degree relatives 522
Pseudomembranous colitis 482
Push enteroscopy 476

Single-balloon enteroscopy 476
Sonomorphology 482
Spondylarthropathy 511
Surveillance in Crohn's disease 584
– programs and guidelines 584
– strategies, problems 584
Systemic therapy 542

Targeted therapies 465
Terminal ileum 560
Therapy 511
Therapy-dependent infections 555
Thiopurines, efficacy 516
Tight junction 443, 450
Topical therapy 542
Transabdominal ultrasound 482
Treatment algorithm(s) 536, 550, 565
Tropheryma whipplei, characteristics 494
Tuberculosis 482

Ulcerative colitis 450, 542
– –, diagnostics 550
– –, joint manifestations 502
– –, pathogenesis 550
– –, Ukraine 550

Whipple's disease 494
– –, cardiac and neurologic involvement 494
– –, clinical features 494
Wireless capsule endoscopy 476

Zinc 450